THE
HEALTH
ECONOMY

The
Health
Economy

VICTOR R. FUCHS

Harvard University Press
Cambridge, Massachusetts, and
London, England   1986

Library of Congress Cataloging-in-Publication Data

Fuchs, Victor R.
　The health economy.

　Bibliography: p.
　Includes index.
　1. Medical economics—Addresses, essays, lectures.
2. Medical policy—Addresses, essays, lectures.
I. Title [DNLM: 1. Health Policy—economics—
United States.　2. Health Services—economics—
United States.　3. Physicians—economics—United
States. W 74 F951h]
RA410.F83　1986　　338.4′73621′0973　　85-16442
ISBN 0-674-38340-0 (alk. paper)

To Sarah Jane, Frances, and Emma

Contents

THE
HEALTH
ECONOMY

Introduction

My work in health economics grew out of research I did on the service industries in the late 1960s, and was motivated in part by a desire to gain a better understanding of the postindustrial society that was emerging in the United States and other developed countries. The growth of a service economy and improved methods of contraception were bringing women into paid employment and dramatically changing gender roles and relationships. Lower fertility and longer life expectancy were transforming the age distribution of the population, and this transformation, along with the fragmentation of the family and the decline of traditional religion, was creating new social and economic conditions. The growing importance of service industries such as health care was affecting the demand for labor, the role of government, the measurement of productivity, and the nature of economic growth.

In this book, which consists of work I did in the 1970s and 1980s, I look at health and medical care in a broad social, political, and economic context. The discussion throughout reflects my desire to use economics to help health professionals and health policy experts develop answers to extremely difficult questions of efficiency and equity. Although economics does not furnish definitive solutions to health problems, the economic point of view is enormously useful in understanding the complexity of current dilemmas.

According to one definition, an economist is "a person who sees something that works in practice and wonders if it will work in theory." My view is somewhat different. Once a problem or puzzle engages my attention, I may use economic theory as a starting point, but then usually move rapidly to an examination of data through statistical analysis and through observation and reflection on the behavior of individuals and institutions. Economic theory helps to frame the questions and to identify the variables that are likely to be of interest; useful answers to the questions only emerge, if at all, from a close study of the particular phenomenon.

In the opening chapters (1 and 2) I try to show the relevance of economics to health problems. The first was written in the early 1970s for a conference on technology, at a time when many were looking for a "technological fix" to improve the health of the population and contain the cost of care. It seemed to me then (and seems now) that the emphasis on technology was overdone. I tried, therefore, to provide a *systemic* view of the problems in this field, with emphasis on the distinctive characteristics of health and medical care and on the difficulty of finding the right mix of market competition, government regulation, and professional control to accommodate these characteristics. The second chapter was written in the early 1980s when there was growing emphasis on improving health through changes in life-style. Life-style *is* important, but programs in health education and promotion, no less than those in therapeutics, will benefit from rigorous economic analysis.

Many of the chapters reflect my desire to emphasize health as well as medical care, and to make clear the difference between the two. When I entered the field I found that medical research, education, and practice were overwhelmingly concerned with the diagnosis and treatment of disease, not with the preservation and enhancement of health. Economic research in this field had a similar bias, as revealed in Herbert Klarman's thorough review of the literature through the early 1960s. Only a few studies dealt with health per se; nearly all of the research concentrated on the demand for and supply of medical care and the economics of hospitals (Klarman, 1965). Health policy, not surprisingly, also emphasized medical care as the primary route to better health; the physical and psychosocial environments and personal life-style did not receive attention commensurate with their importance. I have tried to keep a balance between health and medical care, as evidenced by the chapters that deal with such diverse factors as income, education, time preference, cigarette smoking, radiation, and inspection of motor vehicles.

Though I have often used economic theory as a framework for my research, some studies were sparked by casual observations that cried out for systematic examination. For instance, the study of surgical work loads (Chapter 3) and other research on the economics of surgery grew out of a back-of-the-envelope calculation that showed that the ratio of operations to surgeons in the United States was surprisingly small, but the product of that ratio and the average fee per operation was substantial.

Some studies began with a question—for example, does the correlation between education and health reflect a causal relation? Originally I thought that the answer was clearly yes, that this was another example of education increasing productivity (that is, in the household production of health). I then looked for a data base that would shed light on the question, and turned my attention to cigarette smoking. The results reported in Chapter 12 suggest that a third variable, such as time preference, affects both education and health. Some studies began with an unusual data base, followed by the specification of interesting questions that can be answered with the data. Chapter 7, a comparison of academic and community physicians' case mix, costs, and outcomes, had this genesis.

Sometimes I found a conflict between what standard theory says "ought to be" and what the data seem to be saying. For example, probably the most controversial chapters in this volume (4 and 6) concern the role of the physician in shifting the demand for medical care. There is strong evidence that geographic variation in the physician/population ratio is determined in part by physician preferences unrelated to differences in demand. I believe that there is also evidence (although weaker) that this variation in supply leads some physicians to shift the demand for their services. Many health economists either deny that there is shifting, or believe it is impossible to test for its existence. To be sure, the data are open to alternative interpretations, but I continue to believe that shifting does occur.

Direct involvement in policy debates has not been high on my agenda, but much of my work is, I hope, relevant to policymakers. The reasons for the popularity of national health insurance around the world (Chapter 13), the roles of government, family, and religion in health (Chapter 14), the struggle between physicians and professional managers for control of medical care (Chapter 15), the relation between medical care for the elderly and other aspects of aging (Chapter 16), and the implications of recent changes in the reimbursement of hospitals and physicians (Chapter 17) are some of the topics that have engaged me in recent years.

As I look to the future I am impressed by the changing nature of health problems, by the progress in the basic sciences, and by the current revolution in health care organization and finance. These all have important implications for medical practice, medical education and research, and health policy. They also present exciting opportunities and challenges for health economics.

The last twenty years have witnessed major advances in the health of Americans, including a 60 percent reduction in infant mortality, a 65 percent decrease in the age-adjusted death rate from influenza and pneumonia, and major declines in mortality from heart disease and stroke. These advances, along with social and demographic changes, have markedly altered the nation's burden of illness. Currently, one-third of all health care in this country is devoted to persons over the age of 65; 30 percent of that is spent in the last year of life. Prior to death, the elderly suffer primarily from chronic diseases such as arthritis and diabetes.

For those under 65, substance abuse plays a major role in health problems: drugs (legal and illegal), alcohol, cigarettes, too much salt, too much sugar, too much fat. Between the ages of 45 and 65 heart disease, lung cancer, and chronic liver disease (including cirrhosis) account for almost half of all deaths. Substance abuse is part of a larger problem which is often called mental illness but which might more properly be described as the mental or psychological component of illness. There is a tremendous challenge now to build on new scientific knowledge about the relation between the mind and the body, to integrate the treatment of the mental and physical components of illness.

The health problems of younger people are dominated by trauma: among the 60 percent of the population between the ages of 1 and 40, more than half of all deaths are attributable to suicide, homicide, and accidents. At present medical schools devote very few resources to these problems, and many academic physicians believe that they should be dealt with elsewhere. To accomplish this, however, resources would also have to be shifted elsewhere.

Scientific advances have extraordinary implications for medical practice, medical education, and health policy. For instance, the elucidation of the role of genetic factors in disease will compel much greater attention to populations, to statistics, and to epidemiology—not just for a few diseases, but over a broad spectrum of illnesses. Genetics may prove to be the key that brings together disparate elements of university medical centers in fruitful cooperative efforts. Contributions from basic scientists, clinicians, biostatisticians and epidemiologists, and social and behavioral scientists will be essential if society is to make the wisest use of the new understanding that is unfolding about genetic factors and health.

A widespread desire to slow the growth of public and private spending for health care has led to revolutionary changes in reimbursement in recent years. Medicare's Prospective Payment System based on diagnosis-related groups, state programs to control utilization and charges for Medicaid programs, the expansion of Health Maintenance Organizations, the spread of Preferred-Provider Organizations, and the trend toward deductibles and coinsurance are among the best-known symbols of this new era of health care finance.

The desire to contain the cost of health care has three principal causes. First, the slow growth of the economy in the late 1970s and early 1980s was not accompanied by an equivalent slowing in health spending. Thus the gap between the increase in health expenditures and that of the gross national product jumped to more than 4 percent per annum. Second, health spending now constitutes such a large fraction of public and private budgets that it is questionable whether even the average gap of the past three decades (about 2.7 percent per annum) can be sustained. Third, the large role played by third-party payment has raised doubts about whether the benefits to patients from additional spending are equal to the cost to society of providing the additional care. A fourth reason for the shifts in health care finance, probably less important from a long-run perspective, is that the country is currently in a pause or even a retreat from the thrust toward more equal access to care. Some, but not all, of the cutbacks in funding and changes in method of reimbursement can be interpreted as a weakening of the commitment to provide high-quality care to the poor.

Attention to the cost of health care was long overdue, but a preoccupation with cost may lead to neglect of problems of health and access to care. What is needed, of course, is not simply *cost containment,* but *cost-effective* medicine. Every 24 hours Americans spend more than a billion dollars on health care. Some of it goes for services of extraordinary value—deaths averted, pain relieved, functions restored. Some of it does more harm than good. A significant portion of that expenditure is for procedures, tests, prescriptions, and hospitalizations, the true value of which is virtually unknown.

Consider length of stay in hospital. Diagnosis by diagnosis, average stays in east-coast hospitals are one to two days longer than on the west coast. Do the patients on the east coast benefit from those extra days? If so, by how much? No one knows. Consider hospital admissions. For decades it has been observed that persons covered by conventional health insurance have about 50 percent more hospital admissions than persons of the same age and sex who belong to prepaid group practice plans. Do these extra admissions have any favorable effects on health? If so, how much? We do not know the answer, but this is clearly more than a $64,000 question.

In the past the fragmentation of medical care has made it difficult to study the effect on patients of hospitalization, x-rays, lab tests, prescriptions, and other types of care, but now the potential exists to do better. Through the growth of computerized records and of organized health plans, it is now possible to develop a more detailed, quantitative picture of what happens to patients as they move through the health care system. We can now study with *some* precision (not as much as one would like) the natural history of treated disease. It is now possible to begin to talk about quality of care as reflected in patient outcomes, both short-term and long-term, rather than simply inferring quality from process, or what is even worse, by the amount of money spent.

In the years ahead physicians, health plan managers, hospital administrators, insurance company executives, government officials, judges, and legislators all over the country will be looking for guidance concerning difficult economic, technical, and ethical questions. What should we treat? What should we pay for? What should we require? What should we invest in? What is *appropriate* care?

To answer these questions, some physicians—indeed all physicians to some degree—will need an education that is richer and more varied than in the past. A knowledge of biochemistry and molecular biology is, of course, essential, but the practicing physician cannot pledge allegiance to any single discipline or small group of disciplines. Any skill that will help serve the patient better should be part of medical training, and that may include knowledge of statistics, epidemiology, economics, behavioral sciences, ethics, and decision analysis.

Although I am convinced that the leading medical centers must and will move their research and teaching in this direction, I hope that the new emphasis on building a firmer scientific base for the practice of medicine will not result in a weakening of the traditional commitment of health professionals to the problems and needs of the individual patient. It may—but it does not have to. Exposure to epidemiology doesn't necessarily breed callousness; nor does ignorance of economics guarantee a warm, caring physician. But the danger of the impersonal physician is there, and it is well to be aware of it. *Caring* is still a big part of every physician's and nurse's job—and sometimes it is a major factor in curing.

If these remarks leave the reader with the feeling that the problems of health economics are difficult and complex, I have only one excuse. They *are* difficult and complex. There is much we don't know about the determinants of health and about the behavior of patients, physicians, and other participants in health care. Economics surely won't solve the problems, but society will come closer to solutions if it pays attention to the central messages of economics—the scarcity of resources relative to wants, the importance of achieving a balance between incremental benefits and incremental costs, and the responsiveness of human behavior to changes in incentives and constraints. When supplemented by detailed empirical investigation and by explicit recognition of the role of values in policy formation, health economics should prove to be "cost-effective."

THE ECONOMIC APPROACH

I

1 Health Care and the United States Economic System

Health care affects and is affected by the economic system in so many ways that any attempt at complete enumeration or description is bound to fall short. The objective of this chapter is more modest. I shall assume that the reader is reasonably familiar with health care, its institutions, technology, and personnel, but is less familiar with an "economic system" that is used by economists to describe and analyze economic behavior. Therefore, major emphasis will be given to indicating the place of health care in this system and showing how related economic concepts can contribute to an understanding of problems of health care in the United States. I shall also attempt to indicate some of the limitations of economics in dealing with such a complex area of human activity and concern.

Introduction and Definitions

Health care can be defined as those activities that are undertaken with the objective of restoring, preserving, or enhancing the physical and mental well-being of people. These activities may be aimed at the relief of pain, the removal of disabilities, the restoration of functions, the prevention of illness and accidents, or the postponement of death. Some health care is produced within the "household": for example, the triage, first-aid, and nursing services rendered to children by parents. Some is bought and sold in the "market": for example, physicians' services, hospital services. Most health care is applied to identifiable individuals, but some may be aimed at a population: for instance, fluoridation of a water supply.

The *economic system* consists of the network of institutions, laws, and rules created by society to answer the universal economic questions: (1) What goods and services shall be produced? (2) How shall they be produced? and (3) For whom shall they be produced? (Samuelson, 1970). Every society needs an economic system because *resources* (natural, human, and man-made) are scarce relative to human wants. The resources have alternative uses, and there is a multiplicity of competing wants. Thus, decisions must be made regarding the use of these resources in production and the distribution of the resulting output among the members of society.

Before turning to several important issues concerning health care in relation to the economic system, it will be useful to dispose of two fallacies that have frequently obstructed clear thinking in this area.

1. Resources are no longer scarce. Some people seem to be so inspired, terrified, or confused by automation and other technological advances as to proclaim the end of scarcity. In the late 1950s and early 1960s it was not unusual to find writers prophesying that in ten years no one would have to work because machines would turn out all the goods and services needed. The falsity of such predictions becomes more apparent each year. That inefficiency and waste exist in the economy cannot be denied. That some resources are underutilized is clear every time the unemployment figures are announced. That the resources devoted to war could be used to satisfy other wants is self-evident. But the fundamental fact remains that even if all these imperfections were eliminated, total output would still fall far short of the amount people would like to have. Resources would still be scarce in the sense that choices would have to be made. An economic system would still be needed. Not only is this true now, but it will continue to be true in the foreseeable future. Some advances in technology make it possible to carry out current activities with fewer resources (for example, automated laboratories), but others open up new demands (renal dialysis, organ transplants) that put further strains on resources. Moreover, time, the ultimate scarce resource, becomes more valuable the more productive we become (Becker, 1965; Linder, 1970).

2. Health is the most important goal. Some of those in the

health field recognize that we cannot satisfy all wants, but they seem to believe that health is more important than all other goals and therefore questions of scarcity and allocation are not applicable in this area. It requires only a casual study of human behavior to reveal the fallacy of this position. Every day in manifold ways people make choices that affect health, and it is clear that they frequently place a higher value on satisfying other wants; for example, smoking, overeating, careless driving, and failure to take medicine continue to be prevalent behaviors.

Criteria for an Economic System in Relation to Health Care

What is it that we want the economic system to do with respect to health care? Given the scarcity of resources and the existence of competing goals, we want a system that will result in:

1. An optimum amount of resources devoted to health care.
2. The combination of these resources in an optimal way.
3. An optimal distribution of health care.
4. An optimal allocation of resources between current provision of health care and investment for future health care through research, education, and similar efforts.

The general rule for reaching such optima is "equality at the margin." For instance, the first criterion would be met if the last dollar's worth of resources devoted to health care increased human satisfaction by exactly the same amount as the last dollar's worth devoted to other goals.

The contrast between this view of a social optimum and the notion of "optimal care" as used in the health field can be appreciated with the aid of Figure 1.1. The relation between health and health care inputs can usually be described by a curve that may rise at an increasing rate at first, but then rises at a decreasing rate and eventually levels off or declines.[1] "Optimal care" in medicine would usually be defined as the point where no further increment in health is possible; that is, point A.[2] The social optimum, however, requires that inputs of resources not exceed the point where the value of an additional increment to health is exactly equal to the cost of the inputs required to obtain that increment (point B). It should be noted that point C, where the *ratio* of benefits to costs is at a maximum, is not the optimal point because additional inputs still add more to benefits than to costs. One of the problems with current health care policy is

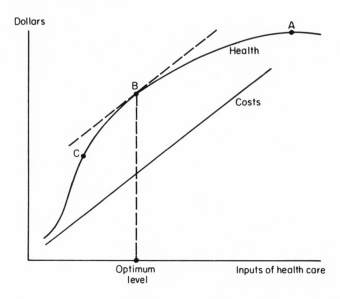

Figure 1.1 Determination of optimum level of health care utilization.

that it frequently fluctuates between trying to drive utilization to A, and then, in frenzied attempts to contain costs, cutting back some programs to point C or below.

Types of Economic Systems

Economists have identified three "pure types" of economic systems—traditional, centrally directed, and market price. Every actual economy is a blend of types, but their relative importance can and does vary greatly. Most primitive and feudal societies rely heavily on a traditional system; the process of decision making is embedded in the total culture—its customs, traditions, and religious rituals. In some ancient empires (Egypt, Babylonia) central direction played a major role. The basic decisions were made by one man or a small group of men who controlled the power apparatus of the society and were in a position to enforce their decisions concerning the allocation of resources and the distribution of output. This system has also been dominant in the Soviet Union since 1928 and in many other countries since World War II. The United States, Canada, and most countries of Western Europe have relied heavily on a market system for the past century or two. Thus a discussion of health care and the U.S. economy requires a close look at the working of a market system. An additional reason for concentrating on this third type of system is for its normative value: under certain specified conditions the results produced by the theoretical market system set a standard against which the performance of any real economy can be evaluated.[3]

The Elementary Model

The elementary model of a market system consists of a collection of decision-making units called *households* and another collection called *firms*. The households own all the productive resources in the society. They make these resources available to firms, who transform them into goods and services, which are then distributed back to the households. The flow of resources and of goods and services is facilitated by a counterflow of money (Figure 1.2).[4] This is called a market system because the exchanges of resources and of goods and services for money take place in markets where *prices* and *quantities* are determined. These prices are the signals or controls that trigger changes in behavior as required by changes in technology or preferences. The market system is sometimes referred to as the "price" system.

In the markets for resources the households are the *suppliers* and the firms provide the *demand*. In the markets for goods and services the firms are the suppliers and the households are the

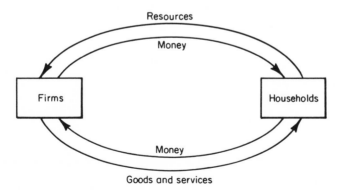

Figure 1.2 Elementary model of a market system.

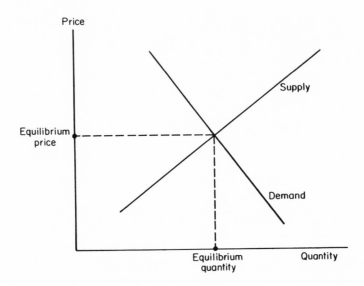

Figure 1.3 A typical market.

source of demand. In each market the interaction between demand and supply determines the quantities and prices of the various resources and the goods and services (Figure 1.3).

The income of each household depends on the quantity and quality of resources available to it (including time) and their prices; the amount of income determines its share of the total flow of goods and services. The household is assumed to spend its income (and time) in such a way as to maximize *utility* (that is, satisfaction). It does this by following the principle of "equality at the margin"; that is, it adjusts its purchases so that marginal utility (the satisfaction added by the last unit purchased) of each commodity is proportional to its price.

It is assumed that firms attempt to maximize *profits* (the difference between what they must pay the households for the use of resources and what they get from them for the goods and services they produce). To maximize profits they too must follow the equality at the margin rule, adjusting their use of different types of resources so that the marginal products (the addition to output obtained from one additional unit of input) are proportional to price.

If the markets are perfectly competitive and if certain other conditions are met, it can be shown that a market system produces an optimum allocation of resources, given the distribution of resources among households and given their "tastes" or preferences. The U.S. economy departs in many respects from the abstract, perfectly competitive market system; this is particularly noticeable in the health care sector. The main body of this chapter is devoted to a discussion of these departures and the problems they pose for health care policy.

Imperfectly Competitive Markets

The essence of a competitive market is (1) that there are many well-informed buyers and sellers, no one of whom is large enough to influence price; (2) that the buyers and sellers act independently (that is, there is no collusion); and (3) that there is free entry for other buyers and sellers not currently in the market. Most health care markets depart substantially from competitive conditions, sometimes inevitably, and sometimes as a result of deliberate public or private policy. A discussion of some of the principal problems follows.

Fewness of Sellers

In most towns and even cities of moderate size, the market is too small to support enough hospitals or enough practitioners in each specialty to fulfill the requirements of a workably competitive market. For instance, most of those who study hospital costs believe there are significant economies of scale in general hospitals up to a size of 200 or 300 beds, and some believe that economies are to be realized in even larger hospitals. Assuming a ratio of 4 beds per 1,000 population, a city of 60,000 could support just one 240-bed hospital. Thus, it would be extremely uneconomical to require numerous competitive hospitals except in large, densely populated markets. These constraints are even more significant when specialty care is considered: it is doubtful that even a population of one million would justify enough independent maternity, open-heart surgery, transplant services, and the like to approximate competitive conditions.[5]

In such a condition of "natural monopoly," the traditional response in our country has been to introduce public utility regulation (electricity, telephone, transportation). The results have not always been satisfactory, however, partly because the regulators often tend to serve the regulated rather than the public and partly because it is inherently difficult to set standards of performance without competitive yardsticks. Many other countries rely on government ownership and control, but the United States experience with government hospitals has not, on balance, been favorable. Another possible solution is the development of what John Kenneth Galbraith has termed "countervailing power" and what the economics textbooks describe as bilateral monopoly. If, for instance, in a one-hospital town all the consumers were organized into a single body for purposes of bargaining with the hospital, at least some of the disadvantages of monopoly would be lessened.

The typical solution in the hospital field has been to emphasize the "nonprofit" character of the hospitals and to assume that therefore the hospital will not abuse its monopoly power. There are two obvious criticisms of this "solution": the absence of a profit incentive may lead to waste, inefficiency, and unnecessary duplication, and the hospitals may be run for the benefit of the physicians (Pauly and Redisch, 1969).

Cooperation (Collusion) among Sellers

Even when numerous sellers of the same health service are in the same market, there may be significant advantages to society if they do not maintain a completely arms-length competitive posture vis-à-vis one another. The free exchange of information, cooperative efforts to meet crisis situations, and reciprocal backup arrangements may help to reduce costs and increase patient satisfaction. Unfortunately, the intimacy and trust developed through such activities may spill over in less desirable directions, such as price fixing, exclusion of would-be rivals, and other restrictions on competition. For 200 years economists have been impressed with the wisdom of Adam Smith's observation (1776, p. 128) that "people of the same trade seldom meet together, even for merriment and diversion, but the conversation ends in a conspiracy against the public, or in some contrivance to raise prices." Pathologists have been found guilty of price fixing, and price discrimination by physicians is not uncommon. The latter practice, which physicians view benevolently as a way of reducing inequality of access to medical care, is viewed by some economists as evidence of the use of monopoly power to maximize profits (Kessel, 1958).

Restrictions on Entry

Probably the most obvious and most deliberate interference with competition in the market for physicians' services is the barrier to entry imposed by compulsory licensure. The case for licensure presumably rests on the proposition that the consumer is a poor judge of the quality of medical care and therefore needs guidance concerning the qualifications of those proposing to sell such care. Assuming this to be true, the need for guidance could be met by voluntary *certification* rather than compulsory licensure. Indeed, the need could probably be better met through certification because there could be several grades or categories, and periodic recertification would be more practicable (and less threatening) than periodic relicensure. Under a certification system patients would be free to choose the level of expertise that they wanted, including uncertified practitioners.

The principal objections that could be raised against such a system are that some patients might receive bad treatment at the hands of uncertified practitioners, and that it might result in an expansion of unnecessary care. The obvious advantages of such a system are greater availability of care and lower prices. For certain health care needs, practitioners with lesser qualifications than present physicians have would clearly be adequate. The existing system results in some persons receiving no care, or being treated by individuals without any medical training (family members, neighbors, friends).

Another example of entry restrictions is the system of limiting hospital privileges to certain physicians. This has been justified in terms of the desire to ensure quality of care (in the institution) and as a way of obtaining free services from the physicians. However, it can also be viewed in an economic context as a way of limiting competition.

In general, the codes of professional ethics that physicians have evolved undoubtedly serve many useful social purposes. But it is well to recall Kenneth Arrow's observation that "codes of professional ethics, which arise out of the principal-agent relation and afford protection to the principals, can serve also as a cloak for monopoly by the agents" (Arrow, 1969, p. 62).

Disequilibrium

One disturbing characteristic of some health care markets is the failure of price to reach an equilibrium level (the level where the quantity demanded and the quantity supplied are equal). For instance, the market for house calls seems to be characterized by excess demand (see Figure 1.4). The "going price," about $20 per visit, is not high enough to bring supply and demand into balance. The quantity (number of house calls) that patients are willing and able to pay for at that price is much greater than the quantity physicians are willing to supply. Some observers, notably Martin Feldstein (1970), believe that the market for physicians' services in general is characterized by excess demand.

The market for general surgery, however, can best be described as an example of excess supply (Hughes et al., 1972; see Figure 1.5). At the going price for most general surgical procedures ($300 for a herniorrhaphy), the quantity that surgeons are willing and able to do is much greater than the quantity demanded. A condition of excess supply is probably also

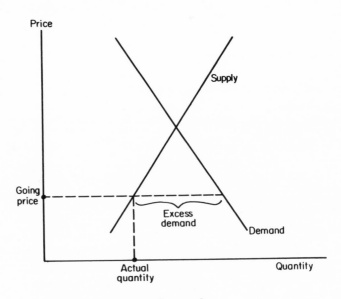

Figure 1.4 Excess demand.

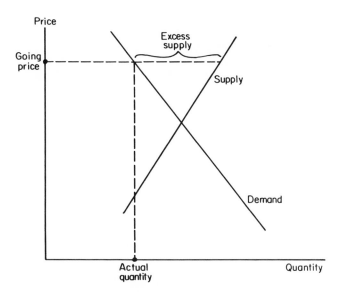

Figure 1.5 Excess supply.

present for many types of specialty surgery (ophthalmology, gynecology).

The persistence of a disequilibrium price is a clear indication that the market departs substantially from the competitive norm. In the case of excess demand, physicians are apparently reluctant to let the price of house calls rise to their equilibrium level; they introduce a form of rationing instead. This may yield certain psychic satisfactions in lieu of the higher income that is clearly possible. In the excess supply example, the price fails to fall either because the individual surgeon does not think it would be to his advantage to cut price or because surgeons have collectively reached this decision. A contributing factor is the option that most surgeons have of using their nonsurgical time for general practice or other income-producing activities.

The alleged shortage of nurses indicates another potentially troublesome health care market. If what is meant by "shortage" is that it would be nice to have more nurses, no analytical problem arises and the point is trivial. In that sense there is a shortage of every type of good or service. If, however, the allegation refers to a shortage in the sense shown in Figure 1.4 (that is, an excess demand for nurses), the failure of nurses' salaries to rise to their equilibrium level must be explained. Some investigators (Altman, 1970; Yett, 1970) claim that it is monopsonistic behavior on the part of hospitals that keeps nurses' salaries from rising to the point where supply and demand would be equal.

Costs of Information

The elementary competitive model assumes that all information relevant to decision making is known by the households and firms—prices, production possibilities, utility to be derived from different commodities. In the real world, of course, such information may be difficult or even impossible to obtain. High information costs are characteristic of many health care markets; frequently the only way a person can know whether he needs to see a physician is to see a physician. The incorporation of information costs into economic analysis is relatively recent,[6] and the theory is far from complete. Many health care markets function poorly because of imperfect information, but there is considerable disagreement as to how to make them function better. One point might have general validity: in situations where the costs of information are increased as a result of public or private policy, reversal of that policy would probably be desirable. For instance, restrictions on the right of physicians to advertise and on the right of pharmacies to advertise prices of prescription drugs ought to be reexamined in the light of the consumer's need to know more about physicians and drugs in order to make intelligent choices. A study of variations in restrictions on advertising by optometrists and opticians found that prices were substantially lower in states that permitted advertising (Benham, 1971).

Externalities

An externality exists when the actions taken by an individual household or firm will impose costs or confer benefits on other households or firms, and when no feasible way exists of arranging direct compensation for these costs or benefits. The presence of externalities indicates that the individual household or firm, in attempting to maximize its own utility or profit, will not make socially optimal decisions.[7] A classic example of an externality is the costs of air pollution imposed on others by the smoke emanating from a factory; another example is the benefit to society that results when an individual decides to be vaccinated or treated for a communicable disease.

One way to deal with externalities is for the state to prohibit or require certain actions. Another is to attempt to modify the prices facing individual firms or households (through taxes or subsidies) so that the price properly reflects the social costs or benefits. In principle, use of the price mechanism will permit a much closer approximation to a social optimum, but practical difficulties may preclude the price approach in some situations.

Externalities are very important to health care in the broadest sense of the term. Consider, for instance, the effects of automobiles on health. The decisions of individual households involving the purchase and use of an automobile, the speed and manner of driving, the amount of maintenance and repair, and even the choice of gasoline have potentially important implications for the health of others, but these implications are not reflected in the prices facing the household. Similar problems arise in connection with many other consumption or production activities that create environmental health hazards.

In seeking to reduce such hazards, a few central points should be kept in mind. First, costs (resources used or wants unsatisfied) are usually associated with the reduction of hazards, and these costs frequently increase at an accelerating rate, the greater the reduction desired. It follows, therefore, that the social goal should rarely be the complete elimination of the hazard, but rather its reduction to the point where the value of a further reduction is less than the cost of achieving it. A major problem for health care policy is to identify these externalities, estimate their effects, and impose appropriate taxes or subsidies so that individual households and firms, in seeking to maximize their own utility or profits, will make socially appropriate decisions.

Medical research is a good example of an activity with large external benefits, and therefore, in the absence of specific public policy, too little will be undertaken. One solution is to permit the discoverer of new knowledge to appropriate the benefits (for example, through patent protection), but with regard to much health research this solution will frequently not be feasible or acceptable. The alternative is for the government to subsidize research. It has done this to a considerable degree; the question is, how much health research is socially desirable? The answer, in principle, is the same as for any other decision regarding the use of scarce resources—the optimum level of research is reached when the incremental value of the prospective benefits is equal to the incremental cost. The more basic the research, the more likely it is to give rise to external benefits, but the more difficult it is to estimate their value or incidence.

In contrast to environmental programs and medical research, medical care today frequently does not involve significant external benefits. For instance, the benefits of most surgery accrue primarily to the patient and his family. This is equally true for treatment of most major diseases, such as heart disease and cancer.[8] The best known examples of externalities arising from medical care involve the prevention and treatment of communicable diseases. Another potentially important source of externalities is the treatment of mental illness, but lack of knowledge concerning causes or cures makes it difficult to reach firm policy conclusions in this area.

One important application of the externality idea has to do with the problem of inequality of access to care. A frequent criticism of the market system is that it results in an unequal and "unfair" distribution of income.[9] Households that are poorly endowed with resources will earn relatively little and will command only a small share of the nation's output. Many people would like to see a reduction of inequality, either in general or with respect to a particular commodity (medical care). To the extent that they are prepared to back their demand for less inequality through voluntary redistribution (philanthropy), no modification of the elementary model is required. We simply note that some households derive utility from giving money to others or from knowing that other households are receiving medical care. They are, therefore, willing to devote a part of their income (or part of their time) for that purpose. The purchase of a good or service for someone else is no different analytically from the purchase of a good or service for one's own household.

The externality problem arises because a philanthropic act by one household confers benefits on all other households that derive utility from observing a decrease in inequality. If each potential philanthropist considers only the psychic benefits *he* derives from reducing inequality, the total volume of philanthropy will be less than warranted by the collective desires of the group.[10]

One solution is compulsory redistribution. Society, working through government, may decide that the distribution of income resulting from the market system is inequitable or otherwise unsatisfactory and may seek to change it through taxation. This requires only a slight modification of the elementary model. The simplest way to do this is to take money away from some households and give it to others; each household is then free to allocate its income as it pleases.

For any given amount of redistribution, the utility of households is presumably maximized by a general tax on the income of some households and grants of income to others rather than by taxing particular forms of spending or by subsidizing particular types of consumption. Mathematical proofs of this proposition are available, and its plausibility is obvious. If a household is offered a choice of either $100 or $100 worth of health care, it will prefer the former because it can use the additional income to buy more health care (if that is what it wants), but usually utility will be maximized by increasing consumption of many other commodities as well. Similarly, if a household is offered a choice between giving up $100 and giving up $100 worth of health care, its utility will be diminished less by the reduction in income.

Despite the obvious logic of this argument, many of the nonpoor seem more inclined toward a reduction in inequality in the consumption of particular commodities (medical care is a conspicuous example) than toward a general redistribution of income (Pauly, 1971). Two reasons may explain this attitude. First, the nonpoor may believe that significant externalities are associated with medical care (in addition to the psychic benefits of observing a reduction in inequality) that are not associated with other commodities. The earlier discussion indicated some grounds for skepticism concerning this belief.[11] A second reason may be that the nonpoor think they know better what will maximize the utility of the poor than do the poor themselves.

A special aspect of the problem arises when the emphasis is put on reducing inequality of access to medical care per se rather than raising the consumption of medical care by the poor. This goal may require rationing the amount available to the nonpoor as well as subsidizing the poor. One economist has argued that the British approach to health care through a national health service can best be understood in these terms (Lindsay, 1969).

Compulsory Insurance

At the extreme, the demand for reductions in inequality takes the form of an assertion that "health care is a right"; that if someone needs health care, society has an obligation to provide it. To the extent that society honors that obligation, the incentive for households to provide for their own health care (as through voluntary insurance) is diminished. Those without insurance—and especially those individuals who prior to their illness could have afforded the normal premium—become, in effect, "freeloaders" on the rest of society. If this behavior is widespread, the only solutions are to make insurance compulsory or to modify the ethical imperative. Thus far the United States has opted for a little of each. Insurance is virtually compulsory for many through their employment contract; on the other hand, free care is made less attractive by means tests, long waiting lines, unpleasant surroundings, and similar inconveniences.

Another argument advanced in favor of compulsory insurance is that it overcomes the problem of adverse selection. If insurance is completely voluntary, it may be impractical to adjust each household's premium to its expected utilization. To the extent that uniform premiums are charged, however, households with lower than average expected utilization have an incentive to drop out, and this process can continue until the plan collapses.

It seems likely that the United States will move further in the direction of compulsory insurance, but this development is likely to create new problems even as it solves others. It increases the incentive to reduce health care in the home and throws more of the burden on collectively provided care. If the money price of market-provided care goes to zero, people will tend to use more than the amount they would like to use if they were free to shift resources to satisfy other wants.

Some Limitations of the Model

It is becoming increasingly evident that many health problems are related to individual behavior. In the absence of dramatic breakthroughs in medical science, the greatest potential for improving health is through changes in what people do and do not do to and for themselves. Household decisions concerning diet, exercise, smoking, drinking, work, and recreation are of critical importance.

It is useful to distinguish between two different classes of decisions. The first consists of those that affect health, but without the decision maker's awareness of these effects. In such instances, public policies are needed to increase information. The question of how much of this activity can be justified can be answered (in principle) along the familiar lines of weighing incremental costs and benefits.

The "Taste" for Health

A more difficult problem is posed by those decisions that are made with full information available, and that, according to economists, reflect the household's "tastes." *Tastes* is a catchall term given by economists to the underlying preference patterns that determine demand at any given structure of income and prices. The overeater, the heavy smoker, the steady drinker are all presumably maximizing their utility, given their tastes. They may be knowingly shortening their lives. Should it be an object of public policy to try to change their tastes—to try to increase people's tastes for health? Economics can provide very little guidance in this area because economists have no way, even in principle, of saying what has happened to utility once tastes have changed. Economists are not, of course, alone in this dilemma; none of the other social sciences has a well-developed theory of preference formation or the capacity to make judgments about the relative merits of different social goals.

The issues involved are extremely complex. Tastes are not acquired at birth or formed in a vacuum. It seems that economists should make an effort to determine how the working of the economic system itself influences tastes, studying the impact of advertising and other sales efforts on demand and trying to determine whether taxation or subsidies of such efforts and counter-efforts are justified. Tastes are also undoubtedly influenced by the information and entertainment media, by the schools, by religious institutions, and by other organizations that are either tax-supported, subsidized through tax exemptions, or regulated by government to some degree.

Another way of thinking about this problem has been proposed by Gary Becker and Robert Michael (1973). In their approach, all households have the same basic wants or "tastes." They try to satisfy these basic wants by producing "commodities" with the aid of purchased goods and services plus inputs of their own time. Households differ greatly in their ability to produce different "commodities," and these differences explain much of the observed differences in purchases of goods and services in the market.

This approach has been developed and applied to health by Michael Grossman (1972a). In his model it is the household, not the physician or the hospital, that produces health. Health care and other goods and services (food, shelter) are used in the production of health, and some goods (for example, cigarettes) may have negative effects. If one pursues this approach, it could be a legitimate aim of public policy to help households become more efficient producers of health.[12] The chief ways of doing this would be through health education and by providing more information about the health care that is purchased in the market. It is interesting to note that the United States government currently assumes more responsibility for informing consumers about the quality of steaks they buy than about the quality of hospitals or physicians they use.

Behavior within Households and Firms

A significant shortcoming of the elementary model in analyzing health care is its treatment of the firm and the household as the basic elements of analysis. In recent years some economists have directed their attention to decision making within the firm (Cyert and March, 1964; Simon, 1962; Williamson, 1970) and within the household (Becker, 1965; Gronau, 1973).

Attention to decision making and allocation within the firm is particularly important if we are to try to understand one of the major institutions in health care, the nonprofit voluntary hospital. It is relatively easy to identify several significant interest groups within the hospital—the board of directors, the management, the full-time medical staff, the attending staff—but it is more difficult to weigh their impact in order to formulate a predictive theory of hospital behavior. When the goals of the various interest groups are similar, the simple theory of the profit-maximizing firm may be adequate, but when they conflict (for example, the selection of cases for admission), such a theory is obviously incomplete.

Decision making and allocation within the household also pose problems that have special relevance to health care. The quantity and quality of health care provided to children by parents differ greatly among households, even among those with equal incomes. The ability of parents to "produce" health for themselves and for their children seems to vary considerably. Society feels an obligation to protect the health rights of minors, but it has found this difficult to do. The health care provided for elderly parents by their children also varies greatly. The decline of family ties tends to shift some production of health care from households to firms, and part of the observed rising cost of health care in recent decades is undoubtedly attributable to such a shift (for example, the growth of nursing homes).

Implications for Technological Change

The basic economic principles concerning resource allocation and utility maximization apply in a world of technological change as well as in a static one. Neither blanket endorsement nor condemnation of technology is rational; every change in technology involves costs and benefits, and wise social policy depends on an accurate assessment of their relative magnitudes.

There is a widespread belief that the health care sector harbors many wonderful technological changes that have not been diffused widely and rapidly enough. An opposing view has been advanced by Richard Nelson of Yale, one of the nation's leading investigators of the economics of technological change. He has written, "In both defense and health there has been a lot of R and D, and technical change has been extremely rapid; but it also has been extremely expensive and poorly screened . . . In health one has the strong impression that one of the reasons for rising health costs has been the proclivity of doctors and hospitals to adopt almost any plausible new thing—drugs, surgical methods, equipment—that increases capability in any dimension (and some for which even that isn't clear) without regard to cost" (Nelson, 1972).

Nelson's view has considerable validity. The tendency toward rapid and indiscriminate adoption of innovations in the medical care field can be attributed in part to efforts of suppliers of the innovation, especially drug companies. Possibly the most important reason is the technological imperative that influences medical choices (Fuchs, 1968b). This is instilled in physicians by their training, and reinforced by present systems of financing health care. It produces the attitude that if something can be done it should be done. Most medical decision makers, be they physicians or hospital administrators, are not trained to weigh marginal benefits against marginal costs. Moreover, present methods of third-party payment and provider reimbursement do not give them any inducement to acquire that ability. To be sure, patient pressure and the ethical imperative to do everything possible for the patient make this a complex problem. But a more rational approach could result in saving more lives and providing greater overall patient satisfaction.

Another popular misconception is that any change in health care technology that reduces labor requirements must be desirable. No such a priori assumption is warranted. A change in technology that is capital-saving and labor-intensive may be more valuable than the reverse, and a change that permits the substitution of two relatively unskilled workers for one highly skilled one may be more valuable than either.

The nature of technological change can have profound effects on resource requirements, and some attention should be paid to this matter in granting funds for research and development. In choosing between two projects, for instance, it is not sufficient to consider only the importance of the problem and the probability of success. The granting agency should also consider what resources will be required to implement the solution if the project is successful (Weisbrod, 1971). Some technological advances, such as the antibiotic drugs, greatly reduced the demand for physicians' services; others, such as organ transplants, greatly increased demand (Fuchs and Kramer, 1972).

Traditional societies resist or inhibit technological change. Our society probably errs in the opposite direction: we seem to be fascinated by technology and often look to it to solve problems when less expensive solutions lie elsewhere. This may be particularly true of health care. It is to be hoped that this emphasis on technology will not serve to obscure other fundamental questions concerning the organization and financing of health care and personal responsibility for health.

Consider the problem of hospital costs. Hundreds of millions are being spent to make hospitals more efficient through new technology, but the return is likely to be small compared to the savings possible now with existing technology through reductions in utilization. Most informed observers believe that on any given day approximately 20 percent of the patients in the average general hospital do not need to be there. Research probably will prove this to be a conservative estimate because it still assumes customary medical interventions, conventional lengths of stay, and so forth.

What, for instance, is the appropriate length of stay after hernia surgery? A British team, in a carefully controlled study, showed that patients discharged one day after surgery did as well as those discharged after six days. Another British team compared surgical repair of varicose veins with injection/compression sclerotherapy. The former method involves expensive hospitalization; the latter is done on an outpatient basis at minimum cost. The outcomes seem to be similar (except that surgical patients lost four times as many days from work), and patients seem to prefer the injection/compression technique (Ford, 1971).

No reasonable person would want to inhibit the development of new technologies or their application to health problems. But everyone concerned with American health care should realize that the most pressing problems are not centered on technology, and their solutions will probably be found in other directions. As this chapter has suggested, we need to make health care markets work better; we need to quantify and control the externalities that affect health; and we need to recognize the importance of individual behavior and personal responsibility for health. Substantial alterations in organization, financing, and education are required to achieve these objectives.

These are the realities. Tomorrow's technology may help to bring about these changes, but let us not underestimate what is possible today if we have the will to do it. Let us not oversell technology. Let us not divert attention and misdirect energies that could be devoted to the complex task of creating a more equitable, more effective, and more efficient health care system.

| 2 | Setting Priorities in Health Education and Promotion |

Most health experts today agree that diet, exercise, cigarette smoking, and other aspects of personal behavior are major determinants of morbidity and mortality. Many experts also agree that health education and promotion can result in modification of these behaviors. A key task in the field of public health is to identify those interventions and behavioral changes that can yield the greatest payoff.

The magnitude of this task is readily evident in *Promoting Health/Preventing Disease*, a publication of the Department of Health and Human Services (U.S. Department of Health and Human Services, 1980). This comprehensive document, a follow-up to *Healthy People,* identifies fifteen major health areas that need attention and provides a rich menu of possible interventions to improve health (U.S. Department of Health and Human Services, 1979). It is, however, extremely circumspect in choosing *among* areas and interventions. For each health problem, it lists a large number of possible programs of education and promotion (as well as treatment), but it is cautious about the relative merits of these programs. Such caution is readily understandable. The government officials who released *Promoting Health/Preventing Disease* may have been reluctant to antagonize important constituencies by designating some problems and programs as more important than others, but even an author who is free of such inhibitions is constrained by the absence of an adequate scientific base on which to build a rational set of priorities.

In this chapter, therefore, I will explore questions that must be answered in order to set priorities rationally. In addition, I will discuss some of the alleged obstacles to health promotion and attempt to appraise their significance. I will conclude with a brief case study of cigarette smoking, which is one of the behaviors that most adversely affects health and one of the most important subjects of health education and promotion efforts.

Stating the Problem

At the formal level, the problem of setting priorities for health education and promotion can be viewed as an aspect of the general problem of allocating scarce resources to satisfy human wants. In short, it is a matter of choice. Some choices are made by individuals and families allocating their income to acquire market-produced goods and services and their time and energy to produce goods and services outside the market (home production). Other choices are made by government and are financed by taxes. The best mix between private and public efforts is a subproblem within this general framework.

To simplify the analysis, let us bypass the question of how much of the nation's productive resources should be allocated to health and how much to other goals; let us assume a predetermined "health budget." Similarly, let us bypass for the moment the question of choosing between education and promotion efforts and other interventions (diagnostic, therapeutic, and rehabilitative) to improve health. I shall return to this particular trade-off later in the chapter. Whatever money, time, and effort are available for health education and promotion permit various possible interventions. A particular intervention, such as an antismoking campaign, can have multiple outcomes, such as reduction in lung cancer and in emphysema. Similarly, a particular outcome, such as reduction in myocardial infarctions, can be the result of several interventions, such as increased exercise and changes in diet.

The problem is to choose the best set of interventions. To do this, we need to identify the costs of each intervention; we need to know the functional relationships between the interventions and the outcomes; and we must place a value on each outcome. Given this information, we could, in principle, allocate the scarce resources among the interventions in order to maximize the value of the outcomes.

Costs of interventions. Among the education and promotion programs that have been attempted or proposed are health courses in the schools, television programs, and home visits by family health workers. It is usually relatively easy to estimate staff salaries and fringe benefits, outlays for materials and supplies, and other direct costs of such programs. However, careful setting of priorities in the public interest will try to take account of all costs, not just those that constitute charges against the budget of the organization setting the priorities. Other kinds of costs may also be incurred by the program participants. Time costs and psychic costs, for example, are much more difficult but equally important to estimate.

Most health education programs make demands on the time of recipients. It is difficult to imagine any educational effort that does not require time input on the part of the person to be educated. Failure to take account of the value of time will result in an underestimation of the overall cost of health education. This failure will also bias choices among programs, and, other things being equal, will result in an underallocation of resources to programs that are less time-intensive. How shall time be valued? Cost/benefit analyses of transportation programs and evaluations of other service activities also confront this problem, but no method of evaluation has been universally accepted. Some analysts consider the value of time equal to the value of the foregone wage—what the individual could have earned if he or she had worked during that time. Others argue that time is worth only a fraction of the wage if, for example, people would rather spend their time in health education than at work, or if the individual has no opportunity to use the time in question for work.

Consider an intervention such as the 55-mile-per-hour speed limit. This limit has unquestionably reduced the number of deaths attributable to traffic accidents, apparently at low cost. One critic of the speed limit, however, argues that the cost per life saved is actually very high (Lave, 1978). He states that the slower speeds result in 459,000 person-years of additional driving time per year. Lave assumes that this time is worth 42 percent of the average wage, yielding a cost of $6 billion in 1977. By dividing this cost by the estimated number of lives saved per year, 4,500, he obtains an average cost per life saved of $1.3 million. Of course, this calculation does not include the value of reductions in nonfatal accidents, of savings in fuel consumption, and other possible benefits of the 55-mile-per-hour speed limit. It does, however, serve as a reminder that the cost of time is relevant to the setting of priorities among health programs.

Another type of cost that needs to be considered is the psychic cost of health promotion interventions. Consider, for instance, a prohibition on the consumption of alcohol. Let us suppose that such a prohibition would unambiguously improve the physical health of the population. Apart from large enforcement expenses and other costly effects, predictable from the experience of the United States with prohibition in the 1920s, such an intervention might impose psychic costs on those who would have to forgo alcohol consumption.

Relationship between interventions and outcomes. One of the biggest problems in setting priorities for health education and promotion is uncertainty about the relationship between interventions and outcomes. This problem has two major components. One is the effect of education and promotion efforts on behavior. For instance, if an antismoking campaign is run on television, how many people will stop smoking, reduce their use of cigarettes, or refrain from starting? The other is the effect of changes in behavior on various measures of health. If people smoke less, will the incidence of lung cancer, heart disease, or emphysema also decrease?

The Stanford Heart Disease Prevention Project, in a three-community study, demonstrated that mass-media interventions aimed at reducing cardiovascular disease led to desired changes in cigarette smoking, weight, systolic blood pressure, and other cardiovascular risk factors (Farquhar et al., 1977). The study did not attempt to measure the effect of changes in risk factors on health outcomes, but a new five-city experiment conducted by the same investigators will address that question.

The recently completed Multiple Risk Factor Intervention Trial (MRFIT) attempted to provide information about both components of the intervention-outcome relationship. The results are ambiguous (Multiple Risk Factor Intervention Trial Research Group, 1982). The special intervention group showed reductions in cigarette smoking, diastolic blood pressure, and plasma cholesterol that were significantly greater than those in the control group, where members received "usual care." However, heart disease mortality and overall mortality were not significantly lower in the intervention group. In short, even a $115 million ten-year study did not provide the kind of solid information needed to set priorities in a systematic manner.

Valuation of outcomes. Knowledge of the relationships between interventions and outcomes is necessary, but not sufficient, for setting priorities. Choices must be made arbitrarily unless values are assigned to changes in health outcomes. The assignment of values to illness and disability—even life itself—is disconcerting to many health professionals. It must be recognized, however, that the act of choosing necessarily involves valuation—implicitly, if not explicitly. Viewing human life as an ultimate value does not eliminate the problem. As Isaiah Berlin (1970) has written, "The need to choose, to sacrifice some ultimate values to others, turns out to be a permanent characteristic of the human predicament."

The task of placing a value on human life may be more acceptable if we regard it not as valuing a whole life directly, but as valuing a change in the probability of survival. For instance, suppose we know with certainty that out of a population of one million, one thousand will die of a given disease during a given time period. Suppose we also know with certainty that as a result of some health promotion program, the number of deaths will fall to 500; that is, the probability of death for an individual would be reduced from 1/1,000 to 1/2,000. How much is that reduction worth? Unless a value can be agreed upon, it is impossible to know whether the intervention should be undertaken, or whether the resources required could be more fruitfully used in some other way.

To derive such values, economists have used two principal methods: "discounted future earnings" and "willingness to pay." The discounted future earnings approach values an intervention that postpones a death from age 30 to age 70 as the sum of the earnings of the individual from 30 to 70, all discounted back to the time of the intervention. A discount rate must be applied to future benefits (and future costs) to obtain their present value because an investment of resources today is warranted only if it can show a positive rate of return. At a 4 percent per annum rate of discount, a benefit of $10,000 eighteen years from now would justify a present cost of no more than $5,000.

This approach raises several thorny questions. One involves

the most appropriate rate of time discount. The choice of a high rate favors interventions that promise a quick payoff (for example, immunization against a lethal disease); conversely, the choice of a low rate favors interventions with long-term benefits (for example, modification of diet).

One way of choosing a rate is to use the rate at which individuals lend and borrow money in private markets. These rates typically include a component that reflects expected inflation and sometimes also reflects risk of nonpayment. The rate should exclude the inflation component if costs and benefits are projected in "real" terms and, according to many analysts, also should exclude the risk component. Some analysts argue that the private rate is higher than is appropriate for collective decisions through government. I disagree. If I base my private choices on a discount rate of 6 percent per annum, I would not want my tax money to support programs that are justified only at 3 percent. Indeed, I believe a government that used a rate much below that which consituents thought appropriate for their own actions would soon be voted out of office.

In attempting to estimate the private rate, analysts must also contend with the fact that the rate paid by borrowers is higher than the net rate received by lenders because of taxes. The borrower's rate presumably influences private decisions about investment, while the lender's rate influences consumer choices between saving and spending. The "social" rate—the one used for decision making about public programs—probably should fall somewhere in between.

Another question is whether the value placed on lives should vary according to the prospective earnings of different categories of individuals. For instance, should programs that save the lives of men be valued more highly than those that affect women? Should programs that address the health problems of the well-educated be valued more highly than those that affect people with less schooling? Most analysts answer this question in the negative, with one exception. Implicit in the discounted future earnings approach is a consensus that programs that postpone death for young people are more valuable than those that postpone death for old people, other things being equal. Figure 2.1 shows some typical value-of-life-age profiles based on discounted future earnings.

Many economists are critical of the discounted future earnings

Value of Life ($000)

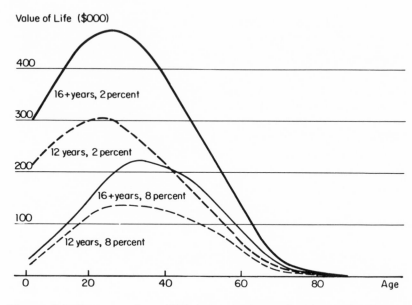

Figure 2.1 Present value of lifetime earnings of white males, by age and years of schooling completed, discounted at 2 percent and 8 percent, 1972. *Source:* U.S. Department of Health, Education and Welfare, Social Security Administration, Research and Statistics Note no. 14-1975, September 30, 1975, tables 2 and 5.

approach; they point out that we do not use it to value other goods and services in the economy. A value of life measure based on "willingness to pay" would rest on stronger theoretical grounds, but it is extremely difficult to obtain reliable empirical estimates based on this approach. Two estimates of the value of life inferred from wage premiums paid to workers in risky jobs differed by a factor of five. One estimate is $200,000, approximately the same figure that could be obtained from a discounted future earnings approach (Thaler and Rosen, 1975); the other is $1 million or more (Viscusi, 1978).

It may be argued that in choosing among interventions the actual value of life is not important, provided it is calculated in the same way for all programs. There is at least one problem with this argument, however. Programs usually have other outcomes (for example, reductions in morbidity, disability, and pain) in addition to their effects on probability of survival. The importance of these outcomes relative to reduced mortality varies from program to program. Thus, if value of life is overestimated, programs that result primarily in reduced morbidity and disability will be underfunded; if value of life is underestimated, these programs will be overfunded.

Obstacles to Health Education and Promotion

The literature on health education and promotion is replete with complaints about the alleged obstacles to more interventions of this type. The whipping boys include health insurance companies, "business interests" such as tobacco growers, the "irrationality" of the public, and fee-for-service reimbursement of physicians. In my view these explanations do not stand up to close scrutiny, although other considerations, such as time preference and uncertainty, do pose major obstacles to health promotion.

Health insurance. According to the conventional wisdom among those interested in health promotion, preventive care is "underfinanced." Breslow and Somers (1977), for instance, assert that "virtually all health insurance discriminates against preventive services, both public and private." They say that "health insurance carriers and programs must be persuaded or mandated to provide coverage for at least a substantial portion of preventive services."

In fact, the case is not as open and shut as they suggest. First, to the extent that preventive services demonstrably "pay for themselves" by reducing expenditures for curative health care, health insurance companies have considerable incentive to cover such services. To be sure, a particular insurance company will suffer some "leakage" of benefits if the recipients of the preventive services are not still covered by that company during the payoff period of lower utilization of health care. In many situations, however, this problem by itself is not likely to deter insurers from covering preventive measures.

More important, expenditures for preventive services are largely predictable for the individual and for this reason are ill-suited for coverage under insurance. The principal purpose of insurance is to protect beneficiaries against unpredictable expenditures, especially expenditures that are large relative to income. It makes no more sense to provide insurance coverage for preventive health services than for shoes, haircuts, or similar items in the budget. (The same argument applies to "first dollar" coverage for ordinary medical expenses. The standard risk-aversion principle that creates a demand for insurance against large losses does not really account for the popularity of such insurance.)

Preventive services are not expensive. Breslow and Somers (1977) estimated that their "lifetime health-monitoring program" would have cost about $15 per capita in 1975, hardly a staggering sum. But it is well known that every insurance policy, either private or public, must raise more in premiums or taxes than it pays in benefits because of administrative costs. Thus, in order to obtain $15 worth of preventive services each year, the average person would probably have had to pay $20 or more per year in premiums or taxes. Even if employers nominally pay the additional premiums or taxes, individuals ultimately bear the costs in foregone earnings, lower benefits in some other area, or higher prices. Thus, consumers are understandably reluctant to pay an extra premium to "insure" against a small, predictable expense.

Although there may be an arguable case for subsidizing or even making compulsory preventive services (for example, immunization for a communicable disease) that provide significant external benefits for others, mandating insurance coverage is not likely to be the most effective way of making sure that everyone gets immunized. At bottom, the case for mandatory insurance coverage of preventive services must rest on an appeal to paternalism. Suppose individuals neither wish to buy these services voluntarily nor seek insurance policies that cover such expenditures. If they can be forced to take out policies that have such coverage, some will be induced to receive the preventive services. The real issue is not finance, but the degree of reliance on voluntary behavior as opposed to compulsion.

"Business" interests. According to health promotion advocates, one of the biggest obstacles to better health is the baneful influence of "business" interests as epitomized by the growers and processors of tobacco. I have no desire to defend tobacco farmers, tobacco subsidies, or cigarette manufacturers, but I doubt that they are the primary obstacle to the elimination of cigarette smoking. This dirty, noxious, expensive habit persists mainly because many people enjoy smoking. Tobacco use plagued the world long before Madison Avenue existed. King James I of

England found that even the death penalty could not eliminate tobacco consumption. The contemporary People's Republic of China has done many wonderful things to improve the health of the population, but it has not attempted to stop the production and distribution of cigarettes—and clearly not because of private business interests.

The "irrational" public. It has frequently been observed (and lamented) that people acting individually or collectively are willing to spend much more to *treat* an illness than to *prevent* it. Such behavior is often characterized as "irrational" and "inefficient."

These characterizations would be justified if the goal of individuals were to maximize life expectancy for any given level of expenditure. It is more plausible, however, to assume that their goal is to maximize utility, and under that assumption so-called irrational behavior could be quite rational. The amount that individuals are willing to pay for a glass of water, for example, undoubtedly depends on how thirsty they are. Other things being equal, willingness to pay varies directly with thirst. Similarly, willingness to pay for a given change in the probability of survival (for example, an increase of .05) probably varies directly with the individual's proximity to death. For instance, if an individual is very sick (let us say the probability of survival is .05), it may be worth a great deal to raise the probability to .10 through some form of treatment (the chance of survival is doubled). On the other hand, if the individual's probability of survival is .90, he is unlikely to value as highly a preventive service that will raise it to .95. In short, when people are healthy they are not eager to spend money to become even healthier, but when they are sick, and especially when they are facing death, they are willing to spend a good deal for even a small chance of improvement.

Fee-for-service reimbursement. Fee-for-service reimbursement has long been blamed for the failure of physicians to emphasize health education and disease prevention. In its crudest form, the argument runs that because physicians make money when their patients are sick, they do not pay enough attention to keeping their patients well. As one who has long advocated capitation methods of reimbursement, I am not about to enter a blanket defense for fee-for-service medicine, but it seems to me that this particular criticism is far off the mark. In the first place, if physicians were motivated only by financial rewards, it would be relatively simple to induce them to emphasize health education and promotion by *paying them* to do so. In fact, neither private patients nor private insurers nor government are willing to pay as readily or as handsomely for prevention as for treatment. Where they are willing to pay, such services are forthcoming.

Second, medical care systems that are not based on fee-for-service, such as those in England and the Soviet Union, place no greater emphasis on health education and promotion than in the United States. Even within the United States, a comparison of a large, well-established, prepaid group practice with a large fee-for-service group practice has revealed that the patients in the latter system actually received more preventive services (Scitovsky et al., 1979).

Finally, fee-for-service reimbursement is even more widespread for dentists than for physicians, but dentists have long been advocates of fluoridation, preventive care at home, and other measures that help preserve dental health. Fee-for-service is not the explanation. More relevant obstacles may be time preference and uncertainty.

Time preference. Health promotion typically involves incurring a current cost in exchange for the chance of some future benefit. In my opinion, this difference in the timing of costs and benefits constitutes one of the major obstacles to more health promotion and disease prevention. If individuals had very low rates of time discount—if they valued future benefits almost as highly as current ones—health promotion might fare better. But many individuals seem to have high rates of time discount, paying high-interest charges for installment credit, personal loans, and the like. Compound interest is a powerful phenomenon. Consider a benefit that will materialize in twenty years. If the value of that benefit is $10,000 (in dollars of constant purchasing power), at a discount rate of 7 percent its present value is only $2,500. At a discount rate of 11 percent, its present value is only $1,250. Thus one important consideration in setting priorities for health education and promotion is to choose programs that yield benefits fairly soon after the costs are incurred.

Uncertainty. Future benefits promised by health promotion efforts are, for the individual, usually highly uncertain. We may know that on average nonsmokers will be less likely to get lung cancer than will smokers, but not all smokers get lung cancer, and not all nonsmokers escape lung cancer. Giving up smoking thus involves incurring a known cost (for example, nicotine withdrawal or the foregone pleasure of smoking) in exchange for an uncertain benefit. Psychologists Kahnemann and Tversky (1979) have shown that most people are risk-averse with respect to gains and risk-preferring with respect to losses. That is, if offered a choice between a guaranteed gain of, say, $500, and an equivalent gamble—a 50 percent chance of getting $1,000 and a 50 percent chance of getting nothing—most people choose the sure $500.

A good way to increase acceptance of health promotion efforts would be to reduce the uncertainty surrounding the benefits. One of the objectives of research should be to enable health experts to pinpoint with greater accuracy who will get what benefit from any given intervention.

Cigarette Smoking: A Case Study

If one were to poll health experts for their judgment concerning the area of highest priority in education and promotion, it is likely that cigarette smoking would be the most frequent response by a considerable margin. Sir George Godber (1981), for instance, has written, "The abolition of smoking would within a short time produce the largest reduction in morbidity and premature mortality that could result from any health-promoting activity open to us." A recent survey of practicing physicians reported that 93 percent regarded the elimination of cigarette smoking as "very important" to the average person. No other behavior was rated as very important by more than 70 percent of the physicians, and most behaviors did not achieve even a 50 percent positive response (Wechsler et al., 1983).

This widespread opposition to cigarette smoking among physicians largely stems from the very strong circumstantial evidence that links cigarette smoking to lung cancer, heart disease, respiratory diseases, and other health problems. Many of these problems affect people at ages when they would normally be highly active and productive. Implicitly, if not explicitly, society is more interested in preventing a death at age 55 than at age 75. The difference in number of deaths between smokers and

Table 2.1 Differential mortality of smokers and nonsmokers, by age, U.S. males[a]

	Smokers: 1,000 males age 35	Nonsmokers: 1,000 males age 35	Excess deaths of smokers
Deaths between 35 and 50	55	18	37
Deaths between 50 and 65	223	94	129
Deaths between 65 and 80	421	315	106

Source: Jeffrey E. Harris, "Ten Expressions for the Mortality Risk of Cigarette Smoking," paper presented at the International Workshop on the Analysis of Actual versus Perceived Risks, National Academy of Sciences, June 1–3, 1981.
a. Death rates were standardized using the 1965–1970 life insurance Male Basic Table; they are appreciably lower than the rates in the U.S. Life Tables.

nonsmokers is particularly large between ages 50 and 65, as Table 2.1 shows. This also illustrates, however, how time preference and uncertainty pose obstacles to antismoking efforts.

Consider the situation of a 35-year-old male smoker. For simplicity, let us assume that the benefit he will derive from giving up smoking will consist of the lower probability of death shown in Table 2.1. (He will undoubtedly receive some immediate benefits as well, such as better breath and more wind. This discussion illustrates a general principle; it is not intended to be a complete evaluation of smoking cessation.) In the years between age 35 and age 50, this benefit is relatively small; not smoking increases his probability of survival from .945 to .982. He will not realize the greatest benefit for fifteen to thirty years after he stops smoking. If he has a high rate of time discount, the current value of that benefit will be quite small.

Furthermore, even in the period of greatest payoff, Table 2.1 does not offer much certainty regarding the benefit. Between ages 50 and 65 most smokers (about 75 percent) will *not* die, while a substantial proportion of nonsmokers (about 10 percent) *will* die. If the individual is strongly risk-averse to gains and risk-preferring for losses (as Kahnemann and Tversky suggest), the uncertainty of its effect makes him perceive the benefit of giving up smoking as even smaller.

Some experts contend that "simply providing information about various substances and their physiological and psychological effects usually produces no reduction in the onset of behaviors like smoking or drinking" (McAlister, 1979). The aggregate statistics on cigarette smoking, however, refute this proposition. Information about the harmful effects of cigarettes on health first became available to the public in 1953 and then again in 1964; each time, releasing the information brought about substantial changes in smoking behavior (Warner, 1977b). These changes are also evident in a cross-sectional multicohort analysis of smoking behavior at ages 17 and 24 that showed a reduction in the probability of smoking among those cohorts who came to maturity after 1953 (Chapter 12; see Figure 2.2).

This study also revealed two important aspects of the change in smoking behavior. First, the reduction in the probability of smoking varied directly and closely with education: the higher the level of schooling, the greater the reduction in the proportion who smoked. Second, the subjects differed in smoking behavior as sharply at age 17 (when they all had completed approximately the same amount of schooling) as at age 24 (when they had completed different amounts). Thus, the additional years of schooling did not *cause* the more educated subjects to alter their smoking behavior. Differences in family background, type of school attended, and other factors probably account for both the choice to remain in school and the choice to refrain from smoking. Of course, both of these choices may be related

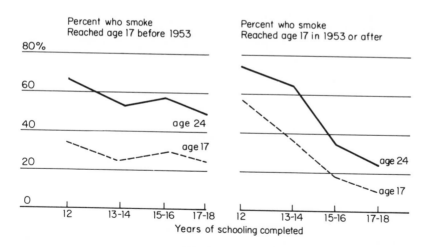

Figure 2.2 Cigarette smoking by men at ages 17 and 24, by years of schooling completed, sex, and cohort. *Source:* Farrell and Fuchs (1982).

to individual time preferences—that is, willingness or ability to incur current costs for future benefits (see Chapter 11). Schooling has long been recognized as a form of investment; decisions about cigarette smoking involve a similar trade-off between current pleasure and future health.

Concluding Comments

This chapter should not be interpreted as a "counsel of perfection." It would be unreasonable and unwise to expect policymakers to refrain from setting priorities until all the relevant information is available. Furthermore, we should not set higher standards for proof of efficacy of preventive programs than we do for diagnostic and therapeutic interventions. Health officials must work with what they have. This chapter has attempted to provide a framework for identifying the necessary data and indicating how they can be brought to bear on the problem of allocating resources to health education and promotion. I have also tried to show why some of the favorite "whipping boys" of health promotion are not the real obstacles, and have discussed two others, time preference and uncertainty, that seem to me to merit more attention. At a time of tight budgets for health agencies, it is becoming increasingly important to ask how tax dollars can be used most effectively to enhance the health and welfare of the population. State and local governments should look closely at the potential payoff from health education, health promotion, and similar interventions that will modify personal behavior. But they must do this in as hard-headed a fashion as possible.

Ten years ago I wrote, "The greatest potential for improving health lies in what we do and don't do for and to ourselves" (Fuchs, 1974a). My views have not changed. But I also still agree with Walter Lippmann (1955) that "a rational man acting in the real world may be defined as one who decides where he will strike a balance between what he desires and what can be done. It is only in imaginary worlds that we can do whatever we wish."

EMPIRICAL STUDIES: PHYSICIANS II

3 | Surgical Work Loads in a Community Practice

Many physicians and laymen believe that the only solution to the alleged "doctor shortage" is a massive increase in the number of physicians (Carnegie Commission, 1970; Journal of the American Medical Association, 1970; New York Times, 1970); other observers, however, have been calling attention to the underutilization of physicians in those tasks which long years of training have equipped them to perform (Ginzberg, 1966; Roemer and Duboise, 1969; Taylor, 1965). With the social cost of college plus medical school now well in excess of $100,000 per student, it is essential that the question of effective and efficient use of medical manpower receive careful study.

One area of medicine that has long been suspected of harboring underutilization is surgery. According to Longmire (1965), "in each community in our country there are a few surgeons who are doing all or more than they humanly can do. Many, though, are working at a pace far below their capacity and this is a tremendous waste of highly skilled talent." Bunker (1970) has hypothesized that in the United States there may be too many surgeons for the needs of the population and has suggested that this may lead to unnecessary surgery. An analysis of aggregate national data (Fuchs, 1969b) showed that even if all operations were done by surgical specialists, their average work load would be below five operations per week, which would fall far below capacity. Maloney (1970) and Owens (1970) have

Written with Edward F. X. Hughes, M.D., John E. Jacoby, M.D., and Eugene M. Lewit.

also presented evidence of work loads in this range—Maloney for university surgeons and Owens for general surgeons. Strickler (1968) and Phillips (1968) have argued the other side of the issue: that there is adequate work for surgeons and even a need for more in certain areas. Riley and associates (1969) provide indirect evidence that such a need may exist.

There have been very few attempts to measure the surgical work load of individual surgeons or of populations of surgeons (LeRiche and Stiver, 1959; Masson et al., 1971; Phillips, 1968), and even fewer attempts to distinguish carefully among different types of surgeons and different types of procedures. This chapter is an attempt to elicit direct evidence about the alleged underutilization of surgeons by quantifying the in-hospital surgical work load of a population of general surgeons. We first develop a methodology for aggregating different types of surgical procedures and then apply it to a population of general surgeons, in private practice, in a suburban community in the New York metropolitan area. No attempt is made here to measure the nonoperative work loads of these surgeons or to evaluate the quality of care they deliver.

Methods

The problem of aggregation. A major problem in measuring surgical work loads is the development of a set of weights to be applied to different procedures so that a meaningful summary index can be calculated. This is a common problem in economics, and the customary solution is to use "price weights." A similar approach could be used for surgical procedures by the application of a relative value scale, such as that developed by the California Medical Association in the 1950s (Committee on Fees, 1960) and subsequently adopted by a number of medical societies (Bureau of Medical Care Insurance, 1965).

The California Medical Association established the relative value scale to assist practitioners in arriving at equitable fees. Practitioners were asked to list their customary fee for a multitude of procedures. After extreme values were discarded, median and modal fees were determined. The median values were then multiplied by a conversion factor in such a way that a small procedure (puncture aspiration of abscess, subsequent) was given unit value and all other procedures expressed as multiples of it.

A surgical relative fee value is intended to encompass all the work associated with a procedure: preoperative and postoperative care as well as the actual operation. The question arises, however, whether the relative fees are systematically related to the amount of work involved in different procedures. To answer this question, the following data were collected for 24 general surgical procedures (of graduated complexity) and three miscellaneous categories. These latter categories were designed to encompass all general surgical procedures not included in the previous 24 and were classified as being of minimal (Class I), moderate (Class II), or considerable complexity (Class III).

1. Operating room (OR) time. The operating room log book of a major New York teaching hospital was examined to obtain the average OR time for each of the 27 categories. OR time, defined as the time from entrance of the patient to the operating room to his leaving that room, was recorded directly from the log. Data were collected for 20 consecutive operations in each category. For the miscellaneous categories, and the unilateral inguinal herniorrhaphy category, 50 operations were recorded. These additional data were collected because of the diversity within the miscellaneous categories and because the herniorrhaphy category is used as an index in our weighting system. The mean for each category was calculated.

2. Length of stay. Total length of hospital stay for each patient whose OR time was recorded was extracted from the hospital discharge record. The mean for each category was calculated.

3. Relative fees. The "1960 Relative Value Studies" of the California Medical Association (Committee on Fees, 1960) was the source of the relative fee value of each procedure.

4. Other data. It was hypothesized that the care of a patient undergoing an operation with a high mortality risk would entail more work than an operation with a lower risk. The lack of comprehensive, comparable data on operative mortality rates, however, precluded the inclusion of this variable in the subsequent analysis.

Table 3.1 and Figure 3.1 reveal an extremely high correlation between the relative fee and OR time ($r = 0.97$). There is a moderate correlation between relative fee and length of stay

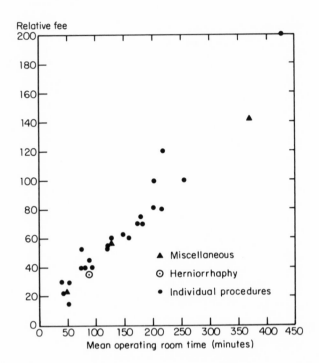

Figure 3.1 Mean operating room time and relative fee, 27 operative categories.

($r = 0.40$). From a regression of relative fee on OR time, the elasticity at the mean values was found to be 0.95, indicating an increase of 0.95 percent in relative fee for each 1 percent increase in OR time. The addition of length of stay to the regression equation has very little effect on either the OR time regression coefficient or the total explanatory power.

This evidence indicates that the relative fee value of a given operation is, in fact, a good reflection of the work associated with the procedure and would serve as a satisfactory weighting scale for comparing different procedures. To simplify our weighting scale, the relative fee value for each category was divided by the relative fee value for an adult unilateral inguinal herniorrhaphy (35.0). The resulting quotient expresses the value of each category as a multiple of a herniorrhaphy (see Table 3.1) and carries the label "hernia equivalents" (H.E.). Thus, a radical mastectomy with a relative value of 70.0, 2.00 times a ble 3.1 Relative fee, operating room (OR) time, and length of stay for 24 rgical procedures and 3 miscellaneous categories

ocedure	Relative fee	OR time (min)	Length of stay (days)	Hernia equivalents		
				Relative fee	OR time	Length of stay
east biopsy	15	50.2	3.7	0.43	0.57	0.44
ctal fistulectomy	22	41.8	7.7	0.63	0.47	0.92
ᵊmorrhoidectomy	30	39.0	5.7	0.86	0.44	0.68
ᵒnidal cyst, excision	30	50.8	6.6	0.86	0.57	0.78
guinal herniorrhaphy, unilateral adult	35	88.4	8.4	1.00	1.00	1.00
ᵈlebectomy, unilateral	40	74.8	1.6	1.14	0.84	0.19
ᵖpendectomy	40	79.5	11.3	1.14	0.90	1.34
ᵖloratory laparotomy	40	93.0	30.2	1.14	1.05	3.60
ᵖlostomy	45.8	87.5	41.6	1.31	0.99	4.95
ᵑputation of leg	52.5	74.8	71.4	1.50	0.84	8.50
guinal herniorrhaphy, bilateral adult	52.5	117.9	8.5	1.50	1.33	1.01
ᵗyroidectomy	55	120.0	6.4	1.57	1.36	0.76
ᵗateral phlebectomy	60	125.5	5.2	1.71	1.42	0.62
ᵖlenectomy	60	155.8	25.1	1.71	1.76	2.99
ᵗolecystectomy	62.5	146.5	19.8	1.78	1.66	2.36
ᵃgotomy and pyloroplasty	70	170.8	12.2	2.00	1.93	1.45
ᵈdical mastectomy	70	179.8	14.2	2.00	2.03	1.69
ᵃstroenterostomy and vagotomy	75	176.0	20.1	2.14	1.99	2.39
ᵃstrectomy	80	214.0	26.6	2.28	2.42	3.17
ᵖlectomy	81.5	198.8	27.2	2.33	2.25	3.24
ᵖbectomy	100	200.0	26.6	2.86	2.26	3.17
ᵖdominal-perineal resection	100	254.5	26.0	2.86	2.88	3.10
ᵊripheral vascular surgery	120	216.2	29.0	3.43	2.44	3.45
ᵒrtic-mitral valve replacement	200	423.8	35.7	5.71	4.79	4.25
ᵃss I	23.7	49.4	12.1	0.68	0.56	1.44
ᵃss II	56.5	125.4	22.6	1.61	1.42	2.69
ᵃss III	141.4	368.1	28.9	4.04	4.16	3.44

herniorrhaphy, is equal to 2.00 hernia equivalents. The unilateral adult inguinal herniorrhaphy category was chosen as the index in our weighting system for several reasons: the procedure is among the most common performed by general surgeons; it is a fairly standard procedure, varying little from surgeon to surgeon or patient to patient; it is in the middle range of complexity; and it holds a position of special importance in the early operative training of a general surgeon. This weighting system was then applied to a population of general surgeons to measure their surgical work loads and the relative complexity of the procedures they performed.

Surgical work load. The study population consisted of 19 general surgeons in private practice who constituted the entire general surgical staff of a medium-sized, voluntary, nonteaching hospital in a suburban community in the New York metropolitan area. The self-designation of these 19 physicians as general surgeons was confirmed by the New York State Medical Directory (Medical Society of New York, 1968–69), the Directory of Medical Specialists (American Board of Medical Specialists, 1970–71), and existing hospital appointments. Two surgeons at this hospital who concentrated on plastic surgery were not included in the study population because their specialized case loads differed qualitatively from the case loads of the general surgeons and did not lend themselves as readily to analysis by our weighting scheme. The case loads of those surgeons performing thoracic surgery and colon and rectal surgery entailed what is traditionally interpreted to be general surgery, and they were included in the study.

A listing of all operating room surgical procedures performed by these surgeons in a recent calendar year was obtained from the index hospital and from seven additional institutions to calculate each surgeon's complete hospital surgical work load. Weights were assigned to each procedure according to the relative fee scale (Committee on Fees, 1960) and expressed in terms of hernia equivalents. Weekly work loads were calculated on the basis of a 48-week year.

The first secondary procedure performed during each operation was recorded and arbitrarily assigned a relative fee value equal to 20 percent of its value as an independent procedure. This 20 percent value was felt to be a reasonable approximation of the additional work entailed in an operation with a secondary procedure. The data were not sensitive to the magnitude of this arbitrary approximation. The relative fee value for this secondary procedure was added to that for the primary procedure to arrive at a total for the operation. Further secondaries were not included.

Data were obtained on the amount of first assisting at operation by these surgeons. Inspection of the data revealed that in the overwhelming majority of cases, first assisting by a general surgeon was not medically indicated, and this work was not included in the calculation of surgical work load (Lohrenz and Payne, 1968).

Results

The 19 general surgeons in our study performed 4,178 operations in the calendar year, a work load that was probably at least as large as that of the national average and substantially above the average for New York State (Fuchs, 1969b). These operations, including 900 secondary procedures, amounted to 3,952 hernia equivalents (H.E.). The mean H.E. per operation was 0.95, and the median operation had a value of 0.94 H.E. Thus, more than half of the operations were less complex than an adult inguinal herniorrhaphy. Variations in complexity will be discussed later in this section.

Variations in work loads. As Table 3.2 and Figure 3.2 show, there was a very large variation in work loads among the 19 surgeons. The busiest surgeon performed 13.0 H.E. per week; the mean weekly work load was 4.3 H.E.; and the median was 3.1 H.E. per week. Thus, half of this population of general surgeons performed less operative work per week than the equivalent of 3.1 inguinal herniorrhaphies. The work was distributed among the surgeons in such a way that the bottom 50 percent of the surgeons performed 25 percent of the work, the upper 25 percent performed 50 percent of the work, and the upper 10 percent performed 25 percent of the work.

The importance of weighting operations is demonstrated by comparisons between surgeons. For instance, surgeons A and B performed almost exactly the same number of operations, but surgeon A's work load measured in hernia equivalents was

Table 3.2 Annual number of operations and hernia equivalents (H.E.) by surgeon

Surgeon	Annual no. of operations	No. of operations with secondary procedure	Annual no. of H.E.[a]	Weekly no. of H.E.[b]	Mean (H.E.)[a] per operation	S.D. of mean	Coefficient of variation
A	569	131	625	13.0	1.10	0.63	56.9
B	562	128	460	9.6	0.82	0.59	72.0
C	451	52	353	7.4	0.78	0.57	73.4
D	275	48	296	6.2	1.08	0.65	60.0
E	300	67	278	5.8	0.93	0.65	69.7
F	274	46	266	5.5	0.97	0.57	58.6
G	249	46	245	5.1	0.98	0.62	63.0
H	177	56	191	4.0	1.08	0.70	64.6
I	178	21	176	3.7	0.99	0.68	68.5
J	121	22	147	3.1	1.22	0.63	52.2
K	165	25	143	3.0	0.87	0.63	72.6
L	139	21	129	2.7	0.92	0.63	68.4
M	133	18	122	2.5	0.92	0.61	66.0
N	121	51	116	2.4	0.96	0.71	73.5
O	127	19	111	2.3	0.88	0.55	62.8
P	136	83	111	2.3	0.82	0.67	81.3
Q	98	23	92	1.9	0.94	0.62	66.7
R	47	8	48	1.0	1.01	0.73	72.4
S	56	35	43	0.9	.77	0.33	42.8
Total	4,178	900	3,952	—	—	—	—
Mean	200	47	208	4.3	0.95	—	—
Median	165	46	147	3.1	0.94	—	—
Weighted mean[c]	—	—	—	—	0.96	—	—

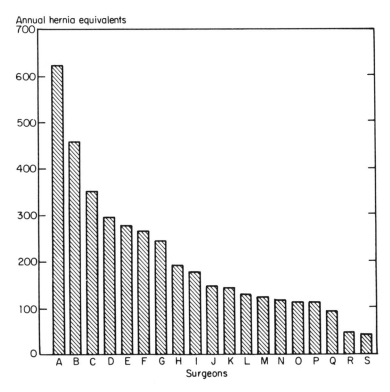

Figure 3.2 Annual hernia equivalents, by surgeon.

more than one-third greater. Surgeon C performed 64 percent more operations than did surgeon D, but his work load was only 19 percent greater.

What characteristics of surgeons are associated with different work loads? Table 3.3 compares groups of surgeons classified by professional accreditation, number of hospital affiliations, and age. Six surgeons were certified by the American Board of Surgery, five were Fellows of the American College of Surgery (FACS; approved residency training without Board certification), six were Fellows of the International College of Surgery (FICS; variable surgical training), and two had no evidence of similar accreditation. No attempt was made to analyze accreditation further in terms of number of years of residency. Board-certified surgeons have a mean weekly work load of 6.0 H.E., two-thirds greater than non-Board-certified surgeons with 3.6 H.E. per week. When non-Board-certified surgeons are cat-

Table 3.3 Work loads of surgeons classified by professional accreditation, number of affiliations, and age

Categories	Annual no. of H.E. per surgeon	S.D.	Weekly no. of H.E.	Mean H.E. per operation per surgeon	S.D. of mean
Professional accreditation					
Board-certified (N = 6)	286	177.6	6.0	0.98	0.10
Non-Board-certified (N = 13)	172	123.2	3.6	0.94	0.12
FACS[a] (N = 5)	148	90.8	3.1	1.03	0.12
FICS[b] (N = 6)	114	45.2	2.4	0.90	0.08
None (N = 2)	406	75.7	8.4	0.80	0.03
Number of affiliations					
2 (N = 4)	156	135.8	3.2	0.92	0.10
3 (N = 5)	143	37.4	3.0	0.96	0.08
4 (N = 5)	211	167.1	4.4	0.94	0.19
≥5 (N = 5)	312	183.7	6.5	0.97	0.08
Surgeon age					
≥65 (N = 2)	95	73.5	2.0	0.99	0.31
55–64 (N = 7)	156	65.4	3.2	0.95	0.07
45–54 (N = 5)	229	164.8	4.8	0.94	0.07
35–44 (N = 5)	305	200.0	6.4	0.96	0.14

a. Fellow of the American College of Surgery.
b. Fellow of the International College of Surgery.

egorized by their respective subgroups, it appears that the most productive group of all is nonaccredited surgeons. On average, the two nonaccredited surgeons performed three times as many H.E.'s as the FICS surgeons, more than twice as many as the FACS surgeons, and 42 percent more than the Board-certified surgeons. Owing most likely to the small sample size (2) of the nonaccredited surgeons, none of the differences between this group and the others are significant at 5 percent by the Mann-Whitney U test. The difference in work loads between the Board-certified surgeons and the FICS surgeons is significant at the 5 percent level.

The volume of surgical work load was inversely related to age of the surgeon. Surgeons aged 35 to 44 years performed twice as much surgery as those aged 55 to 64, and more than three times as much as those over 65. These differences, however, are not statistically significant at the 5 percent level.

The number of hospital affiliations of a surgeon was positively correlated with his work load. Surgeons with five or more affiliations did twice as much work as those with two or three affiliations, and 50 percent more than those with four. Of these differences, only that between those surgeons with three and those with five or more affiliations was significant at 5 percent.

To determine the net influence on annual work load of each of these variables (accreditation, age, and affiliations), a multiple regression technique was employed. The estimated equation was

$$\ln Y = 14.9 + 1.29 \ln X_1 - 2.83 \ln X_2 - 0.809 X_3,$$
$$(0.51) \qquad (1.00) \qquad (0.53)$$

with $\overline{R}^2 = 0.39$ (standard errors of the regression coefficients are given in parentheses). All variables except Board certification are expressed in natural logarithms. Y = annual H.E.; X_1 = number of affiliations; X_2 = surgeon's age; X_3 = dummy variable for Board certification.

The results of this equation are for the most part consistent with the previous findings. The coefficients of affiliation and age are significant at the 1 percent level. In a double log equation of this kind, the coefficients may be interpreted as elasticities; thus a 1 percent increase in a surgeon's age is associated with a 2.8 percent decrease in his annual work load, and a 1 percent increase in the number of affiliations is associated with a 1.3 percent increase in work load. The coefficient of Board certification is not significant at the 5 percent level, and the negative sign is unexpected. This may be the result of a negative correlation between age and certification.

Variations in complexity of operations. Although a few surgeons had a mean H.E. per operation substantially above or below the mean for the group, most recorded very similar values for their average operation and for the standard deviation of the mean (see Table 3.2). The mean operative value for 11 of the 19 surgeons deviated from the population mean by less than 0.10 H.E.

It should be noted that the distribution of operations by degree of complexity departs substantially from a normal distribution for the population as a whole as well as for individual surgeons. As shown in Figure 3.3, the distribution is multipeaked and skewed to the right. Fewer than 1.5 percent of the

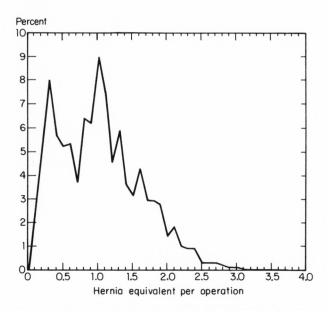

Figure 3.3 Distribution of all operations by complexity. *Note:* Data smoothed by four-term moving average.

procedures are valued at greater than 2.5 H.E., the equivalent of a colectomy. These larger procedures were scattered among surgeons of all degrees of accreditation. Of the 15 surgeons who performed operations of greater complexity than 2.5 H.E., 12 performed fewer than six during the year. The existence of this small number of complex procedures scattered in this population raises questions about surgical training and quality of care, which will be discussed in the following section.

As we saw in Table 3.3, the mean H.E. per operation did not vary much with professional accreditation, number of affiliations, or surgeon's age. Figure 3.4 shows some differences in the overall distribution between Board-certified and non-Board-certified general surgeons: the former have a smaller fraction of their operations in the range of 0.2 to 0.7 H.E., and slightly more from 0.9 to 2.0 H.E. These distributions are significantly different at the 1 percent level by the Kolmogorov-Smirnov test. The distribution of procedures greater than 2.0 H.E. among the two groups, however, is almost identical, with the tail of the curve for the Board-certified surgeons being slightly longer.

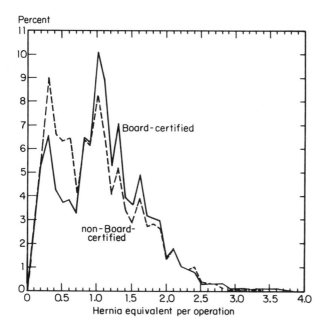

Figure 3.4 Distribution of operations by complexity: Board-certified and non-Board-certified surgeons. *Note:* Data smoothed by four-term moving average.

The data generated about this population of general surgeons permit comparisons of some properties of the surgeons' work in the various hospitals. Table 3.4 shows that the mean H.E. per operation is slightly larger (1.00 H.E.) in acute hospitals with fewer than 100 beds than in acute hospitals with 100 to 200 beds (0.92 H.E.). This difference in size of operations by hospital is confirmed in Figure 3.5, which shows the percentage distribution of operations by hospital size: the hospitals with fewer than 100 beds had less surgery below 1 H.E. and more surgery in the more complex range of 1.5 to 2.5 H.E. than the larger hospitals. These differences are significantly different at the 1 percent level by the Kolmogorov-Smirnov test. It is worthy of note that no surgery of complexity greater than a colectomy was performed in the smaller hospitals.

Table 3.4 shows that the two nonacute government hospitals have a mean H.E. per operation slightly greater than the two acute proprietary hospitals and the four acute voluntary hos-

Table 3.4 Complexity of operations by 19 surgeons in hospitals classified by si
and control

Categories	Annual no. of H.E.[a] per hospital	S.D.	Mean H.E. per operation per hospital	S.D. of mea
Number of beds[b]				
≤100 (N = 2)	65	72.12	1.00	0.25
100–200 (N = 4)	888	665.57	0.92	0.06
Type of hospital				
Proprietary (N = 2)	518	568.51	1.02	0.23
Voluntary (N = 4)	661	792.91	0.91	0.07
Government (N = 2)[c]	134	98.99	1.04	0.20

a. Primaries + 0.2 secondary procedures.
b. Acute hospitals only.
c. Nonacute hospitals.

pitals. The percentage distributions of operations by hospital
type (not shown) confirm the finding that the most complex
surgery is performed in the government hospitals but show that
the proprietary hospitals are doing more complex surgery than
the voluntary. These differences are significant at the 1 percent
level by the Kolmogorov-Smirnov test.

Discussion

The findings in this study of work loads of general surgeons—
the mean weekly work load of 4.3 H.E. and especially the median value of 3.1 H.E.—suggest substantial underutilization of
costly and highly specialized medical skills.

The problem of determining underutilization of surgeons is
complicated by the lack of an adequate standard of what a well-
balanced, productive surgical work load consists of. During this
study, we asked many surgeons in different practice settings
what they considered a desirable surgical work load. Consistently, the surgeons stipulated 10 H.E. per week; they felt that
a work load of this magnitude would provide an adequate technical challenge and still leave time for continuing education and
leisure. Phillips' data (1968) support this standard. Assuming
that the mean operation in his work load had the same H.E.
value as in our population, Phillips and colleagues averaged 10.3

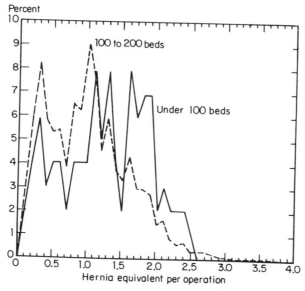

Figure 3.5 Distribution of operations by complexity: hospital size. *Note:* Data smoothed by four-term moving average.

H.E. per week. He felt this work load fulfilled his skills and still left time for other interests. The fact that a work load of 10 H.E. per week is not an unrealistic burden is further suggested by the work of Masson and colleagues (1971), who measured the work loads of two productive surgeons and concluded that a standard of 15 H.E. per week still left time for substantial extramural activities.

In our population, however, only one surgeon had a work load of more than 10 H.E. per week, and only one other approximated that value. The mean work load of the population is less than one-half the standard, and the median about one-third.

Other findings of interest in this study are:

1. Though Board-certified surgeons as a whole had a larger work load than noncertified surgeons, their work loads were smaller than those of the nonaccredited surgeons.
2. Surgeons in the youngest age group had the largest work loads.
3. Board-certified surgeons had slightly more complex work loads than non-Board-certified surgeons, but complex procedures were scattered throughout the population of general surgeons.

4. More complex surgery was being performed in the smaller acute hospitals.

One must be careful not to overgeneralize the results of this study. It was performed on only one population of 19 general surgeons in a state known to have a general surgeon/population ratio that is 64 percent in excess of the national norm (Taylor, 1965). Before generalized conclusions about surgical underutilization can be drawn, further research must be performed on larger and geographically stratified populations. Moreover, this study focuses only on the utilization of a surgeon's operating time. It would be inappropriate to draw conclusions from these data about the utilization of a surgeon's total professional time.

This population of surgeons is the first to have been so extensively studied. The results provide impressive support for the suggestive findings of other investigators. The similarity to results based on national data (Fuchs, 1969b) has already been mentioned. Owens (1970) found that surgical specialists were performing one to four major operations per week. Maloney (1970) found that university geographic full-time surgeons were operating 3.5 times per week, whereas strict full-time surgeons reported 2.2 operations per week. Masson and associates (1971) reported on a population of general surgeons who performed 3.8 operations per week. Subjective evidence of underutilization from surgeons themselves was reported by both Owens and Maloney. In the *Medical Economics* survey (1970), Owens stated, "Most [surgical specialists] felt they could do more—typically, at least five more major operations a week." Maloney (1970) stated that "it was an almost universal complaint among strict full-time surgeons that they had inadequate clinical material to maintain their professional competence." Wolfe and colleagues (1968), in their study of a Saskatchewan group practice, reported that the general surgeon there, earning a very good living, "estimated that he could have handled three times as much work as he actually carried out."

That the problem of underutilization is not universal, however, is illustrated by the work loads of Phillips (1968) and the data generated by Riley and co-workers (1969). The latter study showed that 65 percent of rural family practitioners in upstate New York performed hospital surgery and concluded: "There is significant demand for surgical and obstetrical practice in the rural region of New York State, and at present a large portion of the responsibility for providing these services lies with the family doctor." It appears that geographic distribution of general surgeons may be a factor in determining underutilization.

This investigation raises a number of questions for study for those concerned with the delivery of surgical care in the United States.

1. It appears that there may be widespread underutilization of general surgeons. Is underutilization purely a function of oversupply, or does it stem in part from uneven geographic distribution?
2. Does underutilization of general surgeons jeopardize the quality of care? Do surgical skills atrophy with underutilization? This problem of quality of care is highlighted by the example of a surgeon with a low work load performing one radical mastectomy or portacaval shunt per year.
3. Is a surgeon with a low work load more susceptible to the temptation to operate in equivocal therapeutic situations and run the risk of unnecessary surgery?
4. Is it possible that surgical residency programs are training too many general surgeons and, in addition, are overtraining these general surgeons for the job they will do (mean operation, 0.95 H.E.)? Taylor (1965) has stressed the need for residency reform to prepare for "the job to be done," and Longmire (1965) has actually called for a reduction by 100 in the number of senior residency positions offered in the United States.
5. Since complex procedures were scattered in small numbers throughout the population of general surgeons, could the quality of surgical care delivered by this and other populations of surgeons be improved by a pattern of regional organization in which all complex surgery would be referred to one hospital, and performed by highly trained, full-time surgeons?

This chapter indicates that a group of general surgeons is underutilizing highly trained skills, and other data suggest that this is not an atypical situation. One must be careful not to misinterpret this study, however; it is not a call for more surgery and does not mean to imply that high work loads per se mean high-quality surgery. Academic surgery has emphasized for decades that surgical intervention is only one in an armamentarium of therapies available to the surgeon. It has advocated operating only when precise indications are present and has stressed the importance of preoperative diagnosis and post-operative care. This advocacy has gone far to raise the level of surgical care in this country.

This study shows that there is a need for surgical services in the United States to be further investigated and organized in a more rational way. The American Surgical Association and the American College of Surgeons are now beginning to look at the problems of the delivery of surgical services in this country with the hope of raising the accessibility and quality of surgical care available to all (American College of Surgeons, 1971). It is to the credit of the specialty of surgery that these efforts are being undertaken, and it is to be hoped that they will add credence to Bunker's point (1970) that an "important corrective force . . . (in improving the delivery of surgical services) . . . is the growth and maturity of surgery as a specialty."

This chapter has focused on the field of general surgery. The methodology developed here is applicable to other specialties, and it is hoped that it will be applied. Other surgical specialties and some medical specialties may also evidence underutilization and inefficient utilization of valuable skills.

4 | Determinants of Expenditures for Physicians' Services

$\mathbf{C}$oncern over the cost of medical care is wide-spread. Special attention has been focused on the rapid rise in the price of and the expenditures for physicians' services because it is said that these services are essential, that the price is not determined in a competitive market, and that consumer ignorance gives the physician unusual control over the quantity and type of service provided. Furthermore, the extensive growth of third-party payment, through both private insurance and government programs, is believed to exacerbate inflationary pressures in this area by reducing the net price to the consumer and thus encouraging utilization.

The essentiality argument is a complex one and rests as much on subjective beliefs as on objective evidence. Basically, a service can be considered essential on two grounds. The first applies where the demand for the service is relatively insensitive to changes in income—where it is regarded as so necessary that (in the absence of philanthropy, sliding fee scales, or third-party payment) families with low incomes devote a relatively large portion of their budget to it. Some elements of physicians' services are clearly necessities in this sense (for example, surgery for an inflamed appendix). Many physicians' services, however, ranging from well-baby care through annual checkups to elective surgery, are not so clearly necessities, while still others (like cosmetic surgery) might well be classed as luxuries.

A second criterion of essentiality applies to a service whose

---

Written with Marcia J. Kramer.

consumption involves important external effects. Thus, basic education for all is considered essential in the United States partly because of the belief that the failure to educate some will have serious unfavorable repercussions on others. A similar argument concerning physicians' services could be advanced with respect to the treatment of communicable diseases. At one time such diseases occupied the bulk of physicians' time, but currently they are much less important.

Probably more important than the essentiality argument is the peculiar nature of the market for physicians' services. When a good or service (without significant external effects in either production or consumption) is produced and sold under reasonably competitive conditions, there is usually no special need for public attention or public policy. In such cases, changes in price and expenditures presumably reflect the true cost to society of producing the good or service and the knowledgeable judgment of consumers regarding its value. With respect to physicians' services, the imperfections of competition are numerous and powerful. On the supply side, these include the restrictions on entry created by licensure and professional control of medical education, the limitations on practice implicit in the hospital appointment system, and the absence of price cutting, advertising, and other forms of rivalry. As for demand, the difficulty consumers experience in judging the quality of physicians' services is well known, and it is thought by some that the physician plays a major role in determining the quantity of services to be provided (Barnes, 1970, for example).

The concern over cost among consumers has been reinforced in recent years by that of third-party payers, particularly the government. Open-ended commitments to finance services have been followed by very large increases in price and expenditures; these increases have stimulated efforts to uncover their causes and to develop techniques for moderating them in the future.

This chapter is concerned with the development and testing of a formal model to analyze the behavior of physicians and patients. Cross-sectional (state) data for 1966 are used to gain an understanding of variations in quantity of services per capita, physicians per capita, quantity of services per physician, and insurance coverage. The consequences for health of differences in the quantity of physicians' services are also explored.

The principal limitations of the study are attributable to the paucity of available data. In our analyses we were frequently forced to exclude certain variables that seemed appropriate on a priori grounds, or to include series that were only partially indicative of the variables actually desired. For instance, nearly all of the analysis is limited to physicians in private practice; data on expenditures for services rendered by salaried members of hospital staffs were not available. Even for private physicians, the breakdown of expenditures into price and quantity components is based on indirect estimates rather than precise, direct measures. Finally, it should be noted that this study did not intend to review systematically the literature on physicians' services, although we did consider the views of other observers in the formulation of hypotheses.[1]

Summary of Findings

The most striking finding of this study is that supply appears to be of decisive importance in determining the utilization of and expenditures for physicians' services. This conclusion stands in sharp contrast to the widely held belief that utilization and expenditures are determined by the patient, and that information about income, insurance coverage, and price is sufficient to explain and predict changes in demand.

An examination of variations in demand, holding technology constant, supports the view that the number of physicians has a significant influence on utilization, quite apart from the effect of numbers on demand via lower fees. Indeed, we find that the elasticities of demand with respect to income, price, and insurance are all small relative to the direct effect of the number of physicians on demand. Of course, the emphasis we give to supply does not deny an independent role for demand entirely, especially when the patient is faced with major changes in the net price of care, such as those created by the introduction of Medicare and Medicaid.

Because physicians can and do determine the demand for their own services to a considerable extent, one should be wary of plans which assume that the cost of medical care would be reduced by increasing the supply of physicians. Our analysis suggests that such increases would at best have limited impact on price, though they would result in substantial increases in utilization. In estimating the social value of increased utilization, however, note should be taken of our finding that variations across states in the quantity of physicians' services appear to have little or no effect on either infant mortality or the overall death rate. Of course, an increase in physician supply has other effects that should be considered. The subjective utility derived from the consumption of physicians' services is likely to rise as physicians devote more time and personalized attention to each complaint, and the indirect costs incurred by patients will fall as general access to physicians improves. These subjective and qualitative aspects of physicians' services are not considered in this study.

Given the importance of supply, it is of interest to ask what factors determine it. The cross-sectional analysis throws some light on physicians' locational decisions: they seem to be attracted by higher prices for their services, by medical schools and hospital beds, and by the level of educational, cultural, and recreational opportunities indicated by the average income of the population. We did not find any evidence for the theory that encouraging more state residents to enter medical schools pays off in terms of more physicians returning to practice in their state of origin. Nor do physicians show any special preference for states with low health levels. This absence of what some might regard as "professional responsibility" in choice of location stands in contrast to the behavior of physicians already established in a given location. We find that physicians practicing in states where the physician-population ratio is low *do* provide more services apart from any price considerations. Indeed, given location, there is no evidence to show that higher prices induce additional services from physicians; there is some reason to believe that they may have the opposite effect.

One finding in which we have considerable confidence deserves special mention because it reveals the unusual nature of the market for physicians' services. We refer to the fact that states with high quantity of service per capita (Q^*) have relatively low quantity of service per physician (Q/MD). The coefficient of correlation in 1966 was -0.5. The quantity series is admittedly imperfect, but errors of measurement in that variable would tend to produce a positive correlation between Q^* and Q/MD. There is good reason to believe, therefore, that the true correlation is even more negative than -0.5. Such a relationship is very surprising under either one of the following two interpretations of the Q/MD variable. If it is regarded as a measure of the average size of the "firm,"[2] we would expect a positive correlation with quantity per capita. If we regard it as a partial productivity measure, we would also expect a positive correlation with quantity per capita. These expectations are based on experience with many other industries (Schwartzman, 1969, for example). The negative relationship observed in this industry may be attributed to the behavior of physicians: where they are relatively numerous, they both increase the demand for their collective services and cut back on the amount of service each one individually provides; where they are scarce, the reverse occurs. The result is a strong negative correlation between Q^* and Q/MD.

Having set forth what we believe to be reasonable inferences from the data we have examined, we hasten to present a few caveats. The statistical experiments cannot be regarded as definitive; obvious weaknesses in the data and possible shortcomings in the specification of the model suggest that the empirical findings should be regarded as highly tentative. Given the data limitations, the chief contributions of this study are the development of a comprehensive model of the market for physicians' services and the development of a technique for estimating quantity and price by state.

Additional research is clearly essential in order to predict accurately the consequences of proposed changes in the financing and organization of medical care, and the availability of relevant, reliable data will be of critical importance to the success of that research. Considering the magnitude of health care expenditures, strenuous efforts to make such data available would seem justified.

Differences across States, 1966: An Econometric Analysis

In order to gain an understanding of physician and patient behavior net of technological change, we build and test a cross-sectional model. By examining differences across states at a single point in time we are in effect holding medical technology fairly constant. There may be some lag in the spread of new knowledge from one state to another, but the difference between the frontier of knowledge in the most and least advanced states in any given year is far less than the change that occurs over time.[3]

Another advantage of the cross-sectional approach is that it provides an opportunity to learn something about the factors influencing the supply of physicians. It is widely recognized that there are substantial barriers to entry into medicine, which are partly financial and partly caused by the reluctance of organized medicine to expand the volume of training facilities to the point where all applicants with an ability to pay would be accepted. Moreover, it takes a long time to establish a new medical school, and there is a lag of five or more years between the time a student enters medical school and the time he or she begins to practice. It follows that the total number of practicing physicians in the country cannot be responsive to any important degree to annual changes in price or other market conditions. By contrast, the potential elasticity of physician supply going to any one state is very great. Previous investigators have already demonstrated that licensing procedures pose no significant impediment to interstate migration of physicians (see Benham, Maurizi, and Reder, 1968; Holen, 1965). With entry into the total market effectively limited, the geographic distribution of physicians becomes a matter of particular concern.

A Framework for Analysis

Per capita expenditures for physicians' services vary considerably across states. In 1966, such expenditures were $68.68 in California compared with $26.42 in South Carolina.[4] How are we to explain such large variations in expenditures? By definition, expenditures are equal to quantity multiplied by price. More fundamentally, then, our task is to explain interstate variations in price and quantity. To do this economists employ a general model of demand and supply. In such a model the quantity demanded by consumers depends on price and many other variables, some of which are applicable to any commodity (for example, per capita income), others of which may be relevant only to one or a few commodities (for example, health insurance). The quantity provided by suppliers is also treated as a function of price and other variables. In equilibrium, the quantity demanded is exactly equal to the quantity supplied;

hence, actual quantity and actual price are simultaneously determined through the interaction of the demand and supply functions.

Specification of a model for physicians' services establishes a general framework within which a broad range of hypotheses regarding the behavior of patients and physicians can be investigated. Each structural equation of the model offers an explanation for the determinants of a particular aspect of the market for physicians' services. Our model has one equation dealing with variations in demand, one for the number of physicians, one for physician productivity, and one for the amount of insurance coverage.

Because the variables we wish to explain are not determined independently of one another, it is not possible to test our behavioral hypotheses accurately with ordinary least-squares regression equations. For example, one clear implication of the interdependence among these variables is that we cannot discover the true influence of price on physicians' locational choice simply by relating the total number of physicians practicing in a state to the observed price of physicians' services there. Possibly a demand-induced rise in price does tend to attract many physicians to a state; but this increase in supply will serve to depress price back toward its original level if the population can only be induced to purchase the additional services at a somewhat reduced price.

To cope with this problem, we estimate each of the structural equations of our model by means of two-stage least squares. This procedure allows a statistical disentanglement of the web of mutual causality in order to isolate the specific effect of one variable on another. The first stage of the method consists of obtaining predicted values for each endogenous variable by regressing it on all of the exogenous variables in the model.[5] The second stage consists of estimating the structural equation for each endogenous variable by regressing the actual value of that variable on the predicted values of appropriate endogenous variables and on relevant exogenous variables. With endogenous variables represented by their predicted values, the estimated regression coefficients are not biased by any effect that the dependent variables may have on them.

The model we present in the following section excludes many variables that one might reasonably expect to affect the demand for, or the supply of, physicians' services. The reason for their omission is that tests based on a preliminary model employing 17 exogenous variables revealed that only 5 of these did, in fact, appear in the system.[6] On these grounds we excluded the other 12 exogenous variables from the condensed version of the model presented below, which alone can be considered to possess an unbiased set of first-stage (predicted) endogenous variables. Discussions of the excluded variables and their role in the original model are incorporated into the following section under the appropriate subheadings. A complete list of the variables appearing in each model is presented in Table 4.1.

Table 4.1 List of variables

Final model	Preliminary model	Full title of variable (units)
	Endogenous Variables	
$Q*$	$Q*$	Quantity per capita (visits)[a]
$MD*$	$MD*$	Private physicians per 100,000 population
Q/MD	Q/MD	Quantity per private physician (visits)[a]
AP	AP	Average price (dollars)
$BEN*$	$BEN*$	Insurance benefits per capita (dollars)
NP	NP	Net price (dollars)
—	$INF\ MRT$	Infant mortality rate per 1,000 live births
—	$DTH\ RT$	Crude death rate per 1,000 population
	Exogenous Variables	
$INC*$	$INC*$	Disposable personal income per capita (dollars)
$BEDS*$	$BEDS*$	Short-term hospital beds per 1,000 population
$MED\ SCLS$	$MED\ SCLS$	Number of medical schools
PRM/BEN	PRM/BEN	Ratio of health insurance premiums to benefits
$UNION*$	$UNION*$	Union members per 100 population
—	$EDUC$	Median years of education, persons 25 and over
—	$\%BLK$	Percent black

Table 4.1 *(continued)*

Final model	Preliminary model	Full title of variable (units)
—	%AGED	Percent 65 and over
—	%URB	Percent urban
—	BRTH RT	Births per 1,000 population
—	TEMP	Mean temperature, average of major cities (degrees F.)
—	S&L GOV*	State and local government expenditures for health per capita (dollars)
—	HOSP MD*	Hospital staff physicians per 100,000 population
—	ΔINC*	Change in disposable personal income per capita 1960–1966 (dollars)
—	%PART	Percent of private physicians in partnership practice
—	%SPEC	Percent of private physicians who are specialists
—	MD ORIG*	Physicians originating per 100,000 population[b]

a. G.P. outpatient visit-equivalents.
b. Total of six sample years.

Specification of the Model

The interrelationships among the six endogenous and five exogenous variables of our final model can be summarized by four structural equations and two identities:[7]

(4.1) $Q^*_D = Q^*_D\ (\hat{AP}\ \text{or}\ \hat{NP}, BÊN^*, M\hat{D}^*, INC^*, BEDS^*).$

(4.2) $MD^* = MD^*\ (\hat{AP}, Q\hat{/}MD, MED\ SCLS, BEDS^*, INC^*).$

(4.3) $Q/MD = Q/MD\ (\hat{AP}, M\hat{D}, BEDS^*).$

(4.4) $BEN^* = BEN^*\ (\hat{Q}^*, \hat{AP}, UNIONS^*, PRM/BEN, INC^*).$

(4.5) $Q^*_D \equiv (MD^*)(Q/MD) \equiv Q^*_S.$

(4.6) $NP \equiv \dfrac{\text{Expenditures} - \text{Benefits}}{\text{Expenditures}}\ (AP)$

$\equiv \dfrac{AP{\cdot}Q^* - BEN^*}{AP{\cdot}Q^*}\ (AP).$

These relationships are presented diagrammatically in Figures 4.1 and 4.2.

In this equilibrium model of the market for physicians' services, the quantity of service demanded per capita (Q^*_D) is identically equal to the product of the two supply variables, number of physicians per capita (MD^*), and quantity of service per physician (Q/MD).[8] Because it seems unreasonable to suppose that purchases of medical insurance are unrelated to the price and quantity of the physicians' services covered, medical insurance benefits appear endogenously in the model. Price is represented by two variables: the average price received by physicians for their services (AP) and the net price paid by consumers (NP); AP exceeds NP according to the degree to which insurance benefits pay for the cost of the average visit. The exogenous variables in this system are per capita income (INC^*), number of medical schools ($MED\ SCLS$), hospital beds per capita ($BEDS^*$), labor union members per capita ($UNION^*$), and the ratio of health insurance premiums to health insurance benefits (PRM/BEN).

Both the demand for and the supply of physicians' services are thought to be subject to special forces. Whenever possible,

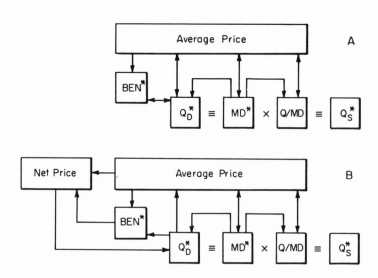

Figure 4.1 Relationships among endogenous variables, alternate specifications.

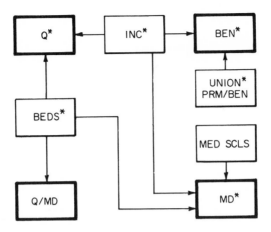

Figure 4.2 Effects of exogenous variables on endogenous variables.

we have attempted to incorporate the unique features often attributed to this market into our model. The following discussion of the four structural equations listed above considers these issues and indicates the range of questions that can be illuminated by a cross-sectional analysis.

Demand (Q^*_D). Prices and income are the customary economic determinants of market demand. How important are these financial considerations to consumers in determining their demand for physicians' services? Is the quantity of service demanded at all sensitive to its own price, and if so, to what extent? Does the quantity demanded vary with income? What is the income elasticity?

What is the role of medical insurance in demand? Some investigators believe that it is a major influence on the quantity of care purchased, yet our analysis of the time-series data yields no evidence indicative of a systematic relationship between changes in benefit levels and changes in Q^*. A related question concerns the mechanism by which insurance operates on demand (if, indeed, it does). In one specification of the model, *NP* replaces *AP* as the relevant demand price variable. The argument for so doing is that the impact of insurance can be entirely attributed to the reduction it effects in the net price of care. The substitution of *NP* for *AP* also implies that patients are indifferent to variations in the average amount collected by physicians so long as they are not personally responsible for financing the differentials. A less restrictive test of the role of insurance in demand retains *AP* as the price variable and adds to the equation the benefits variable, *BEN**. This specification leaves open the manner in which insurance affects demand. It also allows for the possibility that consumers are influenced even by those variations in *AP* which do not translate into variations in *NP*. If price-consciousness is a firmly ingrained consumer trait, changes in the institutional arrangements governing a particular market may not be strong enough to suppress altogether the usual behavior mechanism whereby low-cost goods and services are sought out, regardless of who gets the bill.

Certain services provided by private-practice physicians can only be consumed in hospitals: intensive diagnostic workups and most surgical procedures are common examples. To a limited extent, then, the services offered by hospitals and by private-practice physicians constitute a joint consumption product, hospitalized medical care. If for any reason the supply of hospital beds influences the quantity of hospital care that people purchase, an increase in *BEDS** may affect the demand for physicians' services as well.

The market for physicians' services is characterized by a high degree of consumer ignorance concerning the need for services and the central role of the physician as an authoritative adviser regarding their use. Given these circumstances, we hypothesize that physicians are able to *generate* a demand for their services without lowering price; we therefore include *MD** in the demand equation. When physicians are abundant in a state, they may order care that is not medically indicated (such as unnecessary surgery) or of only marginal importance (for example, cosmetic procedures, numerous postoperative visits, overzealous well-baby care). Alternatively, when physicians are very scarce, patients may lower their expectations and handle minor complaints with a minimum of physician intervention. There is also another reason why the supply of physicians might exercise a direct influence on the demand for physicians' services: a significant part of the cost incurred by the patient is in the form of time spent in travel and in waiting rooms. A reduction in the relative scarcity of physicians is usually associated with both an improvement in their locational distribution and a decrease in waiting-room time. To the extent that the ease or difficulty of seeing a physician is a determinant of demand, we have a second justification for including *MD** in the demand equation. The independent variables in our demand equation thus fall into two categories: economic variables common to any demand analysis (price, income) and institutional factors peculiar to this market (insurance, hospital bed supply, physician supply). Ten additional variables—most of which fall under the heading of "taste" factors—were tested in the preliminary version of the model (see the previous section). Because none proved to be statistically significant or measurably improved the fit of the equations, these were omitted from the final version of the model presented here, since their inclusion would have injected a bias into the first-stage endogenous variable estimates. The rejected demand variables are education (median years of school of persons 25 and over), urbanization, two measures of health status (the infant mortality rate and the crude death rate), percent black, percent elderly, the birth rate, mean annual temperature, per capita state and local government expenditures for physicians' services, and number of hospital staff physicians per capita. The last two variables attempted to measure the availability of alternative sources of supply of physicians' services (services by physicians other than private practitioners, who alone enter our study).

Supply of physicians (MD*). It is hypothesized that one variable influencing physician location is price. *AP* is clearly the relevant supply price variable, since it is of little import to the physician whether payment originates with his patients or with insurance companies.[9] To what extent is the present level of inequality in the distribution of physicians—the number of private practitioners per 100,000 ranges from 60 in Mississippi to 134 in New York—attributable to differences in price?

With price held constant, per capita income serves as a taste factor in this equation. Specifically, *INC** is a proxy here for the level of cultural, educational, social, and recreational opportunities a state has to offer. Because physicians as a group are very high earners, nonpecuniary factors of this sort may be a major consideration in their location decision. Another possible influence on physician distribution is the quality and availability of complementary medical facilities. As a test of this hypothesis we include *MED SCLS* and *BEDS** in the *MD** supply equation. Finally, we investigate the possibility that physicians are disinclined to open a practice in states where the average work load of their would-be colleagues is high. We should observe a negative sign on the endogenous variable $Q\hat{/}MD$ if it is true that physicians shun areas where they might feel under pressure to work long hours or spend less time per patient than they deem optimal.

Originally, we hypothesized that physicians would show some partiality toward their state of origin prior to entry into medical school, but tests with this variable in the preliminary model led to its rejection. In addition, no support was found for the view that physicians are drawn to practice in the medically neediest states, with medical need being measured by infant mortality (an endogenous variable); and therefore health, too, was excluded from this equation in the final model.

Quantity of Service per Physician (Q/MD). The real quantity of services provided by individual physicians varies considerably across states, the coefficient of variation being 15.4 percent. These productivity differences are an important factor in the interstate variations in physicians' gross income, which are quite large in view of the fairly high uniformity of skill among physicians.

Three factors are considered as possible influences on physician productivity. As with the supply variable, the relationship with price is an important matter to investigate. Do physicians respond to higher prices by working more hours and by seeing more patients per hour, or do they display a backward-bending supply curve, cutting back on their work load and maintaining their income while gaining the benefits of additional leisure and a less hectic pace of activity?

An increase in the supply of hospital beds should raise Q/MD if physicians have a tendency to hospitalize patients more readily whenever the necessary facilities are available.[10] This behavior might arise if there is a technological imperative on the part of physicians to practice the most up-to-date medicine within their grasp.

One of the most critical matters to be investigated is whether the situation in areas with a relative scarcity of physicians is partly relieved as a result of higher physician productivity. It is our hypothesis that the average physician, because of the nature of his professional training, feels under some ethical and social compulsion to supply additional services, even at the same rate of remuneration, when he is in an area poorly endowed with physicians. Thus, we anticipate a negative sign on the $\hat{MD}*$ variable in the Q/MD equation.

Two other variables were initially tested in this regression: the degree of physician specialization and the extent of partnership (as opposed to solo proprietorship) practice. Since neither proved to be significant, the two variables were omitted from the final model.

Insurance (BEN*). The argument for treating insurance as an endogenous phenomenon can be made on two grounds. The first is that the amount of insurance purchased depends on the expected level of outlays people are insuring against. Assuming a generally risk-averse population, an increase in expected outlays should call forth the purchase of additional insurance protection. Expected outlays will be highly dependent on expenditures in the recent past, and the best proxy for this in our model is expenditures in the present. The predicted values of both expenditure components, price and quantity, appear as explanatory variables in the insurance equation as a test of this hypothesis. If it is correct, the estimated coefficients of both variables should be (approximately) equal when the regressions are estimated in double-logarithmic form. If risk aversion itself rises (is constant, or falls) with the level of expected loss, the coefficients will exceed (equal, or fall short of) 1.0.

The other rationale for regarding insurance as endogenous lays stress on the cost of insurance itself rather than on the perceived need for the financial protection it offers. The cost of insurance is defined by the relation $PIV = (PRM/BEN)(AP) - AP$. PRM/BEN is the ratio of health insurance premiums to benefits, that is, the average price of purchasing one dollar of health insurance benefits (a figure greater than one). PIV thus represents the average price of insuring one general-practitioner (G.P.) visit-equivalent over and above the price of purchasing it directly. The reason for carrying insurance is that, in the event of extraordinary medical expenses, the return to an individual who expends PRM/BEN will be many times greater than one. Of course, there is also the inherent chance that the return will be as low as zero, but that is the gamble an insured person takes. On the average, an insurance payment of PIV is the nonrecoverable price one pays to be reimbursed for one G.P. visit-equivalent. The cost of insuring a given number of visits is thus seen to depend on two factors, the "fairness" of insurance policies and the price of physicians' services.

PRM/BEN is exogenous in our model, being dependent on such factors as the extent of group coverage compared with individual coverage and the relative importance of policies issued by nonprofit insuring organizations such as Blue Shield. *AP*, by contrast, is endogenous. If *PIV* is found to influence the consumer's willingness to insure, insurance itself is endogenous as a result of this dependence. Because *PIV* is the price of insuring one visit-equivalent and not the price of a dollar's worth of insurance benefits, the dependent variable in this specification should really be the number of insured visit-equivalents, or *BEN*/AP*. For consistency with the financial-protection theory of insurance, which demands a dollar measure of benefits, we maintain the *BEN** form throughout. When we wish to interpret the price coefficient as the price elasticity of demand for insured visits, however, we must first subtract 1.0 from its estimated value.

In addition to *PRM/BEN*, two other exogenous variables enter the insurance function: per capita income and the degree of unionization. The potential effectiveness of unions derives from their role in winning fringe benefits in the form of health insurance policies (which are particularly desirable because of their untaxed status). Unionization should increase the percentage of the population covered by insurance, since the decision to insure is no longer left to the discretion of the individual, and may also increase the mean level of benefits per insured.

In the preliminary version of our model we tested the hypothesis that people are differentially inclined to insure a newly acquired standard of living as compared to one that has been long held. The change in per capita income over the previous six years proved insignificant in the benefits equation, however, and thus was dropped from the final list of exogenous variables. Also rejected on the basis of these early tests was the level of education as a determinant of *BEN**.

The Data

The data used in this analysis come from a variety of sources and are of varying reliability. The critical expenditures and visit series regrettably are not of a kind in which we can place a high degree of confidence. Because interstate variations in these quantities are substantial and move in directions that remain fairly consistent from one year to the next, empirical analysis of the available data does seem justified. Nonetheless, until such time as a better data base has been established, conclusions derived from this study can only be suggestive of the true underlying relationships.

Expenditures. Our study population consists of the 33 states for which expenditures data are available for the year 1966.[11] Most of the omitted states have small populations; their absence does not have much effect on the results because each observation in our model is weighted by the square root of the state population. The 33 states accounted for 90 percent of the total U.S. population. The expenditures data come from the Internal Revenue Service and represent the reported gross receipts from medical practice of all self-employed physicians.

Availability of expenditures data was one of the key factors in our selection of a year for the cross-sectional analysis. When this chapter was written, state data on the gross business receipts of "offices of physicians and surgeons" had been published for only five other postwar years. With the exception of 1949 (for which these figures are obtainable for 48 states), the size of the sample has been limited (27 states for fiscal 1960–1961, 22 for 1963, 28 for 1965, and 26 for 1967). The other controlling factor in our decision was the availability of data on physician visits from the National Health Survey. The choice here was among the periods 1957–1959, 1963–1964, and 1966–1967. The year 1966 was chosen because the requisite data on expenditures were available for a relatively large number of states, and data on visits were also specific to that year.

The accuracy of the expenditures series is not easy to check. The possibility of some underreporting of income is suggested by the fact that the IRS data imply average gross receipts per physician of $46,600, compared with a median of $49,000 reported in *Medical Economics* for the same year. On the other hand, at least some of this disparity is explainable by the fact that *Medical Economics* only surveys full-time, self-employed physicians under the age of 65, while the IRS total includes the smaller average receipts of older physicians and of hospital staff and faculty physicians who devote just a fraction of their working time to private practice. Furthermore, only if the degree of underreporting varied significantly across states would this factor impair the validity of an analysis of variations in expenditures.

Far more serious is the distinct possibility that errors in this series are not uniform across states but have a sizable random component. Our suspicions on this count are based on intertemporal correlations of expenditures per capita across the 26 states for which these data are available for 1965, 1966, and 1967. The correlation coefficient for the 1965–1966 comparison is 0.863, and for 1966–1967, 0.912.[12] Although these figures are high enough to show that there is *something* systematic worth investigating in the pattern of variation in 1966 expenditures, they compare unfavorably with the (weighted) correlation coefficients for per capita disposable income in these states from one year to the next: 0.998 for 1965–1966, and 0.997 for 1966–1967. Closer examination of the official data on expenditures reveals that states with the most extreme jumps in expenditures had parallel shifts in the number of physicians said to be filing business income tax returns. These reported shifts in the number of physicians filing returns show virtually no correspondence to changes in the number of physicians practicing in each state, a statistical series kept by the American Medical Association.[13] To cite two of the most extreme examples, the IRS figures show a gain of 45.1 percent from 1966 to 1967 in the number of physicians filing returns in Wisconsin, and a fall of 25.8 percent in the number filing in Louisiana. According to the AMA, however, the number of practicing physicians in these two states rose by 1.2 percent and 2.0 percent, respectively, over this period.[14] It is apparent that official statistics on health care expenditures are greatly in need of improvement. Changes in nationwide expenditures totals over long periods no doubt provide a fairly accurate indication of changes actually taking place. For specific years or specific states, however, deficiencies in the statistical data now constitute a major impediment to serious research.

Physicians.   The scope of the market for physicians' services relevant to this study does not extend beyond the bounds of private practice. As the official expenditures series is limited to physicians' gross receipts from self-employment practice, so the

MD series we have chosen (our source is the American Medical Association) is restricted to private practitioners. Unlike the IRS count of physicians filing business income tax returns, the AMA data have the conceptual advantage of including salaried physicians in private practice, whose services go to meet the same demand as those of the self-employed and whose contribution to gross receipts may be considerable. The fact that the AMA bases its count on the results of routine questionnaires sent annually to all physicians while the IRS estimate derives from a sample of physicians filing a rather unpopular tax report makes the AMA series superior from a statistical viewpoint. Moreover, as already noted, the extreme instability of the IRS figures calls into question that data-gathering process itself. Unfortunately, neither the AMA nor the IRS series permits us to calculate precisely the number of full-time-equivalent physicians in private practice; the former covers physicians whose *principal* mode of employment is private practice, while the latter covers all physicians with some self-employment income, no matter how small a fraction of their professional time is involved. On balance, however, the AMA series probably more closely approximates the desired figure of full-time-equivalent physicians, since it includes some but not all part-timers and since it it not restricted to the self-employed.

Quantity and average price. Two of the most important series, quantity of service and average price, are not directly available and must be estimated. The quantity series we estimate is a measure of "general practitioner (G.P.) outpatient visit-equivalents," a fairly homogeneous unit across states. Dividing expenditures by quantity then gives us an implicit price series, which represents the average price of a G.P. outpatient visit-equivalent.

The quantity series is derived in the following way. The National Center for Health Statistics has published data on home and office visits per capita for the four census regions in 1966–1967 and for the nine census divisions in 1957–1959. We assume an intraregion per capita visit distribution of the 1966–1967 data based on the distribution that prevailed in the earlier period. The resulting home and office visit figure for each division is then attributed to each state within that division. Next, the number of hospital visits is estimated for each state from the number of patient days spent in nonfederal short-term hospitals.

Our assumption of one visit for each day of stay is supported by *Medical Economics,* which reports that the median number of hospital visits made by private practitioners in 1966 was 22 per week and that the median number of weeks worked per year was 48. If private practitioners in the 33 states of our study conformed to the *Medical Economics* medians, they would have made 177 million hospital visits. In fact, the total number of patient days in these states was very close to this, 185 million. Combining these disparate visit series, hospital inpatient visits are given a weight of 1.71 relative to home and office visits, this being the national ratio of average charges for the two categories of visits, according to Department of Health, Education, and Welfare statistics.[15] A final adjustment takes account of the fact that the distribution of total visits between G. P.'s and specialists varies across states. A visit to a specialist is accorded a weight of 1.93 relative to a G. P. visit, based on the ratio of average gross receipts per visit. In estimating the percentage of total visits made by specialists in each state, we of course make an allowance for the smaller visit load of specialists (0.63 as many visits as G. P.'s).[16]

There are undoubtedly some errors in the resulting quantity series and the price series derived from it, but we are not aware of any systematic biases. Some confirmation of the validity of the overall approach may be found in the fact that the resulting average price for a G. P. visit in our series is $5.75, which is very close to the $5.48 implicit in *Medical Economics* data for the same year.

Other variables. All series pertaining to insurance are based on data in the *Source Book of Health Insurance,* an annual publication of the Health Insurance Institute. The two endogenous insurance variables, *BEN** and *NP*, refer only to insurance coverage for physicians' services, that is, surgical, regular medical, and a share of major medical. The exogenous *PRM/BEN* variable pertains to all forms of health insurance (physician, hospital, and disability).

Information regarding the number of medical schools in each state (*MED SCLS*) is taken from the annual education issue of the *Journal of the American Medical Association. BEDS** represents the bed capacity of short-term, general, and other special hospitals, a series made available by the American Hospital Association. Figures on per capita disposable personal income in each state (*INC**) are published in the *Survey of Current Business*. The *Statistical Abstract of the United States* provides data on labor union membership (*UNION**).

Summary statistics for all variables are presented in Table 4.2. (The sources of data for the tables and figures in this chapter are described in detail in three appendixes in Victor R. Fuchs and Marcia J. Kramer, *Determinants of Expenditures for Physicians' Services in the United States 1948–68*, National Center for Health Services Research and Development, Department of Health, Education, and Welfare, Health Services and Mental Health Administration, December 1972; DHEW Publication no. (HSM) 73-3013. These appendixes also include a complete description of the method developed to estimate Q^*, data tables listing the most important series, and a correlation matrix.)

Regression Results

Table 4.3 presents the results of the second-stage regressions. All of the equations are estimated in double-logarithmic form, the estimated coefficients thus representing elasticities.[17] To avoid problems of heteroscedasticity, each observation is weighted by the square root of the state's population.[18] In computing the *t*-statistics for each variable, we have made those adjustments appropriate for two-stage estimation.[19]

PART A: DEMAND (Q^*)

Income. Estimates of the income elasticity of demand vary over a wide range (0.04 to 0.57), but, taken together, the equations support the findings of previous investigators that physicians' services are considered to be very much of a necessity, with an income elasticity substantially below 1.0. Our results correspond particularly closely with those of Andersen and Benham (1970), even though the units of observation are quite different (1966 state averages in one instance, 1964 family units in the other).[20] Simple regressions with income as the sole independent variable produce elasticities of 0.41 and 0.31, respectively, with both coefficients significant at the 0.01 level. The results for multiple regressions are also similar. In our more successful demand equations (A.6–A.11) we observe considerably lower and much less significant income coefficients (0.20 in A.6, 0.04 in A.7), when indeed income appears at all. Andersen and Benham report a statistically insignificant income

Table 4.2 Summary statistics, 33 states, 1966

Symbol	Full title of variable (units)	Mean[a]	Standard deviation[a]	Coefficient of variation (%)
EXP*	Expenditures per capita (dollars)	44.49	10.66	24.0
Q*	Quantity per capita (visits)[b]	7.71	.72	9.4
AP	Average price (dollars)	5.75	1.16	20.1
NP	Net price (dollars)	3.70	1.16	31.4
BEN*	Insurance benefits per capita (dollars)	16.00	4.29	26.8
MD*	Private physicians per 100,000 population	95.4	22.6	23.6
EXP/MD	Expenditures (gross income) per private physician (dollars)	47,003	5,900	12.6
Q/MD	Quantity per private physician (visits)[b]	8,354	1,290	15.4
DTH RT	Crude death rate per 1,000 population	9.42	.93	9.9
INF MRT	Infant mortality rate per 1,000 live births	23.7	3.2	13.6
INC*	Disposable personal income per capita (dollars)	2,605	418	16.0
MED SCLS	Number of medical schools	3.62	2.82	77.9
UNION*	Union members per 100 population	9.5	4.0	42.4
BEDS*	Short-term hospital beds per 1,000 population	3.78	.53	14.1
PRM/BEN	Ratio of health insurance premiums to benefits	1.27	.08	6.6
%SPEC	Percent of private physicians who are specialists	64.9	5.9	9.0
ΔINC*	Change in disposable personal income per capita, 1960–1966 (dollars)	663	89	13.4
EDUC	Median years of education, persons 25 and over	10.5	.98	9.3
%AGED	Percent 65 and over	9.5	1.4	14.7
%BLK	Percent black	11.2	8.7	78.3
%PART	Percent of private physicians in partnership practice	24.1	8.6	35.5
BRTH RT	Birth rate per 1,000 population	18.5	1.17	6.3
MD ORIG*	Physicians originating per 1,000 population[c]	2.08	.61	29.4

Table 4.2 *(continued)*

Symbol	Full title of variable (units)	Mean[a]	Standard deviation[a]	Coefficient of variation (%)
S&L GOV*	State and local government expenditures for health, per capita (dollars)	34.26	11.41	33.3
HOSP MD*	Hospital staff physicians per 100,000 population	28.4	13.9	49.1
TEMP	Mean temperature, average of major cities (degrees F.)	56.3	7.1	12.5
%URB	Percent urban	70.6	13.8	19.5

a. Each observation weighted by square root of population of state.
b. G.P. outpatient visit-equivalents.
c. Total of six sample years.

elasticity of 0.01 in a multivariate analysis.[21] It should, of course, be stressed that all these values refer to the responsiveness of quantity—not of expenditures—to changes in income. The difference between the two is not trivial, given the tendency of *AP* to rise with income. A simple regression with per capita expenditures as the dependent variable yields an income coefficient of 0.96.

One factor that might possibly contribute to the very low income elasticity of demand is the high correlation of income with earnings, which, in turn, is a good indication of the price of time. Physicians' services are usually time-intensive, and this means that they are more costly to those with high earnings. If we were to estimate the effect of income with earnings held constant, it is likely that a higher elasticity would result.[22] Unfortunately, the requisite state data are not available.

The importance of the earnings factor can be appreciated from Figure 4.3, which shows, for various age and sex classes, the 1966 ratio of per capita physician visits made by persons with family incomes over $10,000 to those made by persons with family incomes under $3,000. Both sexes under the age of 14 display large effects of income on visits; the same holds true for males aged 65 and over. In essence, earnings are held nearly constant (at approximately zero) as family income rises for these groups, allowing us to observe the effect on demand of income alone. The implicit income elasticities of demand are

Table 4.3 Results of weighted, logarithmic regressions, second stage, interstate model, 1966 (N = 33)

Part A: Q* (Quantity per capita)

Equation	$\bar{R}^2$	INC*	$\hat{AP}$	$\hat{NP}$	$\hat{BEN}$*	$\hat{MD}$*	BEDS*
A.1	.515	0.412[b] (5.92)	n.i.	n.i.	n.i.	n.i.	n.i.
A.2	.578	0.571[b] (9.25)	−0.290[b] (−3.58)	n.i.	n.i.	n.i.	n.i.
A.3	.588	0.269 (1.64)	−0.205[a] (−2.25)	n.i.	0.177 (1.99)	n.i.	n.i.
A.4	.585	n.i.	−0.104 (−1.65)	n.i.	0.313[b] (9.97)	n.i.	n.i.
A.5	.566	0.449[b] (9.94)	n.i.	−0.153[b] (−3.24)	n.i.	n.i.	n.i.
A.6	.732	0.199[a] (2.54)	−0.356[b] (−5.28)	n.i.	n.i.	0.388[b] (6.28)	n.i.
A.7	.727	0.042 (0.61)	n.i.	−0.200[b] (−5.55)	n.i.	0.397[b] (6.90)	n.i.
A.8	.735	n.i.	n.i.	−0.201[b] (−5.63)	n.i.	0.428[b] (15.10)	n.i.
A.9	.715	n.i.	−0.297[b] (−4.16)	n.i.	n.i.	0.507[b] (11.22)	n.i.
A.10	.746	n.i.	n.i.	−0.059 (−0.69)	n.i.	0.359[b] (7.34)	0.193 (1.95)
A.11	.752	n.i.	n.i.	n.i.	n.i.	0.335[b] (12.01)	0.252[b] (6.06)

Note: Adjusted *t*-statistics appear in parentheses. n.i. = not included.
a. Significant at 0.05 level.
b. Significant at 0.01 level.

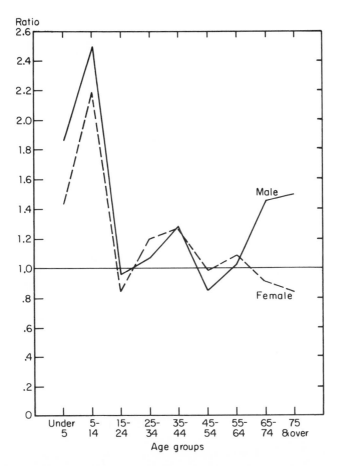

Figure 4.3 Ratio of number of physician visits by persons with family income greater than $10,000 to visits by persons with family income less than $3,000, by age and sex, 1966–1967. *Source:* U.S. Department of Health, Education, and Welfare, "Volume of Physician Visits, United States, July 1966–June 1967," *Vital and Health Statistics,* series 10, no. 49, November 1968, p. 19.

still less than 1.0, but are hardly negligible. By contrast, income exerts no systematic influence on visits of persons aged 15 to 64; the positive effect of income on demand, we believe, is nullified by the negative effect of earnings (that is, the price of time). Also in accordance with our expectations is the fact that among the 25-64 age group, where male labor-force participation rates are roughly twice as large as those for females, income exerts a somewhat greater influence on visits by females than on visits by males. Indeed, only two of the eighteen age-sex categories behave in a contrary fashion to what we would expect under our hypothesis if it were the sole means of explaining age-sex differences in the effect of income on demand.[23]

Omission of quality differences from our quantity measure may also be exerting a downward bias on the estimated income elasticity, but the nature of medical education in this country (all recognized schools must have AMA accreditation, and National Board Examinations are increasingly employed as a state licensure requirement) makes it unlikely that state-to-state quality differences among physicians are an important factor. On balance, we believe that variations in earnings, on the one hand, and patients' *belief* in the essential nature of physicians' services, on the other, are responsible for the low income elasticity of demand.[24]

We should emphasize that problems of multicollinearity prevent any firm conclusions regarding the exact magnitude of the income coefficient. Thus, our income elasticities are consistently larger and generally more significant in the equations that do not consider *MD** as a variable than in those that do. The great improvement in explanatory power that results with the introduction of *MD** (A.6 versus A.2, A.7 versus A.5) and the consistently high *t*-statistic attaching to the physician variable lend credence to the latter specification. It is clear that, of the two variables, *MD** is dominant, with income playing a comparatively minor role. These qualifications notwithstanding, there is nothing in these equations—regardless of what combination of variables we consider—to suggest an income elasticity even approaching 1.0. All the evidence indicates that the demand for physicians' services is quite income-inelastic, though precisely to what degree we cannot accurately say.

Price and insurance. The price elasticity of demand for physicians' services appears to be unusually low. None of the equations reported in Table 4.3A show *AP* or *NP* coefficients exceeding (in absolute value) -0.36. The *t*-statistics on the price variables indicate that a high degree of confidence can be placed in this finding. Our result parallels Paul Feldstein's finding (1964) of a low demand price elasticity of -0.19, also significantly different from zero.[25]

There are three principal explanations for the relative insensitivity of demand to changes in price. First, it should be remembered that the demand for physicians' services is derived from the consumer's demand for health. Michael Grossman (1972a) has estimated the price elasticity of demand for health at -0.5, which seems reasonable, given the absence of any close substitutes for health. The price elasticity of demand for a derived input must be lower than for the final commodity unless there are important possibilities of substitution with other inputs. This leads to the second explanation, namely, that there are many legal and psychological barriers against the substitution of persons without the M.D. degree in the physicians' role, even though such persons might be good substitutes in a technical sense. Similarly, there are many factors other than medical manpower that contribute to the individual's production of health, including diet, housing, recreation, and education. These may, in fact, be excellent alternatives to physicians' services in the long run, but they may not be so regarded by the patient.[26]

Finally, it should be noted that the price paid is only part of the total cost of physicians' services to the patient. In addition to possible inconvenience, the patient must reckon with costs of transportation and, more important, time spent in travel, waiting, and during the visit itself. These indirect costs (IC) vary greatly from individual to individual, though in general we would expect a positive association between them and the direct cost of a visit (AP) because IC is closely dependent on the price of time, AP varies with income, and both income and the price of time are highly correlated with earnings. In the event that IC and AP are perfectly correlated, variations in AP are exactly proportional to variations in the total price of a visit and the AP coefficients we estimate are not biased, despite the omission of an IC variable. If, however, IC tends to rise faster than AP, we are underestimating the true interstate variation in price and thereby overestimating the price elasticity of demand, and vice versa. The direction of possible bias from this source is not ascertainable.

The relevance of insurance to demand is tested in two ways. We first investigate the role of insurance using the BEN^* variable. Unfortunately, strong multicollinearity between income and benefits prevents any conclusions on this score. The $\bar{R}^2$ is essentially unchanged, whether we employ income, benefits, or both in the demand regression (A.2–A.4); although either variable alone is highly significant, both show much lower t values when they appear jointly. It is impossible to infer how much of the observed variation in Q^* is attributable to each of these variables, or what the true coefficients of each are.

NP is superior to BEN^* as a measure of insurance because of its much smaller correlation with INC^* (0.14 versus 0.86). Using NP we may consider all economic influences on demand simultaneously (that is, income, average price, and insurance, the latter two embodied in the NP variable). With insurance thus accounted for, we observe a somewhat smaller but still very significant income elasticity as compared to the case of income and average price considered alone (A.5 versus A.2). The high correlation between AP and NP nonetheless complicates the critical judgment as to whether insurance per se is important to demand. In some instances AP is the stronger variable (A.6 versus A.5), while in others the situation is reversed and NP is stronger (A.8 versus A.9). But in any case, the price elasticity of demand is not much affected by the choice between these two price variables.

What we can say with assurance concerning the role of insurance in demand is that the elasticity of Q^* with respect to BEN^* is, at most, fairly low. That is, even under the extreme assumption that INC^* is of *no* real importance in this relation, the elasticity with respect to BEN^* is only 0.31. The very large t-statistic on BEN^* in A.4 indicates not only that this coefficient is significantly greater than 0, but also that it is significantly less than 0.4. Such a finding is not in line with our prior notions concerning the effect of insurance, despite the fact that in at least one instance comparable findings have been reported in the literature.[27] Some discussion of possible explanations is, therefore, in order.

First, the prevailing impression about insurance is that it induces higher utilization by lowering the price faced by the consumer. Yet if this is the mechanism through which insurance operates on demand, and if demand is price-inelastic, as we have found the case to be, it is to be expected that demand will also be insurance-inelastic. For example, if benefits initially reimburse 40 percent of average price, a 1 percent rise in BEN^* will produce a 0.67 percent fall in NP (from 0.60 AP to 0.596

AP). With a (net) price elasticity of -0.20, this will result in only a 0.13 percent rise in Q^* (close to the 0.18 rise shown by A.3). On the other hand, if demand were highly responsive to price changes, say with an elasticity of -1.50, the same 1 percent rise in *BEN** would call forth a 1.00 percent rise in Q^*. It should be noted that we would expect the effect of insurance on demand to be greater among persons with a very low or negligible price of time (the young, the elderly, the unemployed), because incremental insurance benefits for them result in a much larger percentage change in the full price of a visit.

A second factor is that private insurance for physicians' services is usually heavily biased toward coverage of relatively nondiscretionary care. Surgical procedures and in-hospital care are far more likely to be reimbursed than routine office visits or preventive services (Reed and Carr, 1970). This restriction in coverage may greatly reduce the impact of insurance relative to what it might have been.

Physicians. The highly significant role of *MD** in the demand equation requires some discussion. It cannot be attributed to a supply-induced fall in the physician's fee, because price (*AP* or *NP*) is already held constant. Rather, it seems to be the result of the following forces. First, an increase in *MD** is likely to reduce the average distance separating patient and physician, as well as the average waiting time. The consequent saving in time and transportation expense lowers the total cost of a visit to the patient even if fees are held constant. Given a low price elasticity of demand, however, this factor alone is insufficient to account for the magnitude of the *MD** coefficient. A second possibility is that physicians themselves inflate demand whenever the supply of medical manpower is relatively slack. This thesis is put forth persuasively by Eli Ginzberg (1969): "The supply of medical resources has thus far effectively generated its own demand . . . Much unnecessary surgery continues to be performed . . . There is substantial overdoctoring for a host of diseases, including, in particular, infections of the upper respiratory tract . . . [physicians] usually have wide margins of discretion about whether to recommend that a patient return to the office for one or more follow-up visits." A supply-induced demand change is fully sufficient as an explanation for the role of *MD** in the Q^* equations of Table 4.3A; if verified, its implications for policy are profound. Evidence that the additional physicians' services provided under loose supply conditions are, in fact, of a marginal nature is presented in the discussion of the effect of physicians' services on health in the following section. This much is to be expected if, as Ginzberg also suggests, physicians gravitate toward the more serious cases as their supply becomes taut.

A third possible explanation for the importance of MD^* is the existence of permanent excess demand for physicians' services. This is the thesis advanced by Martin Feldstein (1970), whose time-series analysis of this market yielded positive demand price elasticities (as high as 1.67), inconsistent with an equilibrium hypothesis. Feldstein's negative and significant insurance elasticities and his occasionally negative income elasticities are likewise inexplicable under normal market conditions. In our view, a much simpler interpretation of Feldstein's results is the failure to take account of technological change, which shifted the demand curve to the right over time, and not at a constant rate. Since the cross-section regressions, which essentially hold technology constant, can be readily interpreted under the assumption of market equilibrium, we see no reason to substitute either here or in the time series the less defensible explanation of permanent excess demand.

Hospital bed supply. Introducing $BEDS^*$ into any of the demand equations discussed above seriously affects the conclusions to be drawn regarding price (either AP or NP). A.10 is illustrative: The price coefficient approaches zero (in some equations it actually becomes positive), and the variable loses all statistical significance. Indeed, the "best" demand equation, in terms of sheer explanatory power ($\bar{R}^2$), is one in which price, income, and insurance have all been dropped and only MD^* and $BEDS^*$ appear (A.11). Nevertheless, accepting the results of A.11 on face value may be seriously misleading. To be sure, a rationale is advanced here in support of a causal relationship running from bed supply to demand for physicians' services. That is, the services of hospitals and of physicians are in many ways a joint consumption item, and thus an increase in the former serving to meet a backlog in *its* demand will permit an expanded consumption of physicians' services, desired but previously technically unfeasible because of the unavailability of the requisite hospital facilities. Beyond this, if the frequent allegation is true that the supply of hospital beds tends to create its own demand, it follows that any increase in BEDS*, even if wholly unrelated to the prevailing demand for hospitalization, will (indirectly) raise Q* as well.

The trouble with this explanation for the role of BEDS* in the Q* equation is that it takes no account of the fact that the relationship between these two variables is inherently biased by the very method used to construct Q*. Hospital days per capita constitute one of the three components of the quantity series, and because there is so little interstate variation in occupancy rates, days are almost entirely proportional to bed capacity. In our judgment, BEDS* is probably significant in the Q* equation not so much because it bears a causal relationship to the dependent variable but rather because of the statistical dependence of Q* on BEDS*. Equations in part A that do not include BEDS* are probably more accurate indications of the true determinants of demand for this reason.

PART B: SUPPLY OF PHYSICIANS (MD*)

Medical schools, price, hospital bed supply, and per capita income are the principal factors influencing physicians' locational decisions (Table 4.3B). Collinearity among the last three of these variables makes it difficult to determine precisely the specific effect of each, but the four together account for about 78 percent of the variation in MD*.

The role of the medical school in physician location is twofold. As a center of education, it draws doctors-to-be to the state, and its affiliated hospitals attract interns and residents. Professional contacts are established, and young families take root. As a major medical center, it generally promises superior staff and facilities in its teaching hospitals. Regardless of where they trained, physicians may find it advantageous to have such a complex within close proximity of their practice, since it allows them to arrange referrals and consultations while maintaining contact with the patient. Our estimated coefficient, highly significant in all but two cases, indicates that, on the average, one additional medical school in a state raises the number of physicians practicing there by about 4 percent.

A glance at equations B.2–B.8 makes apparent the presence of collinearity among the three other important location variables. Price is highly significant, with coefficients ranging from

Table 4.3 (continued from p. 90)

Part B: MD* (Physicians per 100,000 population)

Equation	$\bar{R}^2$	MED SCLS[c]	INC*	$\hat{AP}$	BEDS*	$\hat{Q}/MD$
B.1	.521	0.059[b] (5.99)	n.i.	n.i.	n.i.	n.i.
B.2	.754	0.036[b] (4.37)	0.750[b] (5.51)	n.i.	n.i.	n.i.
B.3	.731	0.050[b] (8.46)	n.i.	0.828[b] (6.40)	n.i.	n.i.
B.4	.509	0.061[b] (5.63)	n.i.	n.i.	−0.107 (−0.48)	n.i.
B.5	.775	0.040[b] (4.16)	0.490[a] (2.21)	0.419 (1.64)	n.i.	n.i.
B.6	.784	0.036[b] (8.54)	0.071 (0.40)	1.052[b] (4.26)	0.492[b] (2.86)	n.i.
B.7	.791	0.037[b] (10.34)	n.i.	1.144[b] (14.64)	0.550[b] (7.04)	n.i.
B.8	.755	0.039[b] (4.47)	0.759[b] (5.57)	n.i.	−0.161 (−1.02)	n.i.
B.9	.783	0.032 (0.69)	n.i.	0.994 (0.71)	0.528[a] (2.35)	n.i.
B.10	.776	0.027 (0.36)	0.080 (0.27)	0.752 (0.31)	0.443 (0.92)	−0.199 (−0.11) −0.382 (−0.13)

Note: Adjusted *t*-statistics appear in parentheses. n.i. = not included.
a. Significant at 0.05 level.
b. Significant at 0.01 level.
c. Linear variable.

0.83 to 1.14, in those equations where it appears alone with *MED SCLS* or where *BEDS** is also present (B.3, B.6, B.7), but with *BEDS** dropped and *INC** retained, the price coefficient falls considerably and loses its significance (B.5). In like fashion, *INC** is a significant variable, with an elasticity of 0.49 to 0.76, when it appears alone with *MED SCLS* or in conjunction with either *AP* or *BEDS** (B.2, B.5, B.8), but both its coefficient and its adjusted *t*-statistic plummet when all four variables enter the equation (B.6). Similarly, *BEDS** is significant if, and only if, *AP* also appears in the equation (B.6 and B.7, but not B.4 or B.8). It is with caution, therefore, that we proceed to a discussion of these results.

Our average price measure is clearly superior as a supply variable in this context to physician gross income, the monetary incentive variable employed by Benham, Maurizi, and Reder (1968). In their analysis the two-stage least squares method was utilized to estimate demand and supply equations for the number of physicians in each state in 1950; although physician income had a positive sign in the supply equation, it was not statistically significant. This is as expected: business receipts are positively related to work load as well as to price, and it is surely unreasonable to expect doctors to be attracted to states where they can anticipate little leisure time. If anything, the opposite hypothesis merits consideration, and we investigate this possibility. Unlike the demand equations, where there was some question regarding the specification of the relevant price variable itself (*AP* or *NP*), *AP* is obviously the correct choice in this case, since it matters little, if at all, to the supplier of services who is paying the bills he sends out.

INC* serves in the physician supply equation as a general taste variable rather than as an indication of financial inducements to settlement, since price is also held constant. As predicted, the life-style available in high-income states does appear to exercise some influence over the location of physicians.[28] Hospital bed supply—which is probably a proxy in a more general sense for the whole range of medical facilities and auxiliary personnel— also appears to be an important nonpecuniary consideration in physicians' location decisions.

No support is found for the view that physicians actually shun states where the average physician work load is high. The en-

Table 4.3 *(continued)*
Part C: *Q/MD* (Quantity per physician)

Equation	$\bar{R}^2$	$A\hat{P}$	BEDS*	$M\hat{D}$
C.1	.420	-0.828^b	n.i.	n.i.
		(-3.84)		
C.2	.603	n.i.	n.i.	-0.622^b
				(-3.25)
C.3	.622	-0.297	n.i.	-0.494
		(-0.57)		(-1.50)
C.4	.622	0.012	0.259	-0.672
		(0.01)	(0.39)	(-1.21)
C.5	.635	n.i.	0.252	-0.665^b
			(0.71)	(-2.80)

Note: Adjusted *t*-statistics appear in parentheses. n.i. = not included.
a. Significant at 0.05 level.
b. Significant at 0.01 level.

dogenous $Q/\hat{M}D$ variable bears the anticipated negative sign but never approaches significance, and its inclusion, in fact, only serves to reduce the adjusted R^2 of the regression (B.9 versus B.7, B.10 versus B.6). It is indisputable that certain areas, both rural and urban ghetto, are unpopular with physicians, but fear of overwork does not appear to be a factor in their judgment.

PART C: QUANTITY PER PHYSICIAN (*Q/MD*)

The number of physicians per capita is the only variable tested that clearly has a significant impact on physician productivity; it alone accounts for 60 percent of the variation in *Q/MD* (Table 4.3C). The coefficient of the $\hat{MD}$* variable indicates that about two-thirds of the incremental supply of physicians' services that might be expected to ensue with an increase in the number of physicians practicing in a state will be effectively nullified by a reduction in output of the average practitioner. These results suggest that increases in the number of physicians in a state, whether resulting from shifts in distribution or expansion of the total stock, may actually result in *higher* prices for physicians' services. According to the regressions, a 10 percent rise in *MD** will lead to a 4 percent rise in demand as the new physicians create a market for their services, but the supply of services may rise by as little as 3⅓ percent once resident doctors have adjusted to the decreased urgency of unattended cases and opted for a reduction in their activity.

The price elasticity of supply per physician is probably low. Only a very small degree of confidence can be attached to the initial finding of a negative price elasticity. Some collinearity between AP and MD* is present, as demonstrated by the reduced t-statistic of each when they appear jointly (C.1 and C.2 versus C.3); although C.3, with price included, is superior to C.2, C.4 is inferior to C.5. These results are not unlike those reported by Martin Feldstein (1970): price coefficients in his supply-per-physician equations range from -0.28 to -1.91, with only the higher (absolute) values achieving significance at the 5 percent level. In any case, we find no support for the hypothesis that higher prices induce *additional* services from physicians already located in a state.

Adding BEDS* to the productivity equation with only MD* in it increases the explanatory power by a fair amount (C.5 versus C.2), but the BEDS* coefficient is statistically insignificant and of a low magnitude.

PART D: INSURANCE (*BEN**)

The purchase of insurance for physicians' services, as distinct from the demand for physician care itself, appears to be very sensitive to variations in personal income (Table 4.3D). We find elasticities ranging from 0.76 to 1.61, and in all cases but one they are significant at the 1 percent level (the exception is D.7, where the simultaneous presence of so many independent variables cancels the significance of each and also lowers the INC* elasticity).

Three other hypotheses are investigated relating to the determinants of BEN*. Again, because of high correlations among the independent variables, we test these theories one at a time before assessing their effects in combination. The degree of unionization has a small but important effect on BEN*, raising the $\bar{R}^2$ from 0.74 in D.1 to 0.81 in D.2. This conclusion is weakened when PRM/BEN and AP also appear in the equation, but even then the $\bar{R}^2$ is improved by inclusion of UNION* (D.6 versus D.3). The purchase of insurance seems to be very responsive

Table 4.3 *(continued)*
Part D: *BEN** (Physician insurance benefits per capita)

Equation	$\overline{R}^2$	INC*	UNION*	PRM/BEN	$\hat{AP}$	$\hat{Q}^*$
D.1	.735	1.442[b] (9.47)	n.i.	n.i.	n.i.	n.i.
D.2	.812	0.761[b] (3.39)	0.254[b] (3.70)	n.i.	n.i.	n.i.
D.3	.819	1.465[b] (10.89)	n.i.	−1.576[b] (−5.04)	−0.739[b] (−4.26)	n.i.
D.4	.754	1.270[b] (3.62)	n.i.	n.i.	−0.259 (−0.93)	0.761 (1.43)
D.5	.814	1.605[b] (6.66)	n.i.	−1.691[b] (−5.04)	−0.838[b] (−3.87)	−0.277 (−0.68)
D.6	.823	1.060[b] (3.28)	0.130 (1.48)	−1.116[a] (−2.22)	−0.430 (−1.42)	n.i.
D.7	.820	0.513 (0.77)	0.201 (1.82)	−0.596 (−0.82)	−0.030 (−0.06)	0.634 (0.91)

Note: Adjusted *t*-statistics appear in parentheses. n.i. = not included.
a. Significant at 0.05 level.
b. Significant at 0.01 level.

to its price, *PIV*. This composite variable is dependent on both the average price of physicians' services and the cost of one dollar of insurance benefits. As predicted by this hypothesis, the coefficients of *AP* and *PRM/BEN* are each negative and highly significant in D.3. Deducting 1.0 from the estimated *AP* coefficient allows us to interpret the equation as a representation of the demand for insured visit-equivalents (that is, *BEN*/AP*). We see that the price elasticity of demand, as indicated by both *PIV* components, appears to be quite high, on the order of -1.58 to -1.74.[29] Apparently, the decision to purchase medical insurance is influenced much more by income and price than is the decision to purchase physicians' services. We find no support for the financial-protection theory of insurance, which holds that the amount of insurance people wish to carry varies directly with the level of anticipated expenditures they are insuring against. This theory predicts equal, positive coefficients of approximately 1.0 for both *AP* and *Q**,[30] yet we find in D.4 that the coefficient of *AP* is negative, while that of *Q** is positive but not statistically significant. Dropping *Q** from the regression brings about a slight improvement in the $\bar{R}^2$ (D.7 versus D.6, D.5 versus D.3) and permits a much less ambiguous interpretation of the role of *AP* in insurance purchases. It is only because of its dependence on *AP* that insurance is endogenous to this system.

Because of the many ambiguities complicating the interpretation of most of these regression equations, we feel it wisest to refrain from presenting a reduced-form version of the model.[31] We have seen that two of the exogenous variables, *BEDS** and *INC**, lend themselves to more than one interpretation, depending on the equation in which they appear, but such distinctions would be lost in a reduced form. More serious is the problem of multicollinearity. The consequent instability of coefficient estimates is troublesome enough in the interpretation of individual regression equations, but then at least it is known which variables must be approached with caution. In a reduced form, because of the intricate pattern of substitutions, this instability may be magnified manyfold and its repercussions felt throughout the entire system. Depending on the choice of equations to represent the model, numerous versions of the reduced form are possible, some with sharply contrasting implications. Under the circumstances, it seems preferable to state

Table 4.4 Results of weighted, logarithmic health regressions, ordinary least squares, interstate model, 1966 (N = 33)

Equation	$\bar{R}^2$	%AGED[a]	INC*	%BLK[a]	EDUC	Q*	MD*	EXP*
DTH RT								
DR. 1	.560	0.055[b] (6.41)	−0.008 (−0.12)	n.i.	n.i.	n.i.	n.i.	n.i.
DR. 2	.679	0.061[b] (8.25)	n.i.	n.i.	−0.364[b] (−3.33)	n.i.	n.i.	n.i.
DR. 3	.814	0.060[b] (10.71)	0.333[b] (4.79)	n.i.	−0.823[b] (−6.49)	n.i.	n.i.	n.i.
DR. 4	.811	0.062[b] (9.90)	0.354[b] (4.68)	0.001 (0.73)	−0.780[b] (−5.54)	n.i.	n.i.	n.i.
DR. 5	.804	0.062[b] (9.31)	0.347[b] (3.67)	0.001 (0.71)	−0.779[b] (−5.42)	0.016 (0.13)	n.i.	n.i.
DR. 6	.811	0.062[b] (9.93)	0.404[b] (4.44)	0.001 (0.87)	−0.739[b] (−5.04)	n.i.	−0.057 (−0.99)	n.i.
DR. 7	.815	0.059[b] (8.95)	0.391[b] (4.85)	0.001 (0.88)	−0.658[b] (−3.86)	n.i.	n.i.	−0.079 (−1.24)

Table 4.4 (continued)

Equation	$\bar{R}^2$	%AGED[a]	INC*	%BLK[a]	EDUC	Q*	MD*	EXP*
INF MRT								
IM.1	.796		−0.144 (−1.68)	0.011[b] (6.47)	n.i.	n.i.	n.i.	n.i.
IM.2	.787		n.i.	0.011[b] (6.33)	−0.196 (−1.19)	n.i.	n.i.	n.i.
IM.3	.791		−0.122 (−1.22)	0.010[b] (5.55)	−0.083 (−0.44)	n.i.	n.i.	n.i.
IM.4	.785		−0.089 (−0.73)	0.010[b] (5.43)	−0.090 (−0.47)	−0.079 (−0.50)	n.i.	n.i.
IM.5	.783		−0.132 (−1.08)	0.010[b] (5.38)	−0.090 (−0.46)	n.i.	0.011 (0.14)	n.i.
IM.6	.787		−0.152 (−1.38)	0.010[b] (5.10)	−0.172 (−0.75)	n.i.	n.i.	0.056 (0.69)

Note: *t*-statistics are in parentheses. n.i. = not included.
a. Linear variable.
b. Significant at 0.01 level.

the limitations of our knowledge rather than compound the possibility of error.

The Effect on Health

The degree to which variations in the quantity of physicians' services consumed affect health status, that is, Health = $f(Q^*,$ ...), is a matter of prime concern. A priori considerations suggest that causality might run in the reverse direction as well, from health to demand—that is, $Q^* = g$(Health, ...). If so, two-stage least squares would be the recommended method for determining the effect of quantity on health, with the predicted value of the endogenous Q^* variable entering the health regressions and vice versa. In the preliminary large-scale model described earlier, in the section "A Framework for Analysis," this procedure was adopted. However, tests based on this model lent no support to the hypothesis that variations in health contribute to interstate variations in the demand for physicians' services. Hence, coefficients obtained from ordinary least squares regressions of health on Q^* should not be biased.[32]

Two dependent variables have been chosen to represent health status in these regressions: the crude death rate (*DTH RT*) and the infant mortality rate (*INF MRT*). The independent variables include factors of a general nature—income, education, percent black, and percent elderly (this last only in the *DTH RT* equations)—and factors specifically related to the consumption of physicians' services. In addition to Q^*, we test MD^* and per capita expenditures for physicians' services (*EXP**) in this equation. The first of these is, theoretically, the desired variable, but because of possible measurement errors we do not rely on it exclusively. No two of these physician variables rely on the same data base.

The most important conclusion we can draw from the regressions of Table 4.4 is that, other things being equal, variation in the consumption of physicians' services does not seem to have any significant effect on health, as measured by either the crude death rate or the infant mortality rate. This finding is consistent with the work of previous investigators concerning the relative unimportance of medical care (not restricted to physicians' services) as a determinant of interstate variations in death rates (Auster, Leveson, and Sarachek, 1972).

Higher educational levels are very strongly associated with

lower crude death rates. Education is also negatively related to infant mortality, but this is not statistically significant.[33] Contrary to what many would expect, per capita income is positively related to the crude death rate after controlling for the effect of education. It is, however, negatively related to infant mortality. These results for education and income confirm the findings of Fuchs (1965), Grossman (1972a), and Auster, Leveson, and Sarachek (1972). The "percent black" is positively associated with both death variables, but the effect is much greater with respect to infant mortality.

Conclusion

We have presented a formal econometric model of the market for physicians' services in 1966, using cross-sectional data. Although our findings must be regarded as tentative because of the limited quantity and uneven quality of available data, the demand for physicians' services appears to be significantly influenced by the number of physicians available. The effect exerted on demand by supply appears to be stronger than that of income, price, or insurance coverage. Physician supply, across states, is positively related to price, the presence of medical schools and hospital beds, and the educational, cultural, and recreational milieu. The quantity of service produced per physician is negatively related to the number of physicians in an area, and it does not increase in response to higher fees. The demand for medical insurance, unlike the demand for physicians' services, does appear to be quite sensitive to differences in income. It is also significantly related to the price of insurance and to unionization. Finally, interstate differences in infant mortality and overall death rates are not significantly related to the number of physicians, to the quantity of their services, or to expenditures.

If subsequent research should confirm these findings, the implications for public policy are substantial. According to a widespread view, large increases in the number of physicians will drive down the price of and expenditures for physicians' services, will diminish the inequality in their location, provide a proportionate increase in the quantity of services, and make a substantial contribution to improved health levels. The model and data we have examined do not provide any support for this view.

Studies of medical-care utilization have focused on the determinants of demand (Newhouse et al., 1974; Lave, Lave, and Leinhardt, 1975; Feldstein, 1971; Roemer and Shonick, 1973), on the effects of care on health outcomes (Benham and Benham, 1975a), and on barriers to access to hospitals and physicians (Aday and Andersen, 1975; Davis and Reynolds, 1976; Benham and Benham, 1975b). Particular concern has been expressed about improving access for low-income families, non-whites, the elderly, and people living in rural areas.

This chapter is primarily a description of access to surgical operations, although the results elucidate some of the determinants of demand. Through a detailed multivariate analysis of National Health Interview Survey data, we measured the relation between socioeconomic factors and the utilization of in-hospital surgical care in 1970. In addition, we analyzed changes in surgical utilization between 1963 and 1970, a period that spans the introduction of Medicare and Medicaid, the spread of poverty health clinics, and other efforts designed to improve access for disadvantaged groups.

We examined both overall differentials in surgical utilization and the nature of the differences. If race or residence or income affects surgical utilization, do the differentials vary by procedure according to their complexity, urgency, or necessity? Similarly, if there were significant increases in surgical utilization by dis-

---

Written with Claire Bombardier, M.D., Lee A. Lillard, and Kenneth E. Warner.

advantaged groups between 1963 and 1970, were they uniform across types of operations or larger for some types than for others? It has been suggested, but rarely examined empirically (Rafferty, 1975; Ferguson, Maw, and Wallace, 1976; Warner, 1977a), that utilization of certain types of "discretionary" medical care responds to changes in economic variables, whereas the utilization of "nondiscretionary" care is largely unaffected by such changes. One purpose of this study is to contribute some empirical evidence relevant to these conjectures.

Data and Methods

The data source is the Health Interview Survey (for 1963 and 1970) conducted by the National Center for Health Statistics. The data represent a probability sample of households including all living civilian noninstitutionalized individuals. In 1970 interviews were conducted with approximately 37,000 households containing about 116,000 individuals, and in 1963 with 42,000 households containing 134,000 individuals. Surgical rates were obtained in response to the following questions: "Was the respondent hospitalized at any time during the last 12 months?" and, if an operation was performed, "What was the name of the operation?"

We studied the socioeconomic determinants of the overall utilization of surgical operations[1] as well as those of 11 selected procedures isolated to explore more fully the nature of possible differentials by type of operation. The 11 selected operations are appendectomy, cataract removal, cholecystectomy, dilation and curettage (excluding abortions), hemorrhoidectomy, hernia repair, hysterectomy, lumbar laminectomy for disk, prostatectomy, tonsillectomy, and varicose-vein stripping. Each of the 11 procedures occurs frequently (the sum of the 11 accounts for 42 percent of all nonobstetrical operations), and each represents a well-defined procedure for a reasonably well-defined health condition. The 11 procedures have been scaled on indexes of "complexity," "urgency," and "necessity." The complexity index is based on the California Relative Value Scale (Committee on Relative Value Studies, 1969). The urgency and necessity indexes are based on 93 replies (50 percent response rate) by physicians to a mailed questionnaire. Physicians were asked to indicate for each of the 11 procedures which of the following five statements best characterized their impression of most of the operations being performed:

1. In most situations it is imperative for the safety and comfort of the patient to operate within 24 to 48 hours.
2. The operation is necessary for the safety and comfort of the patient, but can be delayed up to a few weeks.
3. The operation is generally indicated, but can be postponed for convenience with little risk to the patient.
4. There is substantial divergence of opinion concerning the indications for this operation.
5. In my opinion, the operation is probably done too often in this country.

Urgency was measured as the proportion of physicians categorizing the procedure with statements 1 or 2. Necessity was measured as the proportion of physicians *not* categorizing the procedure with statements 4 and 5.

The original unit of observation in the survey is the individual person, but in our analysis individuals have been grouped into cells by year of observation, sex, race (white, nonwhite), residence (in or outside standard metropolitan statistical areas), age (six classes), and education of the head of the household in which the individual resides (five classes). There were potentially 240 cells in each year, but because some cells had zero observations, our final sample consisted of 238 cells in 1970 and 232 in 1963. Although each individual either had an operation of a particular type in the survey year or did not, our analysis focused on the variations in surgical rates (per 1,000 population) among the cells. These rates represent the probability of operation for each individual, given the characteristics used to define the cell.

We applied a linear regression model, with surgical rates in each cell being a function of cell characteristics. The cell characteristics are included in the regressions as dummy variables—variables that take the value 1 or 0 depending on whether or not the characteristic applies to the cell. Weighted regressions were used to correct for heteroscedasticity (that is, unequal variance) due to unequal numbers of observations per cell. Each cell was weighted by the square root of the number of persons in the cell.[2] The mean rate for any aggregate group can be calculated from the regression coefficient of the dummy variable for that group. For example, if race was the only independent variable in the regression, the coefficient of the nonwhite variable was the difference between the crude or unstandardized mean rates for nonwhites and whites: if the regression included age and sex as well as race, the coefficient of the nonwhite variable would then represent the difference in the mean rates of whites and nonwhites standardized for age and sex. The rates adjusted for age and sex obtained by this method were checked against rates obtained by the "indirect" method of age-sex adjustment. The results were almost identical.

In addition to the dummy variables corresponding to the characteristics used to classify individuals into cells, we also regressed on family income in several alternative specifications. When we wished to standardize for family income to see the effects of other variables holding income constant, we entered a series of income dummy variables based on the percentage of individuals in each cell distributed across family-income classes. This was the most general way to enter income into the regression, since it did not constrain the income effect to any particular form. When we wished to determine the relation between the dependent variable (for example, the operative rate) and income, we entered the mean income of each cell and the square of mean income, or, alternatively, we entered the natural logarithm of mean income. Income in 1963 was always adjusted for the Consumer Price Index and expressed in real 1970 dollars.

Although the Health Interview Survey is a rich source of data representative of the nation's population, several shortcomings and biases should be noted. The chief disadvantage of the operation data is that they are based on recall by the individual or proxy respondent. Although hospitalizations and operations are reported with greater accuracy than simple episodes of illness, an overall rate of underreporting of 10 percent remains (National Center for Health Statistics, 1965); moreover, this underreporting is not uniformly distributed among the characteristics used to classify the cells. When deliveries are excluded, there is little difference between rates for male and female reporting, as well as among age groups. Whites, however, report hospitalization more accurately than nonwhites (10 percent and 16 percent underreporting, respectively). Higher education is also associated with more accurate reporting, as is higher income (controlling for education). This underreporting complicates the analysis of operation rates among socioeconomic groups within a given year, but it should not bias the measurement of changes in surgical rate for specific groups between 1963 and 1970 unless the differentials in underreporting changed appreciably between the two years.

A second limitation of the data is that only living noninstitutionalized individuals are included in the survey. This limitation will lead to a slight underreporting of operation rates, mostly among the elderly, who are more at risk of dying or of being institutionalized.

Current family income is the only income variable available in this data set. If income were used to classify individuals by cell this procedure could create a bias in the estimation of the effect of income on surgical utilization since individuals who have undergone operations in the last year may have had their income temporarily reduced. We minimized this problem in our analysis by working with data grouped by characteristics other than income. The number of individuals who have had operations in each cell relative to those who have not is small; we would therefore expect the cell's mean income to be minimally affected.

Results

Surgical Rates, 1970

The results for all operations (except obstetrical procedures) for 1970 are presented in columns 1 and 2 of Table 5.1 in the form of number of operations per thousand population per annum. The overall rate is 55.5 per thousand. Each year in the United States approximately one person in twenty enters a hospital for an operation. Adjusted for age and sex (column 1), the rate is significantly higher for whites and residents of standard metropolitan statistical areas than for nonwhites and those living outside standard metropolitan statistical areas. Though not shown in Table 5.1, a significantly higher rate for females and the elderly than for males and persons under age 65 is also observed. Surgical utilization is greater for individuals in households in which the head has 9 to 14 years of schooling

Table 5.1 Utilization rates for all operations (excluding obstetrical procedures) and 11 selected procedures, by socioeconomic characteristics (operations per 1,000 population), United States, 1970

| Characteristic | All operations standardized for: | | 11 selected procedures standardized for: | |
	Age and sex (1)	Age, sex, race, residence, education and income (2)	Age and sex (3)	Age, sex, race, residence, education and income (4)
All	55.5	55.5	23.4	23.4
Race				
Whites	57.3*	56.2	24.6*	23.6
Nonwhites	42.1	50.2	15.2	21.8
Residence				
In SMSA†	57.1*	56.9	24.1	23.4
Out of SMSA	52.5	52.9	22.0	23.6
Education of head of family (yr):				
≤8	50.0‡	58.3	20.4‡	27.6
9–12	59.1	58.5	25.7	25.7
13–14	58.2	56.6	23.6	21.1
15–16	50.4	43.7	21.5	14.5
17+	52.3	36.0	18.3	5.6

*Difference significant at 0.05 level by t-test.
†Standard metropolitan statistical areas.
‡Differences significant at 0.05 level by F-test.

than for those in households in which the head has less than 9 years or more than 14 years of schooling. Those differentials that are statistically significant by the t-test ($p < 0.05$) are indicated by asterisks. Double daggers mark differences for a group of dummy variables significant by the F-test (also $p < 0.05$)—that is, at least one of the dummy variables in the group is significantly different from one other.

When we also control for race, residence, education, and family income (column 2), the results change appreciably. In particular, the white–nonwhite differential is much smaller and not statistically significant. Since the differential remains significant when we control for everything except income (not shown in Table 5.1), most of the racial differential in utilization appears to be attributable to differences in income and not to color per se. A similar story holds for residence: the urban-rural differential (residents in and outside standard metropolitan statistical areas) becomes nonsignificant when adjusted for income in addition to the other variables. The age and sex differentials remain significant when controlling for the various characteristics.

Standardizing for income eliminates the difference between the two lowest educational classes and also suggests changes in the rates for the higher-education groups. The higher-education groups have higher average income, which tends to raise their utilization rates, but with income held constant, their rates appear to be below average (although the differences are not statistically significant). There is a well-known positive relation between schooling and health. To the extent that surgical utilization depends on health status, this relation would be consistent with lower surgical utilization by those with more schooling. It is also possible, however, that for a given health problem, the better educated are less likely to be operated on because physicians have more confidence in their compliance in nonsurgical treatment and their home conditions are considered more favorable for outpatient care. Facilitating this compliance would be better ambulatory insurance coverage, which may be held by the more highly educated. The suggested negative relation between education and hospital utilization is supported by our finding (not shown) that the higher-education groups also had fewer nonsurgical admissions. This result is even more striking given the decrease in underreporting as education increases.

Some additional insights concerning the relation between education and surgical utilization are obtained by examination of the interactions between education and age (Figure 5.1). We find that with standardization for race, residence, and sex, rates are fairly uniform across education classes for the young and the old. The significantly lower utilization by the more highly educated is concentrated in those 20 to 64 years of age. These results are consistent with the view that education is a proxy for the value of time (that is, the dollar value of an hour away from regular work activity is greater for more highly educated per-

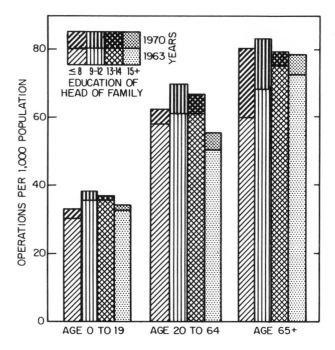

Figure 5.1 Surgical utilization standardized for sex, race, and residence by age and education of head of family, 1963 and 1970.

sons, at least for the head of the family) and that an operation requires much time away from regular activities. The differential value of time across education groups is most important for persons in the prime working ages, and least important for the young and the elderly.

Another strong interaction effect is that between race and residence (Figure 5.2). When data are standardized for age, sex, and education, there is a significant white–nonwhite differential regardless of residence, but this differential is considerably greater outside the standard metropolitan statistical areas. Rural nonwhites report 46 percent fewer operations per thousand population than rural whites. Within standard metropolitan statistical areas, the reported differential between whites and nonwhites in 1970 was only 20 percent. No significant difference is observed between whites residing in and whites residing outside these areas.

Columns 3 and 4 of Table 5.1 present results for the 11 surgical procedures. The overall rate for these operations is 23.4

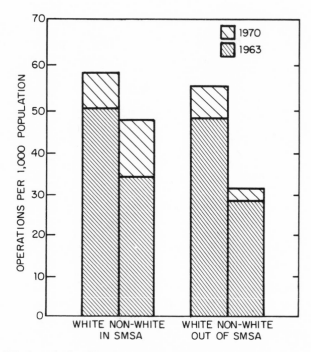

Figure 5.2 Surgical utilization standardized for age, sex, and education of head of family by residence and race, 1963 and 1970. *Note:* In 1970 residence was classified as "in SMSA" (standardized metropolitan statistical area) or "out of SMSA." In 1963 it was classified as urban or rural.

per thousand population. As with all surgical procedures, the differential between whites and nonwhites is very large until standardized for income. It then becomes statistically nonsignificant and is of the same order of magnitude as the probable differential in underreporting. Whether one controls only for age and sex (column 3) or for all the characteristics (column 4), there is no significant difference by residence for the 11 procedures; however, there is a significant difference for the other procedures (that is, operations other than the selected 11—results not presented here). As was true for all operations, the apparent decline in the rate of the 11 procedures as education rises is suggestive though not statistically significant.

Type of Operation, 1970

The results of scaling each of the 11 selected procedures on indexes of complexity, urgency, and necessity are presented in

Table 5.2. There is, of couse, some correlation between the urgency and necessity measures (the coefficient of rank correlation R_S is 0.46), but there are also important differences for particular procedures. For example, most physicians do not rate the removal of cataracts high on the urgency scale, but neither do they believe that it is often done unnecessarily. There is some correlation between complexity and necessity across the 11 procedures ($R_S = 0.20$), but essentially none between complexity and urgency ($R_S = 0.04$).

The mean index of complexity, urgency, or necessity per operation was calculated for each cell, and these indexes were then regressed against the socioeconomic characteristics.[3] Table 5.3 presents the results of these regressions in the form of index

Table 5.2 Indexes of complexity, urgency, and necessity, 11 selected procedures

Operation*	Complexity Value† (CRVS units)	Complexity Rank	Urgency Value‡ (%)	Urgency Rank	Necessity Value‡ (%)	Necessity Rank
Appendectomy	1.12	6	99	1	99	1
Cataract	2.12	3	2	11	96	2.5
Hernia repair	1.00	8	24	5	96	2.5
Prostatectomy	2.21	2	47	4	92	4
Cholecystectomy	1.79	5	48	3	88	5
Dilation and curettage (excluding abortions)	0.52	10	53	2	77	6
Hemorrhoidectomy	0.71	9	12	7	65	7
Varicose-vein stripping	1.06	7	4	10	63	8
Lumbar laminectomy (for disk)	2.88	1	22	6	38	9
Hysterectomy	1.92	4	8	8	28	10
Tonsillectomy	0.45	11	5	9	24	11
Weighted mean values for 11 procedures (1970)	1.16	—	28.7	—	63.9	—

*Listed according to ranking on the necessity index.
†*Source:* California Relative Value Scale (CRVS) Study (1969), expressed in hernia equivalents (hernia repair = 1).
‡*Source:* Questionnaires mailed to California physicians, 93 replies (50% response rate).

Table 5.3 Indexes of type of operation for 11 selected procedures, by socioeconomic characteristics, United States, 1970*

Characteristic	Complexity	Urgency	Necessity
All	100	100	100
Race			
Whites	100	101	100
Nonwhites	99	87	99
Residence			
In SMSA	99	102	100
Out of SMSA	101	97	100
Education of head (yr)			
≤8	102†	94	103
9–12	101	98	99
13–14	94	103	100
15–16	90	105	97
17+	109	125	104
Sex			
Male	104‡	102	111‡
Female	97	98	89
Age (yr)			
0–9	58†	43†	62†
10–19	68	128	88
20–34	102	118	105
35–49	127	98	103
50–64	126	110	126
65+	159	111	146

*Standardized for age, sex, race, residence, education, and income. Each index is normalized separately to mean 100.
†Differences significant at 0.05 level by F-test.
‡Difference significant at 0.05 level by t-test.

numbers. The first column indicates no difference in average complexity between whites and nonwhites or by residence. As expected, there is a significant increase in complexity by age. For these selected procedures the average operation on males is slightly more complex than the average on females. The most unusual result is for education, which shows a slight but significant decrease in complexity with increasing education until the highest-education class, in which there is a sharp upturn in the average complexity.

The most striking result of the analysis of the urgency and necessity indexes is how little difference there is across race, residence, or education groups. Given the lower surgical rates for nonwhites, for example, one might have thought that the average operation performed on nonwhites would be somewhat higher on the urgency and necessity scales than the average operation performed on whites, but this is not the case, at least across the procedures that we have examined. Of course, it is possible that there are systematic differences in urgency or necessity within each procedure; our data do not permit analysis of this possibility. We do observe, however, that the necessity index increases significantly with age and is significantly higher for males than for females.

Changes between 1963 and 1970

Between 1963 and 1970 the number of nonobstetrical operations per thousand population rose from 48.6 to 55.5—a significant increase of 14 percent. AMA data show that during that same period, the number of surgical specialists per hundred thousand population rose from 36.4 to 40.3, an increase of 11 percent. Because there was a decline of 28 percent in the number of general practitioners per hundred thousand, some of whom performed operations, the number of operations per surgical specialist probably rose by several percent from 1963 to 1970. Even so, these figures indicate that the average surgical work load remained light, with the typical surgical specialist performing two or three in-hospital operations per week.

Although the average increase in operations per thousand population was 14 percent, some groups experienced considerably larger changes. Though our analysis did not establish any of these changes as statistically significant, all are consistent with expectations. For example, the elderly (age 65 and over) showed a marked increase in operations performed, no doubt reflecting the effect of Medicare. This increase was most noticeable for the elderly in the lower-education groups (see Figure 5.1). In 1963 there was a positive relation between education and surgical utilization among the elderly, but this association had disappeared by 1970. Among the other age groups the relation between education and utilization in 1970 was essentially the same as in 1963.

Nonwhites experienced larger increases in utilization than

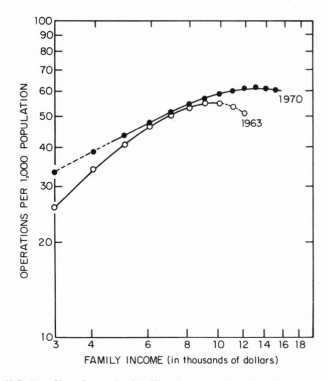

Figure 5.3 Predicted surgical utilization standardized for age and sex as a function of family income, 1963 and 1970. *Note:* Dashed lines represent prediction outside the 90 percent range of mean cell income in each year. Family income for both years is in real 1970 dollars.

whites between 1963 and 1970 in urban areas (see Figure 5.2). There were larger increases in operations performed for persons in families in which the head had 12 years of schooling or less.

A comparison of the complexity, urgency, and necessity indexes in 1963 with 1970 (not shown here) reveals remarkable stability, both overall and by broad socioeconomic characteristics. This is a rather surprising result. For instance, the age-sex-education–adjusted rate of surgical utilization for urban nonwhites rose from 34.2 per thousand in 1963 to 47.0 in 1970, an increase of 37 percent, and their rate for the 11 selected procedures rose from 11.4 to 17.1, a gain of 50 percent. With such a large increase in utilization one might have expected some decrease in the necessity index for the average operation, but we find that the average necessity score for urban nonwhites remained unchanged, 64.0 in both 1963 and 1970. Similarly, the surgical utilization rate for the elderly with eight years of schooling or less jumped from 59.3 to 79.6 for all operations, and from 22.1 to 29.8 for the 11 procedures, but the average necessity score per operation actually increased slightly between 1963 and 1970 — from 86.6 to 88.6.

Surgical Utilization and Family Income

The relation between surgical utilization and family income in 1963 and 1970 is shown in Figure 5.3. These curves represent predicted probabilities of operation obtained from the regressions across cells on mean income and mean income squared, including age and sex as controlling variables. The curves are plotted on a double-logarithmic scale and illustrate the relative change in surgical rates predicted by the regression equation for any given relative change in income. Again, the results are not statistically significant (possibly because of the limited sample size in relation to the surgical rates involved); however, they are suggestive. In 1963 there appears to have been a positive relation between utilization and income, but in 1970 this relation is weakened. When race, residence, and education were also included in the regressions (not shown here), we found that in 1970 differences in utilization by income were not statistically significant.

To obtain a better understanding of the effect of income on utilization, we analyzed separately different age-sex groups, as shown in Figure 5.4. As in Figure 5.3, these curves illustrate predicted probabilities of operation for each age-sex group. In 1963 the increase in surgical utilization with income appears to have been most marked for young age groups (under 20). It was also present for older age groups (65 and over) and for adult females, but not for adult males. When similar curves were drawn for 1970, they suggested that the bulk of the change during this period occurred in the older population and in adult females. In these two groups surgical utilization by low-income persons increased, and the relation between utilization and income was reduced. For males 20 to 64 years of age and the young, the curves in 1970 were similar to those in 1963.

We also looked at the effects of income on type of operation. A priori, one would expect differences in utilization to be as-

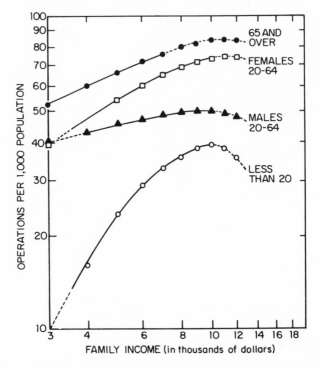

Figure 5.4 Predicted surgical utilization of selected age-sex groups as a function of family income, 1963. Age-sex standardization was done within groups. *Note:* Dashed lines represent prediction outside the 90 percent range of mean cell income.

sociated with a different mix of surgical procedures, with the lower-income groups with low utilization experiencing relatively more of the urgent and necessary procedures. We regressed each of the complexity, urgency, and necessity indexes on income, controlling for age and sex. The complexity and urgency indexes, adjusted for age and sex, did not vary significantly with income; the necessity index, however, showed a slight but significant negative relation with income in both years. It appears that low-income groups do have a higher necessity-index average. This finding, in conjunction with their lower surgical utilization, indicates that the lower-income groups experience fewer of the procedures of low necessity. Do they also experience fewer of the highly necessary procedures? To answer this question, we classified individuals by mean cell income in 1963 and 1970 and calculated surgical rates adjusted for age and sex for different types of procedures by the "indirect" method. The results indicated that, in 1963, persons in cells with low mean income (defined as the poorest 20 percent of the population) had lower surgical rates for all types of procedures, but especially for the least necessary procedures: for the more necessary procedures (appendectomy, cataract, hernia repair, and prostatectomy—see Table 5.2), the rates were 6.0 operations per thousand for the poor and 7.5 for others; for the least necessary procedures (tonsillectomy, hysterectomy, and lumbar laminectomy for disk—see Table 5.2), the respective rates were 3.6 and 9.6. In 1970, the low-income groups had almost the same rates as the rest of the population for the highly necessary procedures (7.3 and 7.8, respectively), but their rates were still lower for the less necessary procedures (5.5 and 9.8). The change between 1963 and 1970 is probably attributable primarily to the impact of public insurance (Medicare and Medicaid) on the demand for operations by low-income persons.

Discussion

In broad outline, the results of this study of surgical utilization are similar to findings concerning overall utilization of hospitals and physicians' services. Large increases in utilization occurred between 1963 and 1970 among the elderly, the lower-educated groups, and nonwhites in urban areas. These changes may be principally a result of the introduction of Medicare and Medicaid during the intervening period. Some differentials by race and residence remain, but they are largely related to income rather than race or residence per se. To be sure, even equality in utilization does not refute the possibility of inequality of access if certain groups have a greater basic need for operations.

Income was found to have a strong positive effect on surgical utilization, although the association was less strong in 1970 than in 1963. The relation between surgical utilization and family income found in this study was greater than that usually reported in studies of physicians' services or hospital utilization. The reason for this may be in part that we could not include data on insurance coverage; in other studies much of the income effect may work through differential insurance coverage, resulting in a negligible net income effect. However, to the extent that there is a positive correlation between income and the gross price of operations (as distinct from insurance coverage), the omission of a gross price variable in our regressions tends to bias downward our results for income.

The positive relation between surgical utilization and family income is strongest for children, fairly strong for the elderly and for females 20 to 64 years of age, and very weak for males 20 to 64. These results appear to be consistent with a "value-of-time" explanation positing that the net effect of an operation is a reduction in time available to the patient and that an operation is thus least attractive to those whose time is most highly priced. The results for the education variables are also consistent with this view. However, factors possibly limiting the force of this explanation are the existence of sick-leave and disability-income provisions and the relatively complete insurance coverage held by prime-age males. An alternative to the "value-of-time" explanation would be the idea that prime-age males are most likely to be heads of families and therefore the "reverse causality effect" (operation leading to lower income) would be strongest for that group. However, our use of group data not classified by income minimizes the bias from this source.

The sharp divergence between the income relation and the education relation should be noted. With other things held constant, higher-income groups tend to have more operations than lower-income groups, but higher-education groups tend to have far fewer operations. This result is consistent with previous findings of a strong positive relation between health and education, and a weak negative relation between health and income (Auster, Leveson, and Sarachek, 1969; Grossman, 1972a).

One surprising finding of this study is the absence of any significant difference in the indexes of necessity or urgency between demographic groups that have significant differences in surgical utilization. It has been speculated that groups that have above-average rates of operation (or above-average rates of increase in operations) would have a mix of operations that, on the average, was lower (or decreased) on the necessity or urgency scales. The absence of such a relation (except for an effect of income) poses a strong challenge to our understanding of the process of care. One possible explanation is that patients' perceptions of urgency and necessity do not conform with those of the physicians who responded to our questionnaire, and it is the patient who initiates the process that leads to operation. Another hypothesis is that the surgical decision is largely determined by physicians, and they do not take into account the patients' overall utilization rate in recommending any particular procedure. A plausible explanation is that both processes are at work, but further research on surgical decision making is clearly needed.

Although we do not observe any relation between surgical rates and the necessity or complexity indexes among the demographic groups, we do find such a relation between necessity and utilization when the cells are grouped by mean income. Individuals in cells with low mean income tend to have fewer operations, and this tendency is most pronounced for procedures rated lowest on the necessity scale. The divergence between these results for income and those for race, residence, age, and education poses a question for further investigation.

The Supply of Surgeons and the Demand for Operations

Inequality in the distribution of physicians across the United States and the possible influence of supply of physicians on the demand for their services are subjects of continuing interest to economists and health policymakers. If physicians choose their locations partly for reasons unrelated to demand, and if, given their locations, they can increase or decrease the demand for their services independently of changes in price, the implications for economic analysis and for public policy are profound. Some economists (Evans, 1974; see also Chapter 4 of this volume) have reported evidence in support of the demand-shifting hypothesis, but others are skeptical (Sloan and Feldman, 1977). Many physicians believe that they have almost unlimited power to shift demand. This belief is based on introspection, clinical experience, and the correlation between supply and utilization, but skeptics offer several alternative explanations for the correlation.

The principal purpose of this chapter is to shed some light on this question through multiequation, multivariate analysis of differences in the supply of surgeons and the demand for operations across geographic areas of the United States. In-hospital operations seem particularly well suited for analysis of demand-shifting because several of the problems that have hampered previous studies can be avoided or minimized.

The Demand-Shifting Hypothesis

Standard economic analysis assumes that the supply and demand schedules in any market are independent. Given an ex-

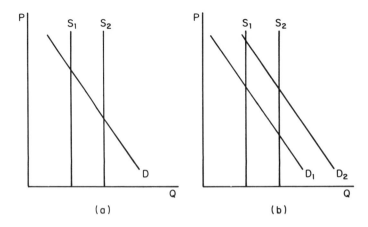

Figure 6.1 (a) No demand-shifting. (b) Demand-shifting.

ogenous increase in supply, a new equilibrium is reached by moving down the (constant) demand curve, as shown in Figure 6.1a. The demand-shift hypothesis asserts that given an exogenous shift in the supply of physicians from S_1 to S_2, the physicians induce a shift in demand from D_1 to D_2 (see Figure 6.1b).

Another way of viewing demand-shifting is presented in Figure 6.2. The benefits from increases in the quantity of medical care, either to an individual patient or to a population, can be assumed to increase at a decreasing rate, hence the falling marginal benefit curve *MB*. For simplicity, let us assume that the cost of medical care to the patient (financial cost, time costs,

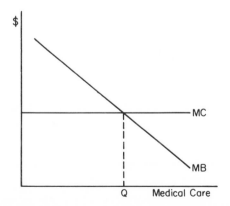

Figure 6.2 Alternative way of viewing demand-shifting.

risk, and so on) increases at a constant rate, shown by the marginal cost curve *MC*. If patients had full information and full control over the quantity of care, they would choose quantity *Q*. The fact that the quantity may be determined by the physician does not in itself imply demand-shifting. The physician, acting as an unbiased agent of the patient, may also choose quantity *Q*. If, however, the physician chooses and the patient accepts a quantity of care greater than or less than *Q*, we would say that there has been demand-shifting.

Note that demand can be shifted either up (to the right) or down (to the left). Let us assume that, other things being equal, physicians prefer to come as close to *Q* as possible, that is, they derive utility from ordering the amount of care that equates marginal cost and marginal benefit for their patients.[1] Let us also assume that physicians derive utility from income and that work (at least beyond some level) is a source of disutility. If the physician/population ratio is relatively high in an area (for reasons unrelated to demand), they may push quantity to the right of *Q* in order to keep prices and incomes from falling drastically. If there are relatively few physicians in an area, and if they cannot or do not raise price to an equilibrium level, they may push quantity to the left of *Q* in order to avoid excessive work. This latter situation, sometimes characterized as "excess demand," has been offered as an explanation for the observed correlation between supply and utilization (Feldstein, 1970). It would be described in Figure 6.1a by a price that is *below* the intersection of S_1 and demand. A shift of supply to the right results in higher utilization because it takes care of some of the excess demand.

Note that the presence of demand-shifting should not be equated with unnecessary care. If "necessary care" is defined as *Q* in Figure 6.2, demand-shifting to the *left* implies that some patients are not getting the care they should, and does not imply that any patients are getting unnecessary care. Moreover, necessary care may be defined differently from the quantity that maximizes the patient's utility (that is, *Q*). If, for instance, it is defined as the quantity that maximizes the patient's health regardless of cost, the optimum would clearly be to the right of *Q*, and such demand-shifting would not necessarily imply unnecessary care.

This study of in-hospital operations provides a sharp test of demand-shifting for several reasons. First, since operations are typically well-defined procedures, it is possible to get a direct measure of quantity. There is some variation in average complexity of operations (as measured by the California Relative Value Scale) across geographic areas; the coefficient of variation for 11 frequently performed procedures is 6 percent. A count of operations, however, is likely to be a much better measure of quantity of medical care than a count of office visits, which may vary greatly with respect to length, number of tests and x-rays, and so on. Furthermore, variations in average complexity can be studied separately.

A second reason for using operations to study demand-shifting is that we can rule out "excess demand" (that is, demand-shifting to the left) as an important explanation for any observed relation between supply and utilization. Excess demand may exist for house calls and other types of services rendered by general practitioners, where price seems to be below its equilibrium level and nonprice rationing is observed, but such phenomena are rare in surgery. Economists and physicians who have studied surgical markets have reported that the average number of operations per surgeon (150 to 200 per year) is far below the level that surgeons consider a "full work load" (about 400–500 per year) (Fuchs, 1969b; Watkins et al., 1976; see also Chapter 3). The average surgical work load is less than half that recorded in group-practice settings such as the Group Health Cooperative (Seattle) and the Mayo Clinic (Rochester, Minnesota), and below the quantity that surgeons would be willing and able to perform at the going price. The data used in this chapter reveal that even in nonmetropolitan areas where the surgeon/population ratio is very low, the average surgeon performs only about 250 operations per year. A recent SOSSUS report noted, "We have failed to identify large or small areas of this country that are significantly under-supplied with personnel suitably qualified to carry out surgery" (SOSSUS, 1976).

The "cost of time" explanation is also likely to be less relevant for operations than for physician office visits. This explanation for the correlation between supply and utilization asserts that equilibrium is achieved by a change in the total price to the patient, including the cost of time. In areas where the physician population is higher, the time costs to the patient of search, travel, and waiting are all reduced, which is equivalent to a decline in price. Thus Figure 6.1a is said to describe adequately the market for physician services if price is correctly specified. There is, therefore, no need to introduce demand-shifting as an explanation. Time costs are undoubtedly important for the average ambulatory visit, but they are likely to be less relevant for in-hospital operations because the psychic costs of surgery and the time costs of hospitalization tend to be large relative to the time costs of search, travel, and waiting. Thus, this study avoids an ambiguity inherent in many previous studies of demand-shifting.

Finally, given widespread insurance coverage for in-hospital surgery (about 80 percent of the population), the absence of accurate price data may cause fewer problems than in studies of demand for outpatient services, which have lower insurance coverage.

Although an interarea analysis focused on surgical operations seems to offer several advantages, there are potential problems as well. First, there is probably a significant amount of "border-crossing" by surgical patients. While most outpatients obtain care from nearby physicians, it is not unusual for patients to travel considerable distances for in-hospital surgery. Such border-crossing is likely to be particularly relevant for residents of non-metropolitan areas who frequently go to metropolitan areas for their operations. According to American Hospital Association (AHA) data (1972), the rate per thousand population of operations (excluding births) in metropolitan area hospitals was 1.75 times the rate in nonmetropolitan area hospitals. Health Interview Survey (HIS) data (1970), based on the *residence* of the patient rather than the location of the hospital, indicate a (nonobstetrical) operation rate for metropolitan residents only 1.10 times the rate for nonmetropolitan residents. Using this information plus the metropolitan/nonmetropolitan population ratio of 2.33, we can calculate that nonmetropolitan residents obtain about 30 percent of their operations in metropolitan areas (assuming no movement of metropolitan residents to nonmetropolitan areas for in-hospital surgery).[2] Thus, if there is an effect of supply on demand, the demand in nonmetropolitan areas may be affected by the supply in the adjacent metropolitan area as well as by the supply in the nonmetropolitan area itself.

There is probably much less unreciprocated border-crossing from one geographic division to another. A comparison of the surgical utilization rates in the HIS data for 1970 with AHA data for 1972 shows four divisions (New England, East North Central–East, South Atlantic–Upper, and Pacific) with rates above the U.S. average for both measures, and five divisions (East North Central–West, South Atlantic–Lower, East South Central, West South Central, and Mountain) with rates below the U.S. average, according to both measures. There are two divisions (Middle Atlantic and West North Central) that show rates above the U.S. average by location of hospital (AHA data) and below the U.S. average by residence (HIS data). This suggests that there may be some unreciprocated border-crossing into these two divisions for surgery. However, it should be noted that both of these divisions had rates above the U.S. average in the HIS data for 1963, so it may be that some of the discrepancy in 1970 is a result of sampling variability.[3]

Another possible source of difficulty is that a significant amount of surgery (fragmentary data suggest about 20 percent; SOSSUS, table 13, p. 39) is performed by physicians who are not "surgical specialists"—primarily general practitioners and surgical residents. The location of surgical residents is highly correlated with that of surgeons, but the location of general practitioners is not, and some attempt will be made to take account of their supply in the analysis.

Not only are some operations performed by "nonsurgeons," but surgical specialists typically do not limit their practice to performing operations. Thus, this study is concerned with only a portion (albeit the major portion) of the demand for surgeons' services and would result in an understatement of demand-shifting if, as seems likely, it is easier and more attractive for surgeons to shift the demand for office procedures and tests than for in-hospital operations.[4]

One perennial problem in attempts to estimate demand-shifting is that of simultaneity. Strong demand for surgery in an area may attract surgeons, rather than surgeons stimulating demand. I will attempt to deal with this problem by using predicted physician supply rather than actual supply. The predictions will be based on a regression incorporating "taste" variables that affect location of surgeons.

Analytical Framework and Data Base

The general framework of this chapter is similar to that used in Chapter 4 to analyze interarea variations in the demand for, and supply of, physicians' services. A demand equation is specified which includes variables usually thought to determine demand (such as demographic characteristics, income, price), and then predicted physician supply is added. This predicted supply is obtained by regressing the surgeon/population ratio on a set of variables believed to determine physician location. The location decision is of interest in its own right, given the wide variation in the physician/population ratio across areas.

Cross-section regressions are run for 1963 and for 1970, and in a few instances the observations for the two years are pooled. The Health Interview Survey (HIS), which is the source for the surgical utilization data, provides information for 22 areas (metropolitan and nonmetropolitan areas in each of 11 divisions)[5] that cover the entire population. These areas are the units of observation for some of the regressions. Other regressions are run on a more detailed breakdown of the HIS data in which individuals are cross-classified by age (six classes), sex, race (white and nonwhite), education of head of family (five classes), and the 22 areas. Regressions across these cells permit much finer control of demographic variables and also permit testing of Pauly's suggestion that demand-shifting might be more important for some groups (for example, the poorly educated) than for others (Pauly, 1980).

The possibility of border-crossing from nonmetropolitan to metropolitan areas is allowed for by including an additional predicted supply variable for each of the nonmetropolitan areas. This variable is based on the ratio of the number of surgeons in the adjacent metropolitan area to the total population of the division. Also, some regressions are run across only the metropolitan areas or only the nonmetropolitan areas. Per capita income and surgical prices are deflated by a general price index for each division, adjusted for metropolitan–nonmetropolitan differences, and all nominal dollar values for 1963 are inflated to 1970 price levels.

The utilization rates were calculated from the Health Interview Survey (for 1963 and 1970) conducted by the National Center for Health Statistics. The data represent a probability sample of households including all living civilian noninstitutionalized individuals. In 1970 interviews were conducted with approximately 37,000 households containing about 116,000 individuals, and in 1963 with 42,000 households containing 134,000 individuals. Surgical rates were obtained in response to the following questions: "Was the respondent hospitalized at any time during the last 12 months?" and, if an operation was performed, "What was the name of the operation?" For each hospitalization, only the first operations were included; the number of second and third operations was small. Deliveries, abortions, and other obstetrical procedures were excluded from the analysis because they are primarily a function of conception rates.

Although the HIS data are representative of the nation's population, they are subject to recall error by the individual or proxy respondent. Hospitalization and operations are reported with greater accuracy than simple episodes of illness, but an overall rate of underreporting of 10 percent remains. Moreover, this underreporting is not uniformly distributed among the population. Whites tend to report hospitalization more accurately than do nonwhites; higher education is also associated with more accurate reporting, as is higher income (controlling for education).

The physician supply data come from the AMA *Distribution of Physicians in the United States* and are reasonably accurate. Most of the other data come from the Bureau of the Census and the Bureau of Labor Statistics. The principal variables (summary statistics in Table 6.1) are as follows.

Endogenous Variables

Q^* Number of operations per 100,000 population.

S^* Number of surgical specialists per 100,000 population. These are office-based patient-care physicians, both Board-certified and non-Board-certified. The physician supply is adjusted to take account of doctors of osteopathy.

$METS^*$ This variable is used only for the nonmetropolitan areas and takes a value of zero for the metropolitan area. It is based on the predicted number of surgeons in the metropolitan area divided by the total population of the division. It is included to allow for the possible effect of the surgeon supply in a metropolitan area on the demand in the nonmetropolitan area in the same division.

Exogenous Variables

INC* Real income per capita (in thousands of dollars). The income data were obtained from *Distribution of Physicians in the United States*. Data for 1969 were used for 1970, and 1965 data for 1963. Nominal per capita income was deflated by a divisional price index derived by Williamson (1980) from Bureau of Labor Statistics data for large metropolitan areas. Prices in nonmetropolitan areas were assumed to be 0.87 of the prices in the metropolitan areas (the cost-of-living differential reported by the BLS). The all-commodity Consumer Price Index was used to adjust for intertemporal change.

HOTEL* Per capita receipts (dollars per person) of hotels and motels in the division.[6] The same value was used for the nonmetropolitan and metropolitan areas in a division. This variable is used as a measure of the "attractiveness" of the area. The "services" component of the CPI was used to adjust for intertemporal change.

NONMET A dummy variable denoting nonmetropolitan area.

NRMET The fraction of the population in a nonmetropolitan area living in counties that were designated as "potential" standard metropolitan statistical areas (SMSAs) or that had population in excess of 50,000. This variable took a value of zero for the metropolitan areas.

%WYTE Percentage of the area's population that is white.

GP* Number of general practitioners per 100,000 population.

In addition to the variables listed here, some attempts were made to use an endogenous price-of-surgery variable. This was based on 1970 AMA data for nine divisions reporting the average price of an initial office visit, a follow-up office visit, and a follow-up hospital visit (all for surgeons). An average of these three prices was calculated and then deflated by the Williamson-BLS divisional price index for all commodities. The surgical

Table 6.1 Summary statistics

Variable	Units	Mean 1963	Mean 1970	Standard deviation 1963	Standard deviation 1970	Coefficient of variation (%) 1963	Coefficient of variation (%) 1970
Q^*	Operations per 100,000	4871	5558	668	567	13.7	10.2
S^*	Surgeons per 100,000	26.9	30.5	10.0	9.5	37.2	31.1
INC^*	$000 per capita	2.97[b]	3.35[c]	0.36	0.33	12.1	9.9
$HOTEL^*$	Dollars per capita	37.4	47.3	10.9	15.1	29.1	31.9
$NRMET$	Fraction	0.139	0.129	0.237	0.232	171.2	179.8
$\%WYTE$	Percent	88.5	87.8	7.6	6.6	8.6	7.5
GP^*	GPs per 100,000	36.4	26.3	6.1	5.2	16.8	19.8

a. Across 22 areas.
b. 1965.
c. 1969.

price index never had any effect in either the demand or location regressions.

A variable measuring the percentage of the division's population with surgical insurance was also tried without any appreciable effect. This variable, obtained from the Health Insurance Institute, is probably not measured accurately.[7]

In the regressions across the cells, dummy variables are included for the demographic characteristics—age, sex, race, and education of head of family—that are used to form the cells.

Regression Results

Location of Surgeons

Table 6.2 presents the results for the surgeon-location regressions.[8] Representative runs for each year across the 22 areas are shown. The fits are extremely good ($\bar{R}^2$ as high as 0.96), and the coefficients are relatively insensitive to changes in specification. The principal conclusion is that the "taste" variables have a very strong influence on surgeon location.

The $NONMET$ dummy variable is highly significant in all

Table 6.2 Results of surgeon-location regressions across states, 1963 and 1970

Year	$\bar{R}^2$	S.E.[a]	NONMET	NRMET	HOTEL*	%WYTE	$\hat{Q}*$	GP*
1970	.93	2.5	−25	14	.16	.24	—	—
			(11.8)	(3.2)	(4.4)	(2.7)		
	—	3.0	−28	18	.17	.27	−.002	—
			(4.8)	(1.9)	(3.6)	(2.2)	(.5)	
	.93	2.5	−25	13	.17	.26	—	−.05
			(9.3)	(2.8)	(4.1)	(2.3)		(.3)
1963	.96	2.1	−24	10	.12	.14	—	—
			(12.7)	(2.7)	(2.7)	(2.2)		
	—	4.3	−28	14	.22	.29	−.005	—
			(4.7)	(1.6)	(1.6)	(1.4)	(.9)	
	.95	2.2	−24	11	.12	.12	—	−.03
			(11.4)	(2.6)	(2.4)	(1.3)		(.2)

Notes: *t*-statistics in parentheses. Regressions weighted by population. Hat over variable indicates predicted value.
a. Standard error of the regression.

runs, with a value usually close to −25. The preference for nonmetropolitan-like areas is also revealed by the NRMET variable, with a coefficient of about 14. This indicates that nonmetropolitan areas with 100 percent of their population in counties that are nearly like metropolitan counties have, ceteris paribus, 14 more surgeons per hundred thousand than nonmetropolitan areas with no population in such counties. The preference of surgeons for metropolitan living may reflect the professional attraction of the "medical environment" as well as their preference as consumers. Potential demand, however, as measured by predicted utilization ($\hat{Q}*$) has virtually no effect on location.

That surgeons live in areas where most people consider it desirable to visit and vacation is demonstrated by the HOTEL* variable. This coefficient (usually highly significant) shows the increase associated with an increase of one dollar per capita in receipts of hotels and motels. The elasticity at the means is approximately 0.2.

The coefficient of %WYTE is always positive and usually statistically significant, but varies somewhat depending on the specification. A value of 0.20 implies an elasticity of 0.6 at the means. The GP* coefficient is not significant and does not have any appreciable effect on the coefficients that are. Some attempts were made to incorporate predicted price into the location regressions. Its coefficient was always insignificant.

Demand

Table 6.3 presents the results for the demand regressions across the 22 areas. Table 6.4 presents similar runs across the cells.

Table 6.3 Results of demand regressions across areas, 1963 and 1970

Year	S.E.	$\hat{S}*$	$MET\hat{S}*$	INC*	%WYTE	GP*
1970	407	60	30	230	—	—
		(3.1)	(2.0)	(.6)		
	419	60	30	223	1	—
		(3.0)	(1.7)	(.5)	(.0)	
	536	—	—	753	2	—
				(2.1)	(.1)	
	412ᵃ	54	26	263	—	—
		(2.8)	(1.7)	(.7)		
	367ᵃ	43	44	801	—	−57
		(2.4)	(2.9)	(2.0)		(2.5)
1963	523	44	41	768	—	—
		(1.4)	(1.7)	(1.4)		
	539	42	37	705	5	—
		(1.3)	(1.3)	(1.2)	(.3)	
	573	—	—	909	16	—
				(2.5)	(.9)	
	524ᵃ	43	41	797	—	—
		(1.4)	(1.7)	(1.5)		
	538ᵃ	42	43	856	—	−6
		(1.3)	(1.7)	(1.4)		(.3)
Addendum		S*	METS*			
OLS						
1970	411	65	34	239	—	—
		(3.8)	(2.4)	(.6)		
	368	55	51	756	—	−54
		(3.4)	(3.5)	(1.9)		(2.3)
1963	520	59	51	633	—	—
		(2.2)	(2.4)	(1.2)		
	535	59	52	676	—	−4
		(2.1)	(2.3)	(1.2)		(.2)

a. GP* added as an instrument.

The latter regressions permit much finer control of the demographic variables but do not, of course, allow for any additional variation in those variables which are only available for the areas. The fits of the demand equations are not as good as those for the surgeon-location equations, and the size and significance of the coefficients are more sensitive to variations in specification. In general, the results support the view that an exogenous change in surgeon supply *does* affect the demand for operations. Each additional surgeon in an area, ceteris paribus, is associated with an increase of between 40 and 60 operations per year. The elasticity at the means for a coefficient of 50 is about 0.28. Use of the two-stage procedure does reduce the relation between supply and utilization. In ordinary least squares regressions (shown at the bottom of Table 6.3), the surgeon-supply coefficient is from 8 to 40 percent larger than in the two-stage runs.

The regressions in part B of Table 6.4 were run across cells with 11 division values instead of 22 area values. The predicted surgeons were obtained from a regression across the divisions of S^* on $HOTEL^*$, $\%WYTE$, and the percentage of the division's population living in metropolitan areas ($\%MET$). The fit was good ($\bar{R}^2 = 0.80$), and the coefficient for $\%MET$ (0.24) was the equivalent of the $NONMET$ dummy coefficient in the area-location regressions. The relative price of surgery was included in the cell-division regressions, but was never significant.

The income coefficient is always positive in the demand equations, but usually not statistically significant unless predicted surgeon supply is omitted. One surprising finding is the statistically significant negative coefficient for GP^* in 1970. One possible explanation is that where general practitioners are numerous, they can provide continuing nonsurgical care for various conditions that might otherwise be treated by surgery. However, this variable was insignificant in 1963. The coefficients for the demographic characteristics are presented in Table 6.5. They are usually very significant and virtually unaffected by the inclusion or exclusion of the area variables.

It is possible that the effect of predicted supply on demand reported in Table 6.3 and part A of Table 6.4 is really the effect of the metropolitan–nonmetropolitan distinction on both supply and demand. To test for this possibility, similar two-stage

Table 6.4 Results of demand regressions across cells, 1963 and 1970

Year	$\hat{S}*$	$MET\hat{S}*$	$INC*$	$GP*$	$PR\hat{I}CE$
Part A (area values)					
1970	62	27	−83	—	—
	(3.4)	(2.2)	(.2)		
	42	44	633	−68	—
	(2.1)	(3.2)	(1.4)	(2.9)	
1963	49	34	300	—	—
	(2.4)	(2.6)	(.8)		
	42	37	550	−18	—
	(2.0)	(2.7)	(1.3)	(1.4)	
Part B (division values)					
1970	29	—	78	—	—
	(1.2)		(.2)		
	33	—	68	—	−2 (−.03)[a]
	(1.0)		(.2)		(.2)
1963	56	—	−40	—	—
	(2.1)		(.1)		
	80	—	−211	—	−9 (−.19)[a]
	(2.1)		(.5)		(.9)

Note: Age, sex, race, education dummy variables included; regression coefficients are presented in Table 6.5.

a. Elasticities at means.

regressions were run for just the metropolitan areas and just the nonmetropolitan areas, with 1963 and 1970 pooled in order to have a reasonable number of observations.[9]

The results for the demand regressions across the areas are reported in Table 6.6, and those for the regressions across cells in Table 6.7. The principal coefficient of interest is for predicted supply ($\hat{S}*$), and we see that this coefficient is generally larger and more statistically significant in these regressions than in those that included both metropolitan and nonmetropolitan areas. For the five metropolitan regressions in the two tables, the median coefficient for $\hat{S}*$ is 82, and for the 10 nonmetropolitan regressions the median is 80. These coefficients imply an elasticity at the means of approximately 0.53 for the metropolitan areas and 0.27 for the nonmetropolitan areas. The difference in elasticity reflects the much lower surgeon/population ratio in the nonmetropolitan areas.

Table 6.5 Regression coefficients of demographic variables in demand regressions across cells (area values)

	1970		1963	
	(1)	(2)	(1)	(2)
Female	710	704	476	475
	(4.6)	(4.6)	(3.7)	(3.7)
Age				
0–9	−1812	−1801	−1488	−1483
	(7.3)	(7.3)	(7.2)	(7.2)
10–19	−2165	−2149	−1917	−1905
	(8.8)	(8.8)	(8.8)	(8.8)
35–49	1490	1487	1202	1188
	(5.8)	(5.9)	(5.6)	(5.6)
50–64	1290	1293	1291	1273
	(4.7)	(4.8)	(5.5)	(5.5)
65+	2526	2512	1441	1432
	(7.9)	(7.9)	(5.3)	(5.3)
Nonwhite	−1498	−1542	−1754	−1733
	(6.2)	(6.4)	(8.6)	(8.4)
Education				
0–8	−627	−472	−673	−510
	(2.1)	(1.6)	(2.5)	(1.9)
9–12	162	183	−140	−112
	(.6)	(.7)	(.5)	(.4)
15–16	−807	−813	−691	−705
	(2.3)	(2.3)	(2.1)	(2.1)
17+	−642	−674	−804	−809
	(1.6)	(1.7)	(2.1)	(2.1)

Note: (1) = no other right-hand-side variables; (2) = INC^*, $\hat{S}^*$, $MET\hat{S}^*$, and GP^* included as right-hand-side variables.

The nonmetropolitan regressions were run with an exogenous $METS^*$ variable, as well as without; this coefficient was not statistically significant. A variable designed to measure the possible impact of border-crossing in metropolitan areas also had no significant effect. The only variable (except predicted supply) that came close to consistently significant results is GP^* in metropolitan areas. The negative coefficient is similar in size to that reported in Tables 6.3 and 6.4 for 1970. In general, the separate

Table 6.6 Results of separate demand regressions across metropolitan areas and nonmetropolitan areas, 1963 and 1970 pooled

Areas	S.E.	$\hat{S}$*	INC*	YEAR	%WYTE	GP*	MET$\hat{S}$*
Metropolitan	463	76	259	404	—	—	—
		(2.1)	(.5)	(1.4)			
	466	91	478	258	-20	—	—
		(2.3)	(.9)	(.8)	(1.0)		
	444	116	1111	-521	—	-47	—
		(2.8)	(1.6)	(.9)		(1.8)	
Nonmetropolitan	466	85	1187	-223	—	—	—
		(3.0)	(2.7)	(.9)			
	468	84	745	-56	16	—	—
		(3.0)	(1.1)	(.2)	(.9)		
	477	82	1311	-330	—	-9	—
		(2.7)	(2.2)	(.7)		(.3)	
	476	79	1107	-189	—	—	9
		(1.9)	(2.0)	(.6)			(.2)
	468	65	424	84	21	—	24
		(1.5)	(.5)	(.2)	(1.1)		(.6)
	489	78	1223	-285	—	-8	7
		(1.8)	(1.7)	(.6)		(.2)	(.2)

Table 6.7 Results of demand regressions across cells, separate for metropolitan areas and nonmetropolitan areas, 1963 and 1970 pooled

Areas	$\hat{S}*$	INC*	YEAR	GP*	MET$\hat{S}*$
Metropolitan	25	98	612	—	—
	(1.0)	(.3)	(3.2)		
	82	1087	−477	−54	—
	(2.6)	(2.3)	(1.1)	(2.9)	
Nonmetropolitan	90	481	35	—	—
	(3.5)	(1.3)	(.2)		
	82	760	−202	−21	—
	(3.0)	(1.5)	(.6)	(.8)	
	65	310	142	—	25
	(1.5)	(.7)	(.6)		(.7)
	58	587	−93	−20	24
	(1.3)	(1.0)	(.2)	(.8)	(.7)

regressions strongly support the demand-shift hypothesis and reject the hypothesis that the metropolitan–nonmetropolitan distinction explains the observed relation between predicted supply and utilization.

Interaction with Education

Mark Pauly has suggested that the ability of physicians to shift demand for their services might vary for different groups in the population. In particular, he hypothesized that the effect might be inversely related to the level of education. Table 6.8 reports the results of regression directed to this question. The regressions are run across the cells grouped by education, with 1963 and 1970 pooled. The effect of predicted supply on demand does seem to be largest for the low-education class and smallest for the high-education class. The differences between the coefficients, however, are not statistically significant.

Complexity, Urgency, and Necessity

Eleven frequently performed procedures[10] that account for 42 percent of all nonobstetrical operations were scaled for "complexity," "urgency," and "necessity." The complexity scale is based on the California Relative Value Scale; the urgency and necessity scales are based on replies by physicians to a mailed questionnaire asking them to choose a statement that best characterizes their impression of the operations being performed in each category (see Chapter 5).

Indexes of complexity, urgency, and necessity were calculated for each cell and then regressed on the demographic dummy variables, income per capita, and predicted surgeon supply, with the results as shown in Table 6.9. There seems to be some positive relation between complexity and surgeon supply, but the coefficient is not statistically significant. The surgeon-supply coefficient in the urgency index regression is large and statistically significant. Each additional surgeon per 100,000 population in an area lowers the urgency index by 1 percent—a large change, given the relatively small variation in the urgency index across areas. The necessity index also shows an inverse relation with surgeon supply, but the effect is smaller than for the urgency index and not statistically significant.

Table 6.8 Results of demand regressions across cells by education, 1963 and 1970 pooled

Years of education	$\hat{S}$*	$MET\hat{S}$*	INC*	$YEAR$
Part A (area values)				
0–8	73	41	−155	442
	(3.0)	(2.5)	(.3)	(1.9)
9–14	54	28	98	497
	(2.9)	(2.3)	(.3)	(2.8)
15+	25	14	462	226
	(.7)	(.6)	(.7)	(.7)
All	56	30	95	433
	(4.2)	(3.5)	(.4)	(3.5)
Part B (division values)				
0–8	41	—	253	434
	(1.2)		(.5)	(2.0)
9–14	49	—	−97	587
	(2.0)		(.2)	(3.5)
15+	8	—	247	365
	(.2)		(.4)	(1.2)
All	41	—	68	503
	(2.3)		(.2)	(4.2)

Note: Dummy variables for age, sex, race, and education (where applicable) included; coefficients not shown.

Table 6.9 Results of regressions of indexes of complexity, urgency, and necessity across cells (area values), 1970

Index	$\hat{S}*$	$MET\hat{S}*$	$INC*$
Complexity	.31	.24	1.3
	(1.4)	(1.6)	(.3)
Urgency	−.98	−.12	12.8
	(2.2)	(.4)	(1.5)
Necessity	−.26	−.01	4.9
	(1.3)	(.0)	(1.3)

Note: Dummy variables for age, sex, race, and education included; coefficients not shown. All three indexes were rescaled to have means of 100. The standard deviations across areas (controlling for age, sex, race, and education) are: complexity, 6.1; urgency, 13.8; and necessity, 4.7.

The Effect of Supply on Price

The effect of predicted supply on quantity (and complexity) provides some evidence in support of the hypothesis that surgeons shift the demand for their services. Confidence in this conclusion would be increased if changes in supply also resulted in changes in price in the same direction. This question is investigated with regressions across the 11 divisions.

The surgical price index is derived from AMA data reporting average fees by specialty and division for initial and follow-up office visits and follow-up hospital visits in 1970. There is reasonably high correlation among these different fees.[11] An average of the three types of fees is taken to be representative of the relative price of surgery across divisions. This index is deflated by the Williamson-BLS divisional price index for all commodities, as shown in Table 6.10.

The surgical price index in both deflated and undeflated form is regressed on predicted surgeon supply and predicted demand and on the observed values of these variables. The predicted values of the endogenous variables are obtained from regressions with $INC*$, $\%MET$, $HOTEL*$, and $GP*$ as instruments.

The results (Table 6.11) reveal a *positive* effect of supply on price; this is clearly contrary to conventional market behavior. By contrast, the effect of demand on price is quite small. A coefficient of 1.5 for supply is equivalent to an elasticity of 0.5 at the means of the variables. Inasmuch as predicted price had no effect in the surgeon-supply equation, we can reject the view

Table 6.10 Divisional price indexes: surgical visits and all commodities (U.S. = 100)

Division	Surgical price index[a] (1)	Williamson-BLS index[b] (2)	Deflated surgical price index (1) ÷ (2) (3)
New England	108.1	107.9	100.2
Middle Atlantic	121.9	107.8	113.1
East North Central	87.5	101.0	86.6
West North Central	86.5	100.2	86.3
South Atlantic	94.2	94.8	99.4
East South Central	83.1	92.6	89.7
West South Central	89.6	91.1	98.4
Mountain	77.8	99.5	78.2
Pacific	111.1	100.9	110.1

a. *Source:* American Medical Association, *Profile of Medical Practice,* 1972, pp. 81, 83, 85.

b. *Source:* Williamson (1977, mimeo version), pp. 79–80. Division values are population-weighted means of Williamson's state data.

that the high correlation between price and surgeon supply[12] reflects a causal relation running from price to supply.

Discussion and Summary

Because of the small number of observations and potential measurement error in some of the data, we must regard the results reported in this chapter as less than definitive. In par-

Table 6.11 Regressions of surgical price on supply and demand across divisions, 1970

2SLS	$\hat{S}*$	$\hat{Q}*$
Deflated surgical price	1.47	.01
	(1.2)	(.3)
Surgical price	1.55	.02
	(.9)	(.6)
OLS	$S*$	$Q*$
Deflated surgical price	2.01	− .01
	(2.7)	(.6)
Surgical price	2.83	− .01
	(3.5)	(.9)

ticular, better price data and a more robust demand specification would serve to increase confidence in the findings. The short-comings notwithstanding, the cumulative impact of the various statistical experiments casts serious doubt concerning the stability of the demand function for operations when there is an exogenous shift in the supply of surgeons. The hypothesis that an increase in the supply of surgeons results in an increase in demand is strongly supported by the following findings.

1. "Predicted" supply consistently has a positive effect on demand in a variety of specifications.
2. The effect is present in both 1970 and 1963 even though the quantity measure is subject to substantial sampling error and the correlation between years is not very high.
3. The effect is present and even stronger when metropolitan areas and nonmetropolitan areas are studied separately.
4. The supply effect on demand is inversely correlated with the level of education.
5. The supply effect is stronger for procedures deemed less urgent and less necessary by physicians.
6. Supply has a positive effect on price, not a negative one.

Can these results be reconciled with "normal" market behavior without recourse to demand-shifting? They can, but it takes some straining to do so. One possible explanation is that surgeon quality is positively correlated with the surgeon/population ratio, and that higher quality induces additional demand much as a decrease in price does.[13]

I agree that quality is probably correlated with quantity, but it seems doubtful that the quality effect would be strong enough to explain the observed differences in utilization or price. One indicator of "quality" is the percentage of surgeons who are subspecialists, such as ophthalmologists, orthopedists, and the like, rather than general surgeons. This percentage is highly correlated with the surgeon/population ratio across divisions ($r = 0.72$), but the elasticity is only 0.15. Let us assume that this captures only half of the quality difference, so that the full elasticity of quality with respect to S^* is 0.3. Let us also assume that the elasticity of demand with respect to quality is 0.3 (about triple the probable elasticity of demand with respect to price). The "quality effect" would then yield an elasticity of demand with respect to supply of 0.09, considerably less than the elasticity actually observed. Furthermore, it should be noted that "better quality" surgeons frequently recommend *less* surgery than do their colleagues with less training.

The results of the econometric analysis can be summarized as follows: Surgeons have considerable discretion in choice of location, and their distribution is determined partly by their preferences as consumers. Thus, geographic areas differ in their surgeon/population ratio for reasons unrelated to the inherent demand for operations. Where surgeons are more numerous, the demand for operations increases. Other things being equal, a 10 percent higher surgeon/population ratio results in about a 3 percent increase in the number of operations and an *increase* in price. Thus, the average surgeon's work load decreases by 7 percent, but income per surgeon declines by much less.

These findings do leave one troublesome question: If surgeons can raise prices where they are more numerous, why don't they raise them even higher where the surgeon/population ratio is lower? One possible answer is that their incomes are already satisfactory because of their higher (but not excessively high) work loads, and they have less incentive to induce additional demand.

The implications of these results for national policy seem striking. If the surgeon/population ratio should increase (this seems likely if no action is taken by government or academic medical centers), the result will probably be higher rather than lower fees, and also more operations. The question of the marginal benefit of these operations relative to marginal cost is not addressed here, but recent studies by physicians raise serious doubts, at least for some procedures (Paradise et al., 1978; Bunker, Barnes, and Mosteller, 1977).

One clear limitation of this study is the omission of that portion of the surgeons' work load unrelated to in-hospital operations. As suggested previously, the ability of surgeons to shift the demand for outpatient services is probably greater than for operations. Thus the total impact of supply on demand may be larger, and the implied difference in income per surgeon smaller, than those observed in this study. Indeed, although the weakness of some of the data and the tentative character of the conclusions need to be stressed, it should also be noted that some of these weaknesses serve to understate rather than exaggerate the extent to which surgeons can shift the demand for their own services.

Prospective payment is a cornerstone of federal and state plans to control health-care costs (Iglehart, 1982). It is also perceived as a threat to the financial viability of academic medical centers, whose costs per admission exceed those of community hospitals (Sloan, Feldman, and Steinwald, 1983; Watts and Klastorin, 1980). Many investigators attribute higher costs to the distinctive mix of patients cared for in teaching hospitals (Ament, Kobrinski, and Wood, 1981). These patients undergo extensive diagnostic investigation, receive more agressive treatment, and stay in the hospital longer—in part because they often present with more complex problems than their counterparts in nonteaching hospitals. Each hospital's case mix changes little from year to year (Lave and Lave, 1971). If academic medical centers continue to serve patients like those they have admitted in the past and to provide them with the same level of care, their revenues will depend on the case-mix adjustment applied to prospective payment.

The case-mix measure that will be applied under Medicare— the use of diagnosis-related groups (DRGs)—is already in use in Maryland and New Jersey (Iglehart, 1983). DRGs are groupings of diagnostic categories drawn from the *International Classification of Diseases* (ninth edition, *Clinical Modification*) and modified by the inclusion of major surgical procedures, age of the patient, and the presence of important complications or concurrent illnesses (Hornbrook, 1982). Currently there are 467 DRGs, chosen to minimize the variance in costs within each

---

Written with Alan M. Garber, M.D., and James F. Silverman, M.D.

group (Thompson, Fetter, and Mross, 1975). Teaching hospitals anticipating DRG-based payment schedules will find little reassurance in previous studies of the relation between hospital costs and case mix; these studies have shown that teaching hospitals have higher costs even when case mix is held constant (Watts and Klastorin, 1980; Becker and Steinwald, 1981; Thompson, Fetter, and Shin, 1978). There has been little discussion of the contribution, if any, of higher costs to better patient outcomes. Both policymakers and hospitals need to know the causes of these cost differences and their implications.

We explored these issues by comparing patients who were admitted to the faculty and community services of a major university-affiliated hospital, measuring the contribution of case mix and other patient characteristics to differences in costs between the two services. We identified subsets of patients with particularly large cost differences and explored the possible causes of those differences. Finally, we investigated whether higher expenditures were associated with differences in outcomes, and explored the implications for hospital costs and performance under prospective payment. By studying differences within a single hospital, we implicitly held constant wage rates, costs of materials and supplies, laboratory fees, pharmacy prices, quantity and quality of nursing, and similar factors that confound comparisons between different hospitals.

Methods

Sample and Data Base

The basic population consisted of all the admissions of patients 45 years of age and over at the Stanford University Hospital during 1981. The sample was limited to admissions of patients whose illnesses placed them in DRGs meeting these criteria: (1) the DRG must have accounted for at least 20 admissions to each of the faculty and community services; and (2) there must have been 10 or more deaths in the DRG in 1981. The second criterion ensured adequate variation in survival for the purposes of analysis of outcome.

Full-time faculty members served as attending physicians for the patients admitted to the faculty service. All other patients were admitted to either the community teaching or the community nonteaching service. Referring community physicians selected cases having particular educational value for the teaching service; these included some of the sickest community-service patients with some of the most complicated diseases. House staff and students cared for these patients under the supervision of community physicians. Their freedom to order tests or diagnostic procedures for these patients was more limited than on the faculty service. The nonteaching service consisted of the two-thirds of community-service patients who received no routine house-staff care. The 43 admissions that lacked a specification of physician type were excluded, leaving a final sample of 1,007 faculty-service and 1,018 community-service admissions in 12 DRGs. These DRGs accounted for 16.2 percent of all admissions and 29.5 percent of all costs of patients 45 years of age and over.

The data were generated from a data base known as the "Care Monitoring System." This system uses discharge data from medical records, including information about patient demographics, physician activity, outcomes, diagnoses, and procedures. The data are classified by DRG, and the medical-record data are merged with the financial record, which assigns charges according to service unit. For this study, the service units were aggregated to form three categories: routine (including room and central service), diagnostic, and therapeutic services. The allocation of charges was made by the hospital chief of staff by review of the cost centers (for example, radiology) and service units (for example, chest x-ray films). Thus, respiratory-therapy charges were assigned to the therapeutic-service category, clinical laboratory studies to the diagnostic category, radiology–chest x-ray films to the diagnostic category, and radiology-angioplasty to the therapeutic category. Costs here refer to patient charges rather than to the actual value of resources used. Because the ratio of resource costs to charges varies according to type of charge, differences in charges may either overestimate or underestimate cost differences if the distribution of charges according to type varies greatly between the faculty and community services. To determine whether this was a serious problem, separate cost/charge ratios were calculated for the routine, diagnostic, and therapeutic categories, and these ratios were applied separately to the faculty and community services in accordance with the distribution of charges in each service. When this result was compared with the actual charge data used, the difference was less than one percentage point for the average DRG and less than one-tenth of one percentage point for the comparison of 51 matched pairs discussed below. Thus, charges are used throughout as an index of costs.

Predicting Hospital Outcome (Survival)

The method of maximum likelihood was used to estimate a multiple logistic equation relating the probability of death during hospitalization to a number of personal characteristics. The dependent variable took the value of 1 if admission terminated in death, and the value of 0 otherwise. Independent variables were age and dummy variables (each observation takes a value of 1 or 0) for sex, urgency of admission, race, area of residence, previous discharge, and each of the 12 DRGs. A predicted probability of death was computed for each patient by applying the estimated logistic equation to the values of the variables for the patient.

Cost and Survival Adjustment

We determined the contribution of patient mix to observed differences in costs and survival by adjusting for DRG alone and for DRGs with personal characteristics. These adjustments are analogous to indirect age adjustments. To adjust costs for DRGs and other characteristics, we first derived a measure of predicted costs. In the first stage, linear regressions were estimated with the natural logarithm of costs as the dependent variable and the following as exogenous variables: dummy variables for sex, religion, type of insurance, urgency of admission, race, location of residence, previous discharge, age category, and DRG. To adjust for DRG alone, we performed similar regression analyses omitting the other variables. The regression coefficients were then applied to obtain the predicted cost for each admission. The geometric means of the ratio of actual to predicted costs (that is, adjusted-cost ratios) were computed for the faculty-service and the community-service patients separately. Finally, the adjusted cost was calculated as the adjusted cost ratio for faculty-service (or community-service) patients multiplied by the mean costs for both groups combined. The formula for adjusted costs for the faculty service was

$$\text{Adj. costs} = \exp\left[\sum_{i=1}^{N_f} \frac{\log C_i - \log \hat{C}_i}{N_f}\right] (\bar{C}),$$

where C_i are the actual costs for ith faculty-service patient, $\hat{C}_i$ are that patient's predicted costs, $\bar{C}$ is the mean cost for faculty-service and community-service patients combined, and N_f is the total number of faculty-service patients in the group.

Outcomes were adjusted in an analogous manner. To obtain the predicted risk of death for an individual patient, adjusting for personal characteristics as well as DRGs, we used the value of the predicted probability of death for that patient. The adjusted-risk ratio for any group of patients was defined as the proportion of the group who actually died divided by the mean predicted probability of death for the group. The adjusted risk was simply the adjusted-risk ratio for either a community or a faculty group multiplied by the percentage of the combined population who died. Statistical significance was determined by testing for differences in means for costs and differences in proportions for mortality, using a two-tailed test.

Matched Observations in Patients with a High Death Risk

All patients whose predicted probability of death was equal to or greater than 0.25 were identified for chart review and follow-up. This included 60 faculty-service and 140 community-service patients. Pairs consisting of one patient from each service were then matched by age, sex, and DRG. Close matches were found for 55 pairs of patients, but 4 pairs were excluded because medical records could not be located for one member of the pair. The remaining 51 pairs were compared for costs and outcomes, their medical charts were reviewed, and their survival status during the year after discharge was ascertained.

Results

Patients admitted to the faculty and community services differed in several important respects, as shown in Table 7.1. The former were much more likely to be admitted for cardiac surgery or treatment of lymphoma or leukemia. A disproportionate number of patients on the community service had diagnoses of cerebrovascular disorders, chronic obstructive pulmonary disease, or heart failure and shock. The faculty-service patients were substantially younger (seven years, on average), less likely to have been admitted on an emergency basis, and much less likely to live within a half-hour's drive of the hospital. The distribu-

Table 7.1 Percentage distribution of admissions according to diagnosis-related group (DRG), patient characteristics, and type of physician

Characteristics	Faculty physicians (%)	Community physicians (%)
DRG		
014 Cerebrovascular disorders	4.6	15.3
082 Respiratory neoplasms	6.1	6.9
087 Pulmonary edema and respiratory failure	2.0	2.3
088 Chronic obstructive pulmonary disease	5.0	10.8
089 Simple pneumonia	2.6	6.2
105 Cardiac-valve procedure	19.2	5.7
107 Coronary bypass	37.2	23.2
127 Heart failure and shock	4.9	14.8
172 Digestive-tract cancer	2.5	4.0
203 Pancreatic or hepatobiliary cancer	2.4	2.8
274 Malignant breast disorders	2.7	2.9
403 Lymphoma or leukemia	11.0	5.0
Emergency status		
Elective	5.1	3.6
Urgent	54.9	28.2
Emergent	40.0	68.2
Discharge within past six months		
Yes	18.6	22.5
No	81.4	77.5
Residence distance[a]		
<30 minutes	12.4	55.3
31–60 minutes	20.2	14.5
61–120 minutes	27.7	18.6
⩾121 minutes	38.0	6.7
Unknown	1.7	4.9
Sex		
Female	34.9	46.6
Male	65.1	53.4
Age		
45–64	57.6	34.7
65–74	31.5	31.2
⩾75	10.9	34.1
Number of admissions	1007	1018

a. Approximate travel time to hospital.

tions (not shown in the table) of patients according to race, religion, and insurance coverage were similar in the two services, except that those on the community side included a larger percentage of Medicare patients, reflecting the difference in age distribution.

Costs

Table 7.2 shows that costs were higher on the faculty service in 9 of the DRGs. The overall cost differential of 59.6 percent was substantially reduced to 10.8 percent (95 percent confidence limits, 3.7 to 18 percent) when costs were adjusted for differences in the distribution of cases across the 12 DRGs. Additional adjustment for the socioeconomic characteristics of the patients had virtually no effect on the overall cost differential of more than $1,200 per case. Similarly, the exclusion of 16 outliers (costs in excess of $100,000) had very little effect on the differential. Adjusted average length of stay did not differ significantly between the two services; adjusted cost per day was significantly higher on the faculty service.

Patients were assigned to four risk categories on the basis of their predicted probability of death. These categories corresponded to values of 0.25 or higher (9.9 percent of the admissions), between 0.15 and 0.24 (22.9 percent), between 0.05 and 0.14 (27.6 percent), and less than 0.05 (39.6 percent). Table 7.3 shows that the cost differential was small and statistically insignificant for patients with low predicted probability of death. It was largest among the most seriously ill patients—those who, at the time of admission, had an estimated probability of death of 0.25 or greater. Among such patients, those treated by faculty had costs that were 70 percent higher (95 percent confidence limits, 33 to 107 percent) than those treated by community physicians, after adjustment for case mix as measured by DRGs. When costs were disaggregated into three major categories, the adjusted percentage differential was greatest for diagnostic costs and smallest for routine costs.

Mortality

Faculty-service patients incurred higher costs, but Tables 7.2 and 7.4 show that they also had better outcomes as measured by deaths per 100 admissions. In-hospital mortality rates were higher for patients on the community service in 11 of the 12

Table 7.2 Cost per admission and hospital mortality according to type of physician

Diagnosis-related group (DRG)	Cost per admission (dollars)		Hospital deaths per 100 admissions	
	Faculty	Community	Faculty	Community
014 Cerebrovascular disorders	9,097[a]	4,865[a]	19.6	21.8
082 Respiratory neoplasms	5,274	4,439	14.8	28.6
087 Pulmonary edema and respiratory failure	13,688[b]	4,903[b]	30.0	17.4
088 Chronic obstructive pulmonary disease	8,872	7,539	6.0	7.3
089 Simple pneumonia	7,630	8,379	7.7	14.3
105 Cardiac-valve procedure	25,054	22,924	4.7	8.6
107 Coronary bypass	19,159	18,075	2.1	3.0
127 Heart failure and shock	5,163	4,364	12.2	14.6
172 Digestive-tract cancer	7,684	4,713	8.0	26.8
203 Pancreatic or hepatobiliary cancer	5,846	4,217	16.7[b]	48.3[b]
274 Malignant breast disorders	4,063	4,259	11.1	26.7
403 Lymphoma or leukemia	9,452	10,341	10.8	19.6
All 12 DRGs	15,313[c]	9,592[c]	7.2[c]	14.9[c]
All adjusted for DRG mix	13,096[a]	11,815[a]	8.6[a]	13.0[a]
All adjusted for DRG mix and other characteristics	13,071[a]	11,840[a]	9.2[b]	12.3[b]

Note: In all tables, "cost" is based on charges; see text.
a. $p < 0.01$.
b. $p < 0.05$.
c. $p < 0.001$.

Table 7.3 Adjusted costs (in dollars) according to type of cost, predicted probability of death, and type of physician

Type of cost	Type of physician	Predicted probability of death[a]				
		<0.05	0.05–0.14	0.15–0.24	≥0.25	All
Total	Faculty	17,781	12,081[b]	7,955	7,976[c]	13,096[d]
	Community	17,048	10,449[b]	7,103	4,697[c]	11,815[d]
Diagnostic	Faculty	3,613	3,408[c]	2,044[b]	1,757[c]	2,985[c]
	Community	3,353	2,506[c]	1,603[b]	843[c]	2,420[c]
Routine	Faculty	9,328	6,131	4,204	4,815[d]	6,795
	Community	9,135	5,495	4,285	3,089[d]	6,529
Treatment	Faculty	4,591	2,697	1,560	1,803[b]	3,209
	Community	4,391	2,386	1,404	973[b]	2,993
Faculty-community differential (%)[e]						
Total		4.3	15.6	12.0	69.8	10.8
Diagnostic		7.8	36.0	27.5	108.4	23.3
Routine		2.1	11.6	−1.9	55.9	4.1
Treatment		4.6	13.0	11.1	85.3	7.2

Note: Costs are adjusted for DRG mix.
a. Estimated with a logistic regression.
b. $p < 0.05$.
c. $p < 0.001$.
d. $p < 0.01$.
e. $100 \times$ (faculty − community) ÷ community.

DRGs. Even after adjustment for DRGs and socioeconomic characteristics, the community-service patients were 34 percent (95 percent confidence limits, 1 to 66 percent) more likely to be dead at discharge. Disaggregation according to predicted probability of death shows that the survival difference was most pronounced for the high-risk patients, the same ones who had the largest differential in costs.

Analysis of the relation between the cost and mortality differentials reveals substantial differences across the 12 DRGs. In one set of DRGs (089, 105, 107, 274, and 403) there was a large mortality differential and virtually no difference in cost. In a second set (082, 172, and 203), there were large differentials in both costs and mortality. And in a third set (014, 087, 088,

Table 7.4 Deaths per 100 admissions according to predicted probability of death and type of physician

	Type of physician	Predicted probability of death[a]				
		<0.05	0.05–0.14	0.15–0.24	≥0.25	All
Unadjusted	Faculty	2.0	8.8	16.1	23.3	7.2[b]
	Community	3.8	9.7	21.4	34.3	14.9[b]
Adjusted for DRG	Faculty	2.1	8.8	16.2	22.8	9.2[d]
and other	Community	4.5	9.6	20.9	34.6	12.3[d]
characteristics[c]						

a. Estimated with a logistic regression.
b. $p < 0.001$.
c. Urgency of admission, age, sex, race, residence, and discharge during the previous six months.
d. $p < 0.05$.

and 127), there was a large cost differential, but adjusted mortality rates were similar on the two services. Interestingly, the distribution of patients according to service and DRG appears to be responsive to these cost–mortality trade-offs. In the first set of DRGs, in which the faculty service had substantially lower mortality with no increase in cost, this service accounted for 63 percent of the admissions. By contrast, in the third set of DRGs, in which the faculty service had substantially higher costs without lower mortality, only 27 percent of the patients were treated by faculty physicians. In the intermediate set of DRGs, admissions were more equally divided, with 44 percent cared for on the faculty service.

Analysis of Matched Pairs

The results of a comparison of matched observations shown in Table 7.5 strongly support the conclusions drawn from the larger sample and offer additional insights concerning the differences between the two services. The 51 admissions to the faculty service were matched by DRG, age, and sex with 51 admissions to the community service. The patients came from the following DRGs (numbers of pairs shown in parentheses): 014 (5), 082 (16), 087 (5), 172 (4), 203 (14), and 274 (7). All patients had a death risk of 0.25 or higher. Within this matched group, the average cost was more than twice as high in the faculty service. Moreover, this difference was not attributable to a few large

Table 7.5 Results of analysis of 51 matched pairs

Characteristic	Faculty physician	Community physician	Faculty minus community[a]	95% confidence limit[a]
Average age (yr)	68.7	69.7	—	—
Average predicted probability of death (%)	31.9	32.8	—	—
Cost per admission ($)	8,809[b]	3,132[b]	5677	±4318
Length of stay (days)	12.2[b]	5.9[b]	6.3	±5.0
Cost per day ($)	797[b]	578[b]	219	±193
Death in hospital (%)	27.5[b]	49.0[b]	−21.5	±19.2
"Do not resuscitate" code (%)	11.8[c]	51.0[c]	−39.2	±18.4
Local residence (%)	41.2[c]	76.5[c]	−35.3	±19.5
Matched by code status (23 pairs)				
Cost per admission ($)	10,756	3,722	—	—
Probability of death (%)	30.2	30.4	—	—
Death in hospital (%)	17.4	34.8	—	—
Matched by residence (22 pairs)				
Cost per admission ($)	11,476	3,570	—	—
Probability of death (%)	29.9	29.8	—	—
Death in hospital (%)	31.8	40.9	—	—
Survival for at least one year (48 pairs) (%)	16.7	16.7	—	—

a. Difference and confidence limits are shown when difference is statistically significant ($p < 0.05$).
b. $p < 0.05$.
c. $p < 0.001$.

outliers. In 41 of the 51 pairs, the patient on the faculty service had the higher costs. Much of the difference in cost per admission was associated with longer stays on the faculty service; however, cost per day was also significantly higher on that service. The difference in outcomes, as measured by status at discharge, was also substantial: the death rate was almost twice as high among patients on the community service.

Although these patients had been carefully matched according to several criteria, review of their medical charts revealed a large difference in the proportion who had a "DNR" ("Do not resuscitate") notation on their charts. Only 6 of the 51 patients admitted to the faculty service had a DNR notation, as compared with 26 on the community service. This could reflect objective difference in the medical condition of the patients that were not accounted for by DRG, age, sex, and predicted probability of death, or it could reflect subjective differences in patient or physician attitudes. In addition, the low use of the DNR code on the faculty service may result from administrative difficulties faced by house officers who must obtain approval from the faculty supervisor in order to put this notation on the chart. The difference in code status is large, but it does not explain the differences in costs and outcomes. For 23 pairs in which the faculty and community patients had the same code status (in 21 the code was "resuscitate"), the faculty–community differentials were similar to those for all the pairs. Among the 23 pairs, 19 of the faculty-service patients had higher costs.

A much higher percentage of the community-service patients were local residents (who could drive to the hospital in less than 30 minutes). We were able to match 22 pairs according to residence zone (19 were in the "local" zone), but this matching did not reduce the cost differential. Among the 22 pairs, 18 of the faculty-service patients had higher costs. The differential in mortality was smaller than for all the pairs, but the faculty-service patients still had lower death rates.

There is no doubt that a higher percentage of the patients on the faculty service were discharged alive, but there is considerable interest in knowing how much longer they lived. The last line of Table 7.5 and Figure 7.1 provide answers to that question. For 48 pairs it was possible to ascertain whether the patient lived for at least one year after discharge or, if not, what the date of death was. The percentage surviving for one year was quite low, and it was equal for the two services. Figure 7.1 shows that there was still a considerable difference in survival rates six months after discharge, but by the end of nine months the difference between the two services had disappeared.

Discussion

Our study, like studies comparing community and teaching hospitals (Becker and Steinwald, 1981; Thompson, Fetter, and Shin, 1978), found that adjustment for case mix eliminated

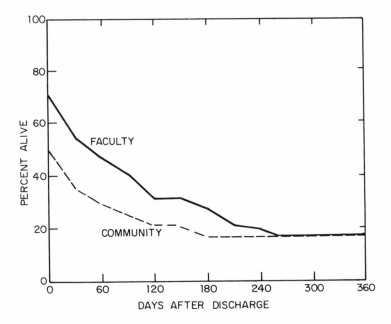

Figure 7.1 One-year survival curves for 48 matched pairs of patients, one of each pair admitted to the hospital's faculty service and the other to its community service.

much of the cost differential between the faculty and community services in this hospital. Nevertheless, admissions to the faculty service generated higher costs within DRGs that could not be explained by other observed patient characteristics. These higher costs were accompanied by lower hospital mortality. Both cost and mortality differences were greatest for the high-risk group of patients.

A number of plausible explanations could be offered for these findings, with distinct and sometimes contradictory implications for health-care financing and for the costs of medical education. These may be divided into explanations based on differences in physician attributes and practice patterns, and those based on differences in patient populations.

Differences among Physicians

The differential in adjusted costs probably reflects in part the greater impact on the faculty service of the hospital's role as a training institution and referral center. House staff and medical students have major responsibilities for the care of patients on the faculty service. They have no role with respect to two-thirds of the patients on the community service, and when they care for community-service patients, house officers have less autonomy than on the faculty service. These trainees, who learn by performing procedures and interpreting diagnostic tests, may order such studies more readily because of their putative educational value. The greater use of diagnostic services by trainees may also reflect their unwillingness or inability to rely as heavily as the more seasoned private physicians on the clinical examination (Martz and Ptakowski, 1978).

Physicians' attitudes toward death may also have contributed to the more aggressive care on the faculty service. An unwillingness to allow patients to die may have driven some house officers to press for more care, even when it led to little or no improvement in patient outcome. Private physicians, who knew their patients better, may have been more aware of the patients' own wishes concerning continued life support. In many cases the patients' preferences may not have been known to the faculty physicians, who would have treated aggressively when in doubt. Finally, the inexperience of house officers and medical students may have led them to provide some services that had few benefits for the patient.

Differences among Patients

Despite efforts to control for diagnosis and other patient characteristics, there may have been systematic differences between the patients on the two services in their medical condition, extent of workup before admission, or attitudes toward death. Chart review suggested that among the seriously ill patients, those admitted to the community service were more frequently admitted for purely supportive care and were less likely to receive extensive diagnostic workups or to be admitted to the intensive-care unit. Since the severity or stage of illness can vary considerably within the high-risk DRGs, control for DRG does not eliminate this source of variation in intensity of service. A single DRG can include both a patient presenting with a metastasis and an unknown primary tumor, who receives an extensive diagnostic workup, and a moribund patient admitted for terminal care. Moreover, physicians on the community service typically cared for patients whom they had followed for long periods before hospitalization; thus, they may have been better able to avoid duplication of tests performed outside the hospital and to minimize other costs associated with the workup of new patients.

Patients' attitudes can also contribute to variation in the type and quantity of services provided. Patients having the same morbidity and the same prognosis will not seek the same care if their attitudes toward death and toward medical intervention differ. A patient who is emotionally prepared to die may not consent to intubation, mechanical ventilation, and cardiac resuscitation, though his equally ill fellow patient may desire such measures. The much higher proportion of "DNR" orders on the community service probably reflects such patient preferences, in addition to possible differences in prognosis and physician attitudes.

Many studies of hospital costs have assumed that hospital output could be represented by the volume of services provided (Sloan, Feldman, and Steinwald, 1983). Such an approach has been justly criticized because inappropriate and ineffective care adds to such "output." Patients seek improvements in personal welfare from a hospital, not the tests and treatments themselves; however, improvement in patient welfare is difficult to measure. Hospital survival is undoubtedly an important component of welfare, and according to this criterion, patients on the faculty service did better. In the matched sample of patients for whom follow-up data were available, the faculty-service patients also had longer out-of-hospital survival. The distribution among DRGs and the variation in other patient characteristics could only partially explain their lower mortality rates. Like the cost differentials, the outcomes deviated most for the group of patients with the highest risk and were likely to reflect differences in practice patterns as well as in the types of patients seen on each service.

The more extensive use of diagnostic procedures and the more intensive care provided on the faculty service may have reduced mortality while generating higher costs. Because the patient populations may have differed, these results do not prove that faculty physicians reduced mortality by providing more care. But if patients on the faculty service were less likely to die simply because they were better risks, why did the faculty service attract them? It is unlikely that chance alone could cause such a marked disparity in patient populations. One possible explanation is that community physicians waited longer to admit their patients to the hospital than did their faculty counterparts. By substituting outpatient for inpatient services, they may have increased the proportion of their patients who were in the final stages of illness, while reducing hospital costs. Just as an all-inclusive measure of costs of illness, including outpatient services, might have shown less discrepancy between the faculty and community services, better control for stage of illness might have reduced the mortality differential.

Patients' perceptions of the difference in practice styles may underlie systematic differences in the patient populations of the faculty and community services. Patients who desired or were likely to benefit from more care may have sought, or may have been referred to, members of the faculty. Not only did differences in underlying disease contribute to the mortality differences, but they appeared to determine what kind of care was appropriate. Notably, in the DRGs that included mainly faculty-service patients, those patients had lower mortality than community-service patients, with similar costs. In the DRGs with mostly community-service patients, those patients had lower costs than faculty-service patients, with similar mortality. It is as if most of the patients were assigned to the service that would provide the best balance of costs and benefits. Neither the faculty nor the community medical practice was necessarily better or worse, merely different. There is no reason to expect or to desire that patients with diverse conditions and attitudes should receive the same care or have the same outcomes.

We have studied only one hospital, and therefore our results may not be generalizable. On the other hand, the differences we observed between the faculty and community services in the same hospital are likely to understate the differences between separate teaching and community hospitals. In the hospital we studied, the same advanced, specialized facilities were available to the faculty-service and community-service patients, and house staff participated in the care of some community-service patients. Furthermore, faculty and community physicians in this hospital undoubtedly interacted more closely than faculty and community physicians in separate hospitals, contributing to a more homegeneous style of medicine. On the other hand, mortality differences in the 12 DRGs we studied were greater than in other DRGs, which had lower death rates.

It is difficult to ascertain whether the aggressive care on the faculty service contributed to the lower in-hospital mortality; it is even more difficult to judge whether the reduced mortality was justified by the cost. In the matched sample of seriously ill patients, more than half were discharged alive, but fewer than one-fifth survived for as long as one year. The absence of relevant data on the postdischarge experience precludes our drawing strong inferences from the survival curves shown in Figure 7.1. We did not investigate the quality of life for the survivors, nor did we ascertain their source of postdischarge care or its cost. Many of the faculty-service patients presumably returned to their home communities after discharge and were cared for by their community physicians.

Even if the extra costs on the faculty service are attributable to the education of house staff and students, without corresponding patient benefits, these activities may be worthwhile. In that case, the question is not whether such care should continue, but whether it should be financed with patient-care revenues. If, on the other hand, these services have few educational benefits and little value to the patient, other methods of training physicians should be investigated. But if more intensive care helps some patients while educating house staff, effort should be devoted to identifying the patients most likely to benefit from such care. These are the patients who are likely to suffer most from prospective payment.

Under a prospective-payment plan, hospitals will have incentives to manipulate discharge diagnoses to fit patients into DRGs with higher payment schedules, to perform surgical procedures that shift patients to other DRGs, to limit hospital stays, and to minimize daily expenditures (Simborg, 1981). Institutions that continue to practice the high-cost medicine that is typical of the faculty service will incur financial penalties. Less aggressive services will become more common. Institutions will face the difficult challenge of both limiting expenditures and continuing to provide costly care to patients for whom it is appropriate. If hospital services become more homogeneous, we may see hospital mortality rise. Undoubtedly, policymakers will closely monitor the effects of prospective payments on expenditures; an important potential consequence of prospective payment will be overlooked if they do not also monitor hospital mortality rates.

EMPIRICAL STUDIES: HEALTH III

8 | Motor Accident Mortality and Compulsory Inspection of Vehicles

The article by Buxbaum and Colton (1966) on the relation between motor vehicle inspection and accident mortality is a pioneering contribution to a subject of considerable interest to economists as well as to public health investigators. The principal economic question is whether the costs of compulsory vehicle inspection are justified by the benefits of such a program. This question is being raised with increasing frequency about many government programs in health and other fields in an effort to secure more efficient allocation of scarce resources in the pursuit of competing national goals (Dorfman, 1965). In this instance an estimate of the effect of inspection on accidents is needed, as well as estimates of the costs of inspection and of the economic value of accident reduction.

This investigation is addressed primarily to the question of the relation between inspection and motor accident mortality. The Buxbaum-Colton study was restricted to men aged 45 to 54; it used groups of states; and it considered only one variable, in addition to inspection, at a time. We extend the analysis by making use of age-adjusted death rates, by using individual states as the units of observation, and by the use of multivariate analysis to test the inspection hypothesis statistically under conditions that more closely approach the desired ceteris paribus assumption. Some dollar estimates of the costs and benefits are also presented.

Written with Irving Leveson.

Methods

This study is concerned with age-adjusted death rates by state during the period 1959 through 1961. The dependent variable, motor accident mortality, is regressed on a number of independent variables believed to affect mortality. An equation of the following form is solved by least squares:

$$X_0 = a + b_1 X_1 + b_2 X_2 + b_3 X_3 \ldots + b_n X_n + u.$$

The partial regression coefficients (b_1, b_2, b_3, and so on) show the relation between each independent variable and motor accident mortality after allowing for the influence of the other variables.

The following variables are included in the analysis.

X_0 = death rate (age-standardized mortality ratio, indirect method, motor vehicle accidents, average 1959–1961, deaths by state of residence). Each state's value is the ratio of its rate to the national average.

X_1 = inspection (a dummy variable). States with compulsory inspection in 1960 are given a value of 1; those without inspection are given a value of 0. A negative regression coefficient for this variable would support the hypothesis that states that require inspection have lower motor accident mortality.

X_2 = motor fuel consumption per capita in 1960. This variable is included to allow for interstate differences in motor vehicle usage. A positive coefficient is expected because greater usage should result in higher death rates, ceteris paribus. This variable is measured in hundreds of gallons per capita.

X_3 = density (hundreds of persons per square mile in 1960). This variable is included because the lower vehicle speeds usually found in densely populated areas would tend to result in lower mortality. (The speed explanation is supported by the high ratio of accidents to deaths in urban areas relative to rural areas.)

X_4 = young drivers. The percentage of the population 18 to 24 years of age in 1960 is used as a proxy for the relative importance of young drivers. The latter are known to have a higher than average motor accident rate, and some of these accidents will result in deaths in other age groups. Ceteris paribus, the more young people there are in a state, the higher will be the motor accident mortality even after standardizing for age.

X_5 = other accidents (age-standardized mortality ratio, other accidents, average 1959–1961, ratio to national rate). This variable is included in an attempt to allow for sociocultural factors that might make the inhabitants of one state more prone to accidents than those of another. It also serves to allow for possible differences in the health services available to deal with accidents. A positive coefficient is expected.

X_6 = percent nonwhites (the percentage of the population that was nonwhite in 1960). This variable is tested because it appears that nonwhites tend to have a higher motor accident rate than whites. A positive coefficient is expected.

X_7 = alcohol consumption per capita (total absolute alcohol content of sales per person of drinking age in 1962). A positive coefficient is expected.

X_8 = age of vehicle (percentage of motor vehicles more than nine years old). A positive coefficient is expected.

X_9 = vision inspection (a dummy variable). States that require vision inspection for license renewal are given a value of 1; those without inspection are given a value of 0. A negative coefficient is expected.

X_{10} = education (median number of school years completed by population 25 years of age and over in 1960). It is expected that education may be associated with attention to safety, ability to read road signs, or other factors, A negative coefficient is expected.

X_{11} = income (median income of families and individuals in hundreds of dollars in 1959). This variable may reflect socioeconomic status, state of repair of vehicle, or type of driving.

The regressions are run in both unweighted and weighted forms. In the former each state is, in effect, given equal weight; in the latter each state is weighted by its population. The advantage of the latter form is that it reduces the possibility of random influences in a small state significantly affecting the regression coefficients. However, the unweighted run serves as a useful check against the possibility that the inspection coefficient in the weighted run is dominated by the results in a few very large states. In addition to the linear form, the logarithms of the independent variables were regressed on the motor vehicle mortality ratio. The coefficients in those equations indicate the percentage of change in mortality per percentage of change in the independent variable at the average level of mortality.

Results

The regression results are presented in Table 8.1. Two steps are shown for each run. In the first step, only the inspection dummy variable is entered. The regression coefficient, -0.298 (linear unweighted run), is a measure of the gross difference between the states with and without inspection with respect to the dependent variable, the age-adjusted mortality ratio. Since the latter has a mean of 1.0, the regression coefficient may be interpreted as a percentage; that is, the states that require inspection, on the average, have death rates 29.8 percent below those of the states without inspection. The figures in parentheses under each regression coefficient are the t values (the regression coefficient divided by its standard error). Values of t greater than 2.03 indicate that if the true regression coefficient is zero, there would be less than 5 chances in 100 of obtaining a coefficient as large as that actually shown on a two-tail test.

The use of tests of significance when states are the unit of observation can be understood by considering the following example. For the inspection coefficient, the difference in mean death rates between 15 states with inspection and 33 without is compared with its standard error when other variables are held constant. If we had no problem of holding constant other variables, we would use the analogous procedure of testing the significance of the difference between the mean death rates of the group of states with inspection and the group of states without. In the latter case, the standard error of the difference enables us to determine the probability that we would observe such a large difference between means in repeated sampling of groups of 15 and 33 states from the population of all possible groups of 15 and 33 states.

Step 2 shows the results when all the independent variables have been entered. The other variables contribute greatly to the explanation of interstate differences in motor accident mortality; the adjusted coefficient of multiple determination ($\bar{R}^2$) rises from 0.13 to 0.83 for the linear unweighted run. The results when the logarithmic form is used and when the regressions are weighted are very similar. The inclusion of the other variables sharply reduces the differences between the states with and without inspection. The coefficient for the inspection dummy remains negative, but is not consistently significant. In the

Table 8.1 Results of regressing age-adjusted motor accident mortality ratio on vehicle inspection and other variables in 48 states in 1960

Regression	Step	$\bar{R}^2$	$S_{y.x}$	Inspection coefficient	
				b	t
Linear					
Unweighted	1	0.130	0.337	−0.298	(−2.84)
	2	0.834	0.147	−0.096	(−1.46)
Weighted	1	0.242	0.238	−0.288	(−4.00)
	2	0.843	0.108	−0.058	(−1.27)
Logarithmic					
Unweighted	1	0.130	0.337	−0.298	(−2.84)
	2	0.884	0.123	−0.068	(−1.35)
Weighted	1	0.242	0.238	−0.288	(−4.00)
	2	0.878	0.095	−0.065	(−1.86)

Note: Inspection coefficient in last step is not significantly different from zero ($p < 0.05$ on two-tail test) on any runs.

linear unweighted run, the effect of inspection is reduced from 29.8 percent to 9.6 percent; in the linear weighted run the reduction is from 28.9 percent to 5.8 percent. This means that more than two-thirds of the gross differential in age-adjusted mortality between the states with and without inspection cannot be attributed to inspection, but is explained by these other variables.

Table 8.2 presents the regression coefficients for the remaining variables. Population density and gasoline comsumption are the only variables whose coefficients are consistently and significantly different from zero. The less significant variables are included because we may not be able to differentiate effects of interrelated factors which as a group contribute to the explanatory power of the equations. Yet we do not wish to attribute the effects of such factors to motor vehicle inspection.

Number of inspections. Eight of the states that do require inspection require two inspections annually; seven require only one. Table 8.3 provides an answer to the question of whether the number of compulsory annual inspections has any systematic relation to mortality. The regression results suggest that the answer is yes. Two inspection dummies are used: $X_{1.1}$ for those

Table 8.2 Results of regressing age-adjusted motor accident mortality ratio on vehicle inspection and other variables in 48 states in 1960

Other variables	Linear		Logarithmic	
	Unweighted	Weighted	Unweighted	Weighted
Gasoline consumption	0.296[a]	0.260[a]	1.563[a]	1.234[a]
Population density	−0.005[a]	−0.004[a]	−0.369[a]	−0.320[a]
Young drivers	0.075	0.032	0.768	0.541
Other accident mortality	0.453[a]	0.216	0.540	0.091
Nonwhite	−0.003	0.001	0.089	0.115
Alcohol	−0.029	−0.059	−0.293	−0.370[b]
Age of car	0.002	0.002	−0.184	0.067
Vision inspection	0.070	0.085[b]	0.064	0.084[b]
Education	−0.031	−0.003	−1.067	−0.064
Income	0.003	−0.002	0.717	0.341

Note: Degree of freedom = 36.
a. Indicates statistical significance at 0.01 level of confidence on two-tail test for last step.
b. Indicates statistical significance at 0.05 level of confidence on two-tail test for last step.

states that require one annual inspection and $X_{1.2}$ for those that require two. When only the two inspection dummies are entered (step 1), no benefit from multiple inspection is apparent. This is similar to the results shown by Buxbaum and Colton for white men aged 45 to 54. After other independent variables are entered (step 2), the coefficient for the states requiring two inspections is larger than that for the group requiring only one in the linear but not in the logarithmic runs. The coefficients of determination are virtually the same as when X_1 was used.

Interaction with inspection effect. Although many variables do not show any significant relation to motor accident mortality in the multiple regression runs, they may have some relevance through an interaction with vehicle inspection. For instance, it is possible that inspection has more effect in low-income than in high-income states if persons with higher incomes are more likely to make repairs voluntarily. We would also have to examine interactions with education and differentiate those from effects of income.

The hypotheses of interaction between inspection and income or education are tested in the following way. The states are

Table 8.3 Results of regressing age-adjusted motor accident mortality ratio on number of vehicle inspections and other variables in 48 states in 1960

Regression	Step	One inspection ($X_{1.1}$)		Two inspections ($X_{1.2}$)	
		b_1	t_1	b_2	t_2
Linear					
Unweighted	1	−0.374	(−2.66)	−0.231	(−1.73)
	2	−0.064	(−0.86)	−0.147	(−1.70)
Weighted	1	−0.289	(−3.29)	−0.288	(−2.83)
	2	−0.024	(−0.47)	−0.110	(−1.92)
Logarithmic					
Unweighted	1	−0.374	(−2.66)	−0.231	(1.73)
	2	−0.075	(−1.30)	−0.054	(−0.73)
Weighted	1	−0.289	(−3.29)	−0.288	(−2.83)
	2	−0.060	(−1.50)	−0.076	(−1.48)

Note: Inspection coefficient in last step is not significantly different from zero ($p < 0.05$ on two-tail test) on any runs.

ranked from the highest to lowest by income (or education) and divided into two equal groups of 24 states each. For each group the same regressions as those reported in Tables 8.1, 8.2, and 8.3 are run. The partial regression coefficients for inspection and for the number of inspections shown in Tables 8.4 and 8.5 reveal the relation between mortality and inspection after holding constant the effects of all the independent variables. The coefficients for the latter variables, which are not shown, are generally within sampling variability of those reported in Tables 8.1, 8.2, and 8.3.

The inspection coefficients in Table 8.4 reveal a strong interaction between the level of income and the effect of inspection. This is particularly clear when the number of inspections is taken into account. In each case the second inspection is associated with much lower mortality in the states of low income than in the high-income states. Unexpectedly, states with high education reveal a greater effect of inspection than do states with low education. Once interaction effects are taken into account, we find some benefits from multiple inspection, especially in states with low income, but the difference between one and two inspections is not statistically significant.

Table 8.4 Results of regressing age-adjusted motor accident mortality ratio or vehicle inspection and other variables in states grouped by income in 1960

Regression	Income	$\overline{R}^2$	Inspection (X_1)	$\overline{R}^2$	One inspection $(X_{1.1})$	Two inspection $(X_{1.2})$
Linear						
Unweighted	High	0.917	0.015	0.918	0.079	−0.045
			(0.19)		(0.77)	(−0.45)
	Low	0.443	−0.210	0.458	−0.135	−0.367
			(−1.46)		(−0.87)	(−1.87)
Weighted	High	0.919	0.036	0.924	0.094	0.001
			(0.60)		(1.28)	(0.01)
	Low	0.316	−0.098	0.359	−0.070	−0.272
			(−0.78)		(−0.56)	(−1.53)
Logarithmic						
Unweighted	High	0.946	−0.042	0.941	−0.056	−0.022
			(−0.78)		(−0.83)	(−0.28)
	Low	0.507	−0.083	0.497	−0.032	−0.220
			(−0.64)		(−0.23)	(−1.08)
Weighted	High	0.917	−0.044	0.909	−0.038	−0.051
			(−0.89)		(−0.63)	(−0.76)
	Low	0.370	−0.049	0.363	−0.040	−0.194
			(−0.45)		(−0.37)	(−1.03)

Note: N = 24 in each regression. Other variables that were run with inspection dummies are mo▮ fuel consumption per capita, population density, percentage of young drivers, alcohol consumpti▮ per capita, percentage of cars more than nine years old, vision inspection dummy, percent nonwhi▮ median income, median years education, and age-adjusted death rates from other accidents. I▮ pendent variable is always linear.

Comments

The results reported here provide some support for the hypothesis of a negative relation between motor accident mortality and inspection, but the size of the effect of inspection is considerably smaller than that found by Buxbaum and Colton. Most of the gross difference between states with and without inspection is accounted for by the effects of other variables. The effect of inspection was found to be larger for states with more than one inspection per year than for those with only one.

A significant interaction was noted between inspection and income: states with low income reveal a large effect of inspection, while states with high income reveal almost none. One possible explanation is that owners in high-income states maintain their cars with or without compulsory inspection. The finding that the effects of inspection are greater in states with high education than in states with low education is surprising. If more educated people are more likely to bring their cars in for repairs voluntarily, the opposite would have been found.

The regression equations typically explain about 85 percent of all interstate variation in age-adjusted motor accident mortality, but note should be taken of possible biases in the results. Compulsory inspection may reflect a strong desire in a state to reduce motor vehicle death rates, and it may be accompanied by other programs such as more stringent traffic regulations, better roads, or stricter control of drivers' licenses. If this is the case, the reduction in motor vehicle death rates from inspection

Table 8.5 Results of regressing age-adjusted motor accident mortality ratio on vehicle inspection and other variables in states grouped by education in 1960

Regression	Education	$\bar{R}^2$	Inspection (X_1)	$\bar{R}^2$	One inspection $(X_{1.1})$	Two inspections $(X_{1.2})$
Linear						
Unweighted	High	0.905	−0.304	0.922	−0.170	−0.481
			(−2.80)[a]		(−1.40)	(−3.57)[b]
	Low	0.920	−0.017	0.955	0.076	−0.117
			(−0.31)		(1.49)	(−2.23)[a]
Weighted	High	0.896	−0.216	0.904	−0.081	−0.372
			(−1.89)		(−0.56)	(−2.40)[a]
	Low	0.896	−0.067	0.966	0.073	−0.146
			(−1.11)		(1.66)	(−3.88)[b]
Logarithmic						
Unweighted	High	0.918	−0.246	0.914	−0.207	−0.314
			(−2.22)[a]		(−1.59)	(−1.99)
	Low	0.919	−0.035	0.918	−0.010	−0.084
			(−0.68)		(−0.18)	(−1.16)
Weighted	High	0.897	−0.204	0.893	−0.126	−0.279
			(−1.90)		(−0.82)	(−1.87)
	Low	0.941	−0.035	0.955	−0.002	−0.098
			(−0.86)		(−0.06)	(−2.15)

Note: N = 24 in each regression. Other variables that were run with inspection dummies are motor fuel consumption per capita, population density, percentage of young drivers, alcohol consumption per capita, percentage of cars more than nine years old, vision inspection dummy, percent nonwhites, median income, median years education, and age-adjusted death rates from other accidents. Dependent variable is always linear.
a. Indicates statistical significance at 0.05 level of confidence on two-tail test for last step.
b. Indicates statistical significance at 0.01 level of confidence on two-tail test for last step.

is overstated because the observed reduction is probably attributable in part to these other programs. Other programs may be associated with independent variables such as education; such association would affect interaction tests in addition to biasing the estimate of the average effect of inspection. On the other hand, there would be an opposite bias if states with high motor vehicle death rates were prompted to enact inspection laws because the death rates are high. It would be desirable to examine death rates in states that have changed their inspection laws, but unfortunately, there have been too few changes in inspection status to permit any rigorous statistical analysis along these lines. The few states that we have examined yield mixed results.

In our judgment, the regression results should best be interpreted as indicating an effect of inspection in the range of 5 to 10 percent. What is the economic value of reducing motor accident mortality by this amount? A precise answer to this question is impossible, but it is possible to get some notion of the order of magnitude.

By discounting future expected earnings at various ages, an age-value profile can be constructed which shows the potential gross national product (GNP) lost by the death of a man at various ages (Rice, 1966). This profile can then be applied to age-specific death rates by cause of death to calculate the loss of potential GNP by cause. This approach shows that the economic cost to the nation of motor accident fatalities is much greater than that implied by the death rate, because a disproportionate number of deaths from this cause occur at younger ages.

Dorothy Rice (1966), using a discount rate of 6 percent per annum, has estimated the economic cost of all injuries in 1963 at $9.9 billion. Most of this ($6.4 billion) is attributed to mortality; the balance is attributed to morbidity ($1.8 billion) and direct medical and hospital expenses ($1.7 billion). Motor vehicle deaths in 1960 accounted for 29 percent of deaths from all injuries in 1963. Earnings were about 10 percent lower in 1960 than in 1963; on the other hand, the economic loss implied by the average death from motor accidents was about 27 percent higher than the average death from other accidents because of the different distributions of age at death. Putting all this information together, we estimate the 1960 cost of motor accidents at approximately one-third of Rice's estimate of the 1963 cost of all injuries. This yields a cost of $2.1 billion for mortality alone and $3.3 billion for mortality, morbidity, and direct costs.

The National Safety Council (1961, p. 5) estimates the economic cost of motor accident mortality, morbidity, and direct medical expense at $1.8 billion in 1960. They estimate property damage of $2.2 billion and the overhead costs of insurance at $2.5 billion, making a total cost of $6.5 billion. One other relevant statistic is the premium for automobile insurance, which was $6.4 billion in 1960 (U.S. Bureau of the Census, 1966). Since there are many costs not covered by insurance, this would seem to be an underestimate of the total cost of motor accidents.

What do these figures suggest about the economic value of vehicle inspection? If we assume an effect of 5 percent, the value in 1960 would have been about $100 million for mortality alone and about $300 million to $400 million for all costs. (This assumes that the effect of inspection on motor accidents in general is the same as on motor accident mortality.) With a 10 percent inspection effect, the benefits would be doubled.

How does this compare with the cost of compulsory inspection? In 1960 there were approximately 70 million vehicles registered in the United States. Annual inspection costs ranged from 50 cents to $2 per vehicle, depending on the fee and frequency of inspection. Furthermore, there are costs borne by the car owners in the form of lost time, inconvenience, and additional repairs, and costs to the taxpayers of administration and enforcement of the program. Taking everything into account, we estimate the cost per vehicle at $3 to $4. This yields an annual cost in 1960 of $210 million to $280 million if all vehicles were inspected.

These calculations suggest that the expected value of the total economic benefits of inspection might well exceed the estimated costs, but the margin may not be extraordinarily large. Moreover, the benefits are not statistically significantly greater than the costs, which means that we cannot reject the null hypothesis that the rate of return is less than or equal to zero. The margin is probably higher in 1967 than in 1960 because of the rate of growth of motor accidents and motor accident mortality has been more rapid than that of the number of vehicles. Moreover, the gain from extending inspection to all states may be understated by the average inspection coefficient, because more of the states without inspection were in the low-income group where the effect of compulsory inspection seems to be greater.

It should be noted that the reduction in mortality alone was probably not sufficient to justify compulsory inspection. The reader who might object that the saving of life is worth any cost should recall that the choice need not be between saving lives and not saving them, but between alternative programs. The $250 million annual cost of a compulsory vehicle inspection program could be used in other, perhaps more effective, life-saving programs such as stricter licensing procedures, enforcement of speed limits, elimination of road hazards, and so forth. We second Buxbaum and Colton's conclusion that the techniques and experience of many disciplines are needed to deal with the complex socioeconomic factors relevant to motor accident mortality.

Some Economic Aspects of Mortality in Developed Countries

Death is the result of a complex set of interacting physiological, behavioral, and environmental factors; its social and economic consequences are frequently profound. In most countries considerable resources are devoted to postponing death, and the success achieved in developed countries over the past two centuries is generally regarded as one of the outstanding benefits of economic development. It is well to recall that, at the beginning of the eighteenth century, life expectancy in Western Europe was scarcely higher than it had been under the Romans; not one infant in ten could expect to reach the biblical "three-score and ten." Today, in developed countries, close to three-fourths of the female and over half of the male infants can expect to reach the age of 70.

Despite its importance, economists have not had much to say about death. At one time the problem may have appeared too trivial; mortality rates depended on per capita income and not much else. Now the problem may be too complex. Variations in mortality across and within developed countries are still substantial, but their relationships to economic variables are not well understood.[1]

It is widely believed that increased life expectancy is an inevitable consequence of economic growth. Over the broad sweep of economic development there is ample justification for this belief. Among developed countries currently, however, some new bits of evidence suggest that the negative association between mortality and income is disappearing. Three types of data—cross section within countries, cross section among countries, and some time series—do not reveal the expected association. Thus, a major subject of interest in this chapter is the relationship between mortality and income. How has it changed over time? Why has it changed? In the course of the inquiry, consideration is also given to the role of medical care and scientific advances. Some additional insights concerning economic aspects of mortality are obtained by an examination of differentials associated with sex, marital status, and way of life.

Income Per Capita

It seems intuitively reasonable to assume that "life" is a normal good, and to predict a negative relation between mortality and real income per capita. For about two centuries, from the middle of the eighteenth to the middle of the twentieth century, there was ample confirmation of that prediction. Indeed, it is now believed that until this century most of the reduction in death rates was a result of increases in real income rather than improvements in medical care.[2]

In 1963 Irma Adelman seemed to go so far as to argue that the role of real income in life expectancy increases as income rises. She wrote: "Once the major benefits from these improvements [basic public health measures] have been reached it may well be that economic conditions play the primary role in determining the subsequent rate of progress in mortality, for it stands to reason that such factors as better nutrition, improved housing, healthier and more humane working conditions, and a somewhat more secure and less careworn mode of life, all of which accompany economic growth, must contribute to improvements in life expectancy" (1963, p. 324).

In 1965 I reported that income no longer seemed to have any favorable effect on interstate mortality differentials for U.S. whites except at young ages (Fuchs, 1965). This finding was confirmed by Auster, Leveson, and Sarachek (1969), who used a much more comprehensive model employing both ordinary least squares and two-stage least squares estimating procedures. Michael Grossman (1972a) provided additional insights concerning income and health using survey data on individuals instead of state averages, and measuring ill health by disability days and restricted-activities days instead of by mortality.

More important, Grossman developed a model of the demand

for health which shows how rising income could lead to higher death rates. The essence of his argument is that the consumption of some goods (such as rich foods or automobiles) may adversely affect health. If the income elasticity for such goods is very high, the "shadow price" of health rises, and the quantity of health demanded falls. Rising incomes could, therefore, actually raise mortality. Grossman's model shows how this might happen but does not predict that it will, or even that the favorable effect of income diminishes as income rises. The following discussion indicates why there is a tendency for this to occur.

Let us suppose that the elasticity of mortality with respect to income varies for different causes of death. For instance, the death rate from malnutrition or tuberculosis is likely to have a large negative income elasticity, while the death rate from aircraft accidents is likely to have a small elasticity, or may even be positively related to income. The overall elasticity of mortality with respect to income is a weighted average of the elasticities for different causes, where the weights are the fraction of deaths accounted for by each cause.[3] As income rises, ceteris paribus, the causes with small negative elasticities or positive elasticities become relatively more important, and the overall elasticity *must move toward zero or even turn positive*. Assuming initial values and constant mortality functions of income for each cause, the overall elasticity at any subsequent time is a function of the level of income. The following analysis of cross-sectional differences in infant mortality provides a good illustration of this process at work.

Infant Mortality

Age of death is usually reported more accurately than cause, and in infant mortality there is a rough correspondence between time of death and cause. Neonatal deaths (within 28 days of birth) are usually attributable to congenital anomalies, prematurity, and complications of delivery. Post-neonatal deaths (after 28 days but within one year) are frequently the result of infectious diseases or accidents, although, admittedly, correspondence between time and cause is not perfect. Separate regressions of the form $\ln M = a + b_1 \ln Y$ were fitted across states of the United States and across developed countries for 1937 (average of 1936–1938) and 1965 (average of 1964–1966) for neonatal and post-neonatal mortality. Because of data limitations, the country set includes only 15 developed countries with market-type economies. The income series in 1965 are the United Nations estimates of GNP per capita in U.S. dollars. For 1937, Colin Clark's (1960) estimates of "international units" are converted to U.S. 1965 dollars by the U.S. GNP price deflator. (Summary statistics are presented in Table 9.1.)

The results presented in the top section of Table 9.2 show that the income elasticity for neonatal deaths is significantly lower than for post-neonatal deaths. Within each category, the elasticities do not vary as much as they do between states and countries or between time periods. There is some tendency for the elasticities to fall over time, probably for the same reason that the overall elasticity tends to fall as income rises. An attempt was made to fit a curvilinear function by adding $(\ln Y)^2$, but this

Table 9.1 Means and standard deviations of variables in country and state regressions reported in Table 9.2

	1937		1965	
	Mean	Standard deviation	Mean	Standard deviation
Countries (N = 15)				
Income per capita (1965 dollars)	1,024	375	1,954	623
Neonatal mortality (per 1,000 live births)	29.41	6.72	14.52	3.32
Post-neonatal mortality	32.63	18.09	6.45	2.94
Death rates per 1,000				
Males 15–19	2.69	1.66	1.05	0.17
Males 45–49	8.70	2.55	5.66	1.22
Males 65–69	42.33	8.07	38.74	5.36
Females 15–19	2.35	1.82	0.34	0.06
Females 45–49	6.55	1.27	3.34	0.48
Females 65–69	32.96	4.28	21.33	2.39
States (N = 48)[a]				
Income per capita (1965 dollars)	1,589	457	2,880	401
Neonatal mortality	29.38	2.80	15.95	0.80
Post-neonatal mortality	19.83	6.94	5.30	0.74

Sources: See Table 9.2.
a. State variables weighted by population.

Table 9.2 Regression of neonatal and post-neonatal mortality on income per capita across states and countries, 1937 and 1965

Units of observation	Year[a]	Neonatal		Post-neonatal		
		Income elasticity b_1	Standard error of b_1	Income elasticity b_1	Standard error of b_1	N
States	1937	−0.17	(0.04)	−0.53	(0.11)	48
States	1965	−0.19	(0.04)	−0.49	(0.12)	48
Countries	1937	−0.24	(0.13)	−1.03	(0.27)	15
Countries	1965	−0.02	(0.18)	−0.49	(0.33)	15

		Income elasticity b_1	Standard error of b_1	Shift coefficient b_2	Standard error of b_2	Effect of change in knowledge[b] %	N
Neonatal							
States	1937 and 1965	−0.18	(0.03)	−0.50	(0.02)	−39	96
Countries	1937 and 1965	−0.15	(0.11)	−0.60	(0.11)	−45	30
Post-neonatal							
States	1937 and 1965	−0.52	(0.08)	−0.96	(0.06)	−62	96
Countries	1937 and 1965	−0.82	(0.21)	−1.02	(0.21)	−64	30

Note: All state regressions weighted by population.
Sources: Country data: Colin Clark, *The conditions of economic progress* (London, Macmillan, 1960); United Nations, *Demographic yearbook* for 1967, 1966, 1957, 1951; United Nations, *Statistical yearbook* (1967). State data: U.S. Bureau of the Census, *U.S. census of population*, vol. 1, part 1 (1960); U.S. Bureau of the Census, *Vital statistics of the U.S.* (1937, 1938); U.S. Bureau of the Census, *Vital statistics rates in the U.S., 1900–1940* (1943); U.S. Department of Commerce, Office of Business Economics, *Personal income by states since 1929* (1956); U.S. Department of Health, Education, and Welfare, Public Health Service, *Vital statistics of the United States, vol. II: Mortality,* for years 1964, 1965, and 1966.
a. Death rates based on three-year averages centered on year shown.
b. Equals (antilog $b_2 - 1$) (100).

term was never significant. Given the size of the standard errors we cannot, with confidence, reject the null hypothesis that the elasticities within each category were the same in 1965 as in 1937.

Advances in Knowledge

Assuming constant elasticities for 1937 and 1965, we can pool the observations for the two time periods and obtain an estimate of the shift in the mortality-income function with regressions of the form $\ln M = a + b_1 \ln Y + b_2 T$, where T is a dummy variable with a value of 1 for 1965 and 0 for 1937.

This shift can be attributed to the advance in knowledge of medical science per se, plus other knowledge that contributes to a reduction in infant mortality. To be sure, the shift coefficient is also affected by variables other than income that are related to infant mortality and that changed between 1937 and 1965. Where data were available, the number of physicians per capita and years of schooling were tried in the single-year regressions, but their inclusion did not have any significant effect on the results.

The bottom part of Table 9.2 shows the income elasticities (b_1) obtained with the pooled regressions and the shift coefficients (b_2). By taking the antilogarithm of b_2, subtracting 1, and multiplying by 100, we obtain the percentage decline in mortality that can be attributed to advances in knowledge. The results for the states and countries are quite similar. They indicate that, holding income constant, the neonatal death rate declined about 40 percent and the post-neonatal declined about 60 percent. The differences between the two shift coefficients are statistically significant. These shifts are very substantial relative to the gains that can be attributed to the increase in income alone. They suggest that between two-thirds and three-fourths of the decrease in infant mortality between 1937 and 1965 was due to shifts in the mortality-income function, and only between one-fourth and one-third to movement along the function.

It should be noted that differential shifts in the functions also affect the income elasticity of total infant mortality by changing the relative importance of the different causes (see note 3). As it happens, the differential shift due to advances in knowledge and the difference in elasticities both work in the same direction: namely, to decrease the weight of post-neonatal deaths in total infant mortality over time. If the shift differential were the opposite of the elasticity difference, the prediction of an overall elasticity that constantly approaches zero or becomes positive as income rises would have to be modified.

It is possible to predict the income elasticity of total infant mortality in 1965 given the elasticities and the shift coefficients for neonatal and post-neonatal mortality reported in the bottom section of Table 9.2. This prediction can then be compared with the actual elasticities obtained from regressions. The predicted value for the states is the same as the observed value. A sharp decline is predicted for the countries, but it falls short of the observed decline because the prediction assumes constant elasticities within each category over time, whereas in fact these also tended to decline.

Income elasticity of infant mortality

	1937	Predicted 1965	Actual 1965
States	−0.32	−0.27	−0.27
Countries	−0.64	−0.37	−0.17

Adult Mortality

In 1936–1938, other age-specific death rates were also negatively related to income per capita, as indicated by the regression results presented in Table 9.3. The elasticities were particularly high for adolescents and tended to decline as age increased. By 1965 the negative relation had disappeared. Although there is still considerable variability in age-specific death rates (coefficients of variation are around 15 percent), income is no more useful in explaining variability across developed countries than it is in explaining variability of U.S. whites across states.

Because the elasticities change so much over time, we cannot measure the effect of advances in knowledge by pooling the

Table 9.3 Regression of age-specific death rates on income per capita across developed countries, 1937 and 1965 (N = 15)

		1937[a]		1965[a]	
	Age	Income elasticity b_1	Standard error of b_1	Income elasticity b_1	Standard error of b_1
Males	15–19	−0.72	(0.21)	+0.12	(0.13)
	45–49	−0.32	(0.17)	+0.05	(0.17)
	65–69	−0.18	(0.11)	−0.01	(0.12)
Females	15–19	−0.93	(0.23)	+0.04	(0.12)
	45–49	−0.19	(0.11)	+0.05	(0.12)
	65–69	−0.13	(0.08)	−0.06	(0.09)

Sources: See Table 9.2.
a. Death rates based on three-year averages centered on year shown.

data and looking at the shift coefficient. If it were possible to divide death rates into different causes, however, we might find some consistency in elasticities over time. Once these are identified, shift coefficients could be estimated for each cause.

Within developed countries, the relationship between mortality and income for adults is also tending to disappear, except for those at the lowest income levels. This can be seen in the data for English male mortality by social class and occupation presented in Table 9.4. For the first four social classes there is no systematic relation between class and mortality for males 20–

Table 9.4 Male mortality indexes, England and Wales, 1949–1953 (all = 100)

	Age-adjusted 20–64	
Social class	All causes	Coronary disease, angina
I	98	147
II	86	110
III	101	105
IV	94	79
V	118	89
VI	124	60

Occupation	Ages 35–44	Ages 45–54	Ages 55–64
Higher administrative, professional and managerial	80	92	102
Other administrative, professional and managerial	73	85	88
Shopkeepers	91	97	104
Clerical workers	115	119	104
Shop assistants	85	86	84
Foremen	74	77	91
Skilled workers	97	100	107
Semiskilled workers	103	98	96
Unskilled workers	134	125	112
Personal service	135	122	106
Farmers	78	66	68
Agricultural workers	79	71	72

Sources: Top section: S. J. Kilpatrick, Occupational mortality indices, *Population Studies* 16 (November), 1962; Bottom section: United Nations, *Demographic yearbook* (1967).

64, age-adjusted. The bottom two classes do show slightly higher rates, but at least part of this relationship probably reflects a causality running from health to occupation (and, hence, to social class) rather than the reverse. Mortality from coronary disease actually increases with social class, providing a good example of a death rate with a positive income elasticity. Across occupations the relationship between income and age-specific death rates is also very mixed, with several comparisons showing a positive correlation.[4]

Medical Care

The extent to which medical care affects mortality is a subject of considerable controversy. A realistic appraisal requires distinguishing between changes in the quantity of medical care, holding the state of the art constant (movement along the mortality–medical care function), and improvements in the state of the art (downward shifts of the function). A further complication arises because these improvements do not come at a steady rate through time, nor are they some simple function of the volume of resources devoted to medical research.

Studies at the National Bureau of Economic Research on interstate differences in mortality (Auster, Leveson, and Sarachek, 1969; Fuchs, 1965; Grossman, 1972a; see also Chapter 4) all show that variations in the number of physicians per capita, expenditures for physicians' services (deflated or not), and other medical care inputs have only slight effect on mortality, frequently fading into insignificance. Inclusion of the number of physicians per capita in the age-specific mortality regressions across developed countries in 1956 produces similar results. In the absence of contrary evidence it would seem that the marginal contribution of medical care to reductions in mortality, holding the state of the art constant, is small in developed countries.[5]

Changes over time in what medical care can do, however, have had a very large effect on mortality. This was particularly true for the period beginning in the 1930s and extending through the 1950s. The acceleration in the rate of decrease in mortality after 1930 can be seen clearly in Figure 9.1, which shows the average annual percentage rate of decline by age and sex for the periods 1900–1930 and 1930–1960. For every age-sex group, the rate of decrease was greater in the more recent

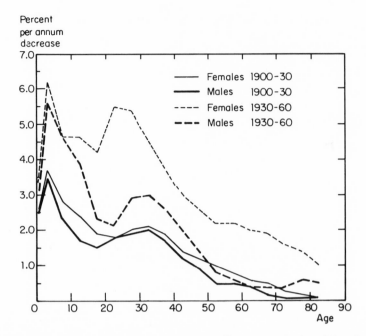

Figure 9.1 Rates of decrease in mortality rates, U.S. whites by age and sex, 1900–1930 and 1930–1960. *Source:* Calculations by the author made from data in U.S. Department of Health, Education, and Welfare, Public Health Service, *Vital statistics of the U.S., 1968*, vol. 2, sec. 5, Life tables.

decades. According to Walsh McDermott (1969), this was attributable to the development in medicine for the first time of a "decisive technology." Medical improvements in those years took many forms, the most noticeable being the discovery of sulfonamide, penicillin, and the modern antibiotics. The broad picture portrayed in Figure 9.1 of a more rapid decrease after 1930 than before, more rapid decreases for females than for males, and a tendency for the rate of decrease to be smaller at older ages is characteristic of the pattern in developed countries generally.

Recent Trends

By 1960 the really effective improvements in medicine were widely diffused throughout developed countries. Subsequent advances, such as organ transplants and other complex types

Table 9.5 Recent changes in male death rates (percent per annum)

Age	United States[a] (whites)	Sweden[b]	Norway[c]
25–29	+0.9	+0.1	−2.0
30–34	+0.8	+0.1	+0.2
35–39	+0.5	+0.2	+0.7
40–44	+0.3	+0.2	+1.0
45–49	−0.2	+0.1	+1.5
50–54	−0.4	+0.1	+0.7
55–59	+0.3	0	+0.8

Sources: Calculations by author made from data in Central Bureau of Statistics of Norway, *Statistical yearbook of Norway* (1969); U.S. Department of Health, Education, and Welfare, Public Health Service, *Vital statistics of the United States, vol. II: Mortality* (1967, 1968); *Statistical Abstract of Sweden* (1971).
a. 1959–1961 to 1967–1968.
b. 1959–1961 to 1967–1969.
c. 1956–1960 to 1967–1969.

of surgery, seem to have had only a small impact on death rates and in some countries have actually been offset by adverse changes in the environment and in personal behavior. In most countries adult death rates are leveling off, and in the United States, Sweden, and Norway age-specific death rates for males 25–60 have actually been rising slowly since about 1960 (see Table 9.5). This adverse trend could be reversed at any time, but such a reversal is not likely to come about simply from the growth of income per capita or the allocation of more resources to medical care. If it does come, it is likely to be a result of the application of new knowledge or a profound change in behavior.

Recent trends in infant mortality show precisely such a reversal. Consider the following average rates of change in U.S. infant mortality (percent per annum):

	Neonatal	Post-neonatal	Total infant mortality
1935–1950	−3.0	−6.6	−4.3
1950–1965	−1.0	−1.4	−1.1
1965–1971	−3.6	−5.9	−4.2

After a drastic leveling off from 1950 to 1965, infant death rates started to drop dramatically again, achieving rates of decline equal to the record decreases of 1935–1950.

The reasons for this recent rapid decline are not known. Some observers believe that special programs of maternal and child care aimed at disadvantaged groups are the principal explanation. Without denying that these programs may have had some effect, it seems to me that improvements in birth control (the pill, intrauterine devices, and liberalized abortion laws) probably deserve a great deal of the credit. The infant mortality rate for "unwanted" children is undoubtedly many times higher than for wanted children.

A related point is the sharp drop of births of higher order in recent years. Babies of birth order four or higher are at greater risk than those of lower order. Between 1950 and 1965 the higher-order birth rates actually increased by 17.5 percent, while the lower-order birth rate declined by 15.5 percent. Since 1965 the lower-order birth rates have continued to decline moderately, but the birth rates of fourth order or above have dropped drastically, probably by as much as 50 percent by 1971, although the detailed statistics are not yet available. To be sure, the change in the distribution of births by order is not, in itself, large enough to explain the huge decrease in infant mortality since 1965, but it is indicative of the general improvement in birth control that has been achieved in recent years.

One piece of relevant evidence is that rapid decreases in infant mortality after 1965 were experienced in most developed countries. In half of them, the rate of decrease was more rapid than in the United States. The special maternal and infant health programs were the result of U.S. legislation, whereas the pill and the IUD became available generally in developed countries.

Way of Life

If mortality in developed countries is relatively independent of income, and if the marginal contribution of medical care is small, what does make a difference? In brief, the *way* people live has considerable effect on *how long* they will live.[6] Both the "demand" for life and the ability to "produce" life (that is, to postpone death) seem to vary considerably among individuals and groups. The differentials examined in this section are suggestive of the importance of such variation.

Sex

In all developed countries, male death rates are considerably higher than those of females of comparable age. At young ages the differential is of the order of one-third and seems to be fairly constant for different developed countries and for different parts of the United States, suggesting that some inherent biological difference is the primary explanation. After age 15, however, the size of the differential varies considerably, both within the United States and among developed countries. This variation is probably related to an interaction between biological and socioeconomic factors.

Some idea of the extent of the sex differential in mortality, and how it varies with age and from one population to another, can be obtained from Figure 9.2. In the United States among young white adults, the male death rate is triple the female rate; in Sweden the ratio is only 2.3:1. Again, in the age group 45–65 the ratio is appreciably lower in Sweden than for U.S. whites. In both cases the high ratio for the U.S. whites is attributable to relatively high death rates for males, while female rates approach those found in Sweden. Among young males, the excess deaths in the United States over Sweden are primarily the result of accidents. For the 45–65 age group, the excess is primarily due to heart disease. Although attempts are frequently made to link the lower mortality in Sweden to that country's system of medical care, it seems unlikely that this system acts differentially for males and females, or that it plays a significant role in the lower incidence of accidents and heart disease among Swedish men.

Among U.S. whites, the largest sex differentials are in small southern towns and the smallest in the suburbs of large northern cities. For the group 15–64, age-adjusted, the male excess is 137 percent in nonmetropolitan counties of the South Atlantic division, and only 82 percent in metropolitan counties without a central city of the Middle Atlantic division. Again, it is extremely unlikely that the *difference* in the differential is related to medical care, income, or the like. The most promising hypothesis is that sex-role differentiation in production and con-

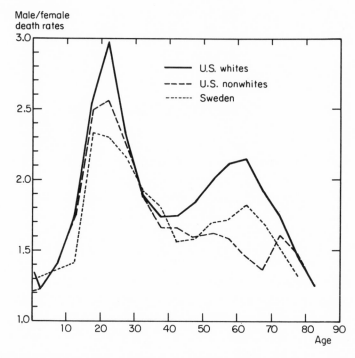

Figure 9.2 Male/female death rate ratios, 1967–1968. *Source:* Calculations by the author made from data in U.S. Department of Health, Education, and Welfare, Public Health Service, *Vital statistics of the United States, 1967* and *1968*, vol. 2: *Mortality. Statistical Abstract of Sweden,* 1971.

sumption varies from one population to another, with significant implications for mortality.

Marital Status

Another type of mortality differential which is common to all developed countries is that associated with marital status: at all ages the unmarried have substantially higher death rates than the married. This may be the result of a selective marriage market, with the causality running from health to marital status. Alternatively, it may be that life is produced more efficiently in a husband-wife household. Finally, it may be that married persons have a stronger demand for life. An examination of variations in the differential may help to shed a little light on these competing (but not mutually exclusive) hypotheses.[7]

Table 9.6 presents unmarried/married death-rate ratios and

percentage unmarried by sex for thirteen developed countries, ca. 1965. The males are ages 45–54, while the females are ages 45–64, a comparable group from the point of view of death rates. The table shows that the mortality differential associated with marital status is much greater for men than for women in every country. This may be viewed as giving some support to the "production of life" hypothesis, if it is assumed that life is primarily produced by nonmarket activities and that the female tends to specialize in such activities. It may also be viewed as supporting the selectivity argument because unmarried males are a much smaller fraction of their age cohort than are females, and might be presumed to be more atypical with respect to health. For males there is a slight negative correlation between percentage unmarried and the unmarried/married mortality ratio, again suggesting some selectivity at work. No such correlation is evident for females.

Table 9.6 Mortality indexes and percentage unmarried, developed market countries, ca. 1965

| Country | Unmarried mortality index[a] (married = 100) | | Percentage unmarried | |
	Males 45–54	Females, average of 45–54 and 55–64	Males 45–54	Females 45–54
Japan	349	174	4.3	30.6
Canada	235	139	10.7	24.6
West Germany	227	129	7.1	34.8
United States	223	146	13.2	28.7
Australia	201	124	15.0	26.2
Sweden	198	138	18.3	25.8
France	194	124	15.9	29.0
Finland	183	138	14.7	37.2
Netherlands	174	130	8.6	22.2
Denmark	167	130	15.9	26.8
New Zealand	160	111	17.0	26.3
Norway	155	123	18.9	26.0
England and Wales	153	129	11.1	25.2
Median	194	130	14.7	26.3

Source: Calculations by author made from data in United Nations, *Demographic yearbook* (1967).

a. Weighted average of death rates for single, widowed, and divorced persons with weights equal to U.S. distribution in 1970.

Within the unmarried male category there is a fairly consistent pattern, with divorced men showing the highest death rates, widowed the next highest, and single men coming closest to the married rate. Compared to the death rates of married men, the median ratios for the thirteen countries are 221, 187, and 167, respectively. This pattern is also evident in Table 9.7, which shows marital-status mortality ratios for U.S. white males of ages 45–54 by cause of death.

Why should the rates of widowed and divorced males be so much higher than for single men? One hypothesis is that of adverse selection; it has been suggested that widowed and divorced males (who do not remarry) constitute an "inferior" group. An examination of earnings and hours of work by marital status shows that such men do earn less and work fewer hours than do married men (holding color, age, and schooling constant) (see Table 9.8). Compared to single men, however,

Table 9.7 Marital status mortality indexes, U.S. white males 45–54, by cause of death, 1959–1961

Cause of death[a]	Single	Widowed	Divorced	Widowed	Divorced
	(married = 100)			(single = 100)	
Arteriosclerotic heart disease	136	164	211	121	155
Malignant neoplasms, respiratory	114	174	263	153	231
Malignant neoplasms, digestive	148	162	199	109	134
Vascular lesions—CNS	201	224	274	111	136
Other accidents	253	299	540	118	213
Suicide	174	352	395	202	227
Motor accidents	157	292	393	186	250
Cirrhosis of liver	276	508	784	184	284
Diabetes mellitus	221	188	298	85	135
Leukemia and aleukemia	107	101	129	94	121
Tuberculosis	520	669	1,062	129	204
Homicide	195	269	721	138	370

Source: U.S. Department of Health, Education, and Welfare, National Center for Health Statistics, Mortality from selected causes by marital status, United States, Part A. *Vital and health statistics,* series 20, no. 8A (1970).

a. Listed in descending order of importance.

Table 9.8 Earnings and hours, U.S. white employed 45–54, by sex, marital status, and years of schooling, 1959

Variable by years of schooling	Indexes for males (married = 100)			Indexes for females (married = 100)		
	Married	Single	Widowed and divorced	Married	Single	Widowed and divorced
Hourly earnings						
5–8	$2.60	90	81	$1.43	109	97
9–11	2.85	79	81	1.62	111	100
12	3.22	75	78	1.81	113	98
Annual hours						
5–8	2,044	93	91	1,566	118	108
9–11	2,142	90	95	1,617	119	118
12	2,219	92	91	1,603	124	118
Annual earnings						
5–8	$5,313	83	74	$2,239	129	104
9–11	6,103	71	77	2,617	132	118
12	7,152	68	71	2,900	141	115

Source: Calculations by author made from U.S. Bureau of the Census, *U.S. census of population and housing, 1960.* 1/1000 sample.

there is no support in the earnings and hours data for the adverse-selection hypothesis. There is, apparently, some extra factor raising mortality for the widowed and divorced that does not as strongly affect single men. This may well be a weaker demand for life.

When we compare mortality ratios for widowed and divorced men to single men by cause of death, the highest ratios are recorded for suicide, motor accidents, cirrhosis of the liver, homicide, and lung cancer. These are all causes in which a self-destructive behavioral component is very significant. At the other end of the scale, the widowed and divorced death rates come closest to the single rates for vascular lesions, diabetes, leukemia and aleukemia, and cancer of the digestive organs—all causes in which identified behavioral decisions play a smaller role.

A Tale of Two States

A startling illustration of the mortality differentials that can result from differences in way of life can be found in a comparison of Nevada and Utah, two contiguous western states. Infant mortality is 40 percent higher in Nevada, and comparable differentials exist at most other ages for both males and females (see Table 9.9). The states are similar in many respects, including availability of medical care, schooling, and climate. Income is slightly higher in Nevada. Why, then, the huge differential in mortality? The most likely answer is that Utah is inhabited primarily by Mormons, who eschew tobacco and alcohol and, in general, lead a quiet, stable life. Nevada, by contrast, is a state with high rates of cigarette and alcohol consumption, as well as very high indexes of marital instability and geographic mobility.

This comparison points up some confusion in contemporary economic thought about mortality. In an interesting paper, Dan Usher (1971) argued that an imputation should be made for increases in life expectancy to be added to the conventional measures of economic growth. If such an adjustment is justified for intertemporal comparisons, it would presumably also be appropriate for cross-section comparisons. According to this view, we should significantly scale down the estimates of real income per capita in Nevada relative to Utah.

But what if the mortality differentials are the result of deliberate, informed choices by all parties concerned? What if Nevadans place a higher value on tobacco and alcohol and a smaller value on longevity than do the people in Utah? Or, to put the matter even more strongly, suppose someone discovers or invents a new activity or a new good which affords a great deal of pleasure but has unfavorable implications for life expectancy? If a substantial number of people avail themselves of the new opportunity, and average life expectancy falls, it would be absurd to say, ceteris paribus, that real income has fallen. There is, however, a case for adjustment for mortality differentials when the differential is attributable to the way income is produced. If the inhabitants of one state have more hazardous occupations, an adjustment would be in order, just as if hours of work were much longer in one state than in the other.

As a practical matter, it is exceedingly difficult to separate consumption patterns from production. Are bartenders heavy drinkers because of their occupation, or do they become bartenders because they like alcohol? Consumption and production are frequently linked, and for the present we fall back on the more comprehensive, albeit general, notion of "way of life."

Table 9.9 Mortality indexes and related variables, Nevada and Utah

| Age | All causes | | Cirrhosis of the liver and malignant neoplasms of the respiratory system | |
	Males	Females	Males	Females
	Nevada Mortality Indexes (Utah = 100)			
<1	142	135	—	—
1–19	116	126	—	—
20–29	144	142	—	—
30–39	137	148	690	543
40–49	154	169	211	396
50–59	138	128	306	305
60–69	126	117	217	327

Related Variables	Nevada	Utah
Median income	$10,942	$9,356
Physicians per 10,000	11.3	13.8
Percent rural	19.1	19.4
Paramedicals per 1,000	16.1	18.0
Median schooling	12.4	12.5
Percent 20 + born in the state	10	63
Percent 5 + in same residence 1970 and 1965	36	54
Percent males 35–64 unmarried or not married to first spouse	47.4	25.5

Sources: Calculations by the author made from U.S. Department of Health, Education, and Welfare, Public Health Service, *Vital statistics of the United States, vol. II: Mortality,* for years 1964, 1965, 1966, 1967, 1968; American Medical Association, Department of Survey Research, *Distribution of physicians in the United States, 1970* (Chicago, 1971); U.S. Bureau of the Census, *Census of population, 1970,* U.S. Summary, *General social and economic characteristics* and *Detailed characteristics,* vol. 30 (Nevada), vol. 46 (Utah).

Concluding Comment

At one time economic growth was both a necessary and a sufficient condition for increasing life expectancy. Now it is neither. Although substantial differences in mortality persist within and between developed countries, they are the result, primarily, of differences in the demand for life and the ability to produce life, which are unrelated to income. A major task for health economists is to gain a better understanding of these demand and production functions.

Low-Level Radiation
and Infant Mortality

The accident at Three Mile Island has rekindled interest in questions concerning the effects of low-level radiation on health. These questions received considerable attention in the late 1960s, especially in several articles by Ernest J. Sternglass (1969a, 1969b) that alleged that radioactive fallout from nuclear weapons tests had a highly significant effect on infant mortality in the United States. Sternglass presented a variety of data, but the crux of his argument was that the periods of heaviest fallout (the late 1950s and early 1960s) coincided with a marked slackening in the rate of decrease in infant mortality (see Figure 10.1), a slackening that has not been satisfactorily explained on other grounds (Shapiro et al., 1968).

Sternglass's conclusions were rejected by many critics, largely on the basis of internal inconsistencies, unexplained selectivity in choice of observations, mathematical errors, and inattention to questions of statistical significance (Tompkins and Brown, 1969; Lindop and Rotblat, 1969; Sagan, 1969). Almost all the critiques concentrated on pointing out shortcomings in Sternglass's work; they did not undertake independent, large-scale, systematic tests of his hypothesis. Thus, the most thorough examination concluded: "We cannot support Dr. Sternglass's conclusions and ascribe changing patterns in infant and fetal mortality to the cause and factors invoked by Dr. Sternglass—certainly not with the conviction or certainty required by most epidemiologists and statisticians. It is clear from a review of all the data that certain gaps in the knowledge of how environmental levels of ^{90}Sr may affect the genetic materials of indi-

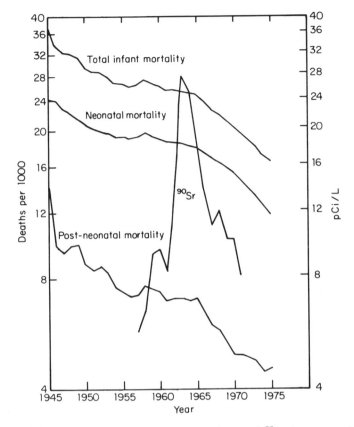

Figure 10.1 U.S. infant mortality, 1945–1975, and ^{90}Sr in pasteurized milk in New York City, 1957–1971.

viduals still exist and further studies in this direction are probably warranted" (Mills, 1969).

This chapter reports the results of an attempt to test systematically for possible effects of radioactive fallout on infant mortality in the United States. Annual data from 1960 to 1970 for each of the 48 contiguous states are analyzed in a variety of ways to determine whether interstate differences in mortality experience were associated with differences in ^{90}Sr or ^{137}Cs. The answer seems to be that they were not. Many different tests were run, and typically the null hypothesis of no effect of fallout on infant mortality could not be rejected. In a few instances a statistically significant association was observed, but the sign of the relationship is negative more often than it is positive.

Data and Methods

The most comprehensive and consistent data available on radiation are the U.S. Public Health Service measures of radioactivity in pasteurized milk. Beginning in 1960, at least one sample city is available in 45 states (Alabama, North Dakota, and South Dakota are missing), and in all 48 by 1962. For those states that had samples for more than one city, a population-weighted average was calculated. States with no sample city were assigned the unweighted average of the surrounding states. Considerable variation in radioactivity is observed over time (depending on the timing of the nuclear weapons tests) and across states at a single point in time (depending on precipitation and other meteorological factors). For instance, the average level of ^{90}Sr rose from 7.6 pico Curies (pCi) per liter in 1960 to 22.7 in 1964, and then fell to 9.4 by 1968. The variation in the biologically shorter-lived ^{137}Cs was even greater—from 8.1 to 133.3 to 12.2 pCi/liter over those same years. In 1964 ^{90}Sr was as high as 54.0 in North Dakota but was only 4.0 in Arizona, while ^{137}Cs ranged from 255 in Massachusetts and New Hampshire to 27.5 in Arizona. Infant mortality data are taken from the vital statistics of the United States and measured in deaths per 1,000 live births.

The mortality and radiation data are analyzed in the simple two-variable case and also in more complex multivariate models. Because there is no unanimity as to how low-level radiation might affect infant mortality (for example, somatic effects, genetic effects), some tests treat mortality as dependent on current levels of radiation while others specify a lagged or cumulative impact of radiation on mortality.

Results

The high point of radioactivity for nearly all states was recorded in either 1963 or 1964. The first test examines whether changes in infant mortality from 1960–1962 to 1963–1964 (simple two-year averages are used to reduce the influence of random fluctuations) or from 1963–1964 to 1966–1967 were correlated with changes in radioactivity across states. In Figure 10.2 the change in the natural logarithm of the infant mortality rate (a measure of relative change) in each state is plotted against the change in ^{90}Sr. No systematic relation is observed during either the pe-

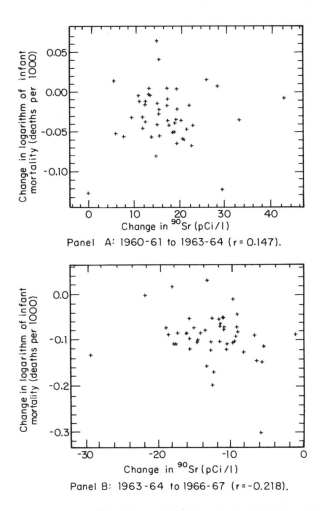

Figure 10.2 Scatter diagrams of changes in infant mortality and ^{90}Sr by state, 1960–1961 to 1963–1964 and 1963–1964 to 1966–1967.

riod of sharp increases in ^{90}Sr (panel A) or the period of sharp decreases (panel B). The statistically insignificant ($p > 0.05$) coefficients of correlation (state observations are weighted by number of births to reduce heteroscedasticity), $r = 0.147$ and $r = -0.218$, confirm the inference based on visual inspection of unweighted observations.

A second test compares mortality changes for the 12 states with the highest levels of radioactivity in 1963–1964 to the 12 states with the lowest levels (see Table 10.1). For the 1960–1961 to 1963–1964 period the two sets of states have similar changes in infant mortality, as indicated by the sum of ranks. For the 1963–1964 to 1966–1967 change, the states with the small de-

Table 10.1 Changes in infant mortality, 1960–61 to 1963–64 and 1963–64 to 1966–67, in states with highest and lowest levels of radioactivity in 1963–64

	1960–61 to 1963–64			1963–64 to 1966–67		
		Change in infant mortality			Change in infant mortality	
State	Change in ^{90}Sr (pCi/liter)	(percent)	(rank)[a]	Change in ^{90}Sr (pCi/liter)	(percent)	(rank)[a]
Highest levels						
North Dakota	+42.8	−0.63	19	−29.5	−14.18	4
Louisiana	+33.0	−3.51	13	−18.8	−9.02	14
South Dakota	+29.4	−12.86	2	−22.0	−.01	23
Arkansas	+28.2	.88	22	−17.9	−11.20	8
Mississippi	+25.8	1.67	24	−17.5	−8.72	16
Tennessee	+22.8	−4.17	10	−17.6	−11.32	7
Massachusetts	+22.5	−6.77	3	−18.4	1.82	24
North Carolina	+22.0	−1.56	16	−14.6	−10.27	11
Kentucky	+21.4	−4.69	8	−16.2	−8.56	17
Minnesota	+20.8	−6.06	4	−12.8	−4.93	20
New Hampshire	+20.6	−6.04	5	−15.2	−7.40	19
Georgia	+20.2	−3.54	12	−12.8	−10.63	10
Total			138			173

Table 10.1 (continued)

| | 1960–61 to 1963–64 | | | 1963–64 to 1966–67 | | |
	Change in ^{90}Sr (pCi/liter)	Change in infant mortality (percent)	(rank)[a]	Change in ^{90}Sr (pCi/liter)	Change in infant mortality (percent)	(rank)[a]
State						
Lowest levels						
Illinois	+13.2	−.49	20	−9.8	−.69	22
Kansas	+12.9	.50	21	−9.4	−9.39	12
Michigan	+12.2	−3.71	11	−9.2	−4.03	21
Texas	+12.2	−1.10	18	−8.3	−13.08	5
Colorado	+11.6	−4.61	9	−9.8	−10.80	9
Wisconsin	+11.5	−3.15	15	−9.1	−8.33	18
Virginia	+10.8	−1.14	17	−6.5	−15.32	3
Florida	+9.2	−3.21	14	−5.5	−11.70	6
California	+7.4	−5.68	6	−6.8	−9.09	13
New Mexico	+5.8	−5.40	7	−5.8	−15.51	2
Nevada	+5.2	1.46	23	−5.9	−35.00	1
Arizona	−0.2	−13.49	1	−1.2	−8.97	15
Total			162			127

a. Largest decrease is ranked first.

clines in radioactivity actually had, on average, larger decreases in infant mortality, but the difference is not large enough to reject the hypothesis that the two groups of states were drawn from populations with the same median, according to the Wil-

Table 10.2 Rate of change in infant mortality, 1960–70, in states with the highest and lowest levels of radioactivity in 1963–64

State	Rate of change[a] (percent per annum)	(rank)[b]
Highest levels		
North Dakota	−4.88	2
Louisiana	−2.83	16
South Dakota	−3.27	9
Arkansas	−2.97	14
Mississippi	−2.94	15
Tennessee	−3.40	8
Massachusetts	−1.98	22
North Carolina	−2.70	17
Kentucky	−3.49	7
Minnesota	−2.45	20
New Hampshire	−2.50	19
Georgia	−3.55	6
Total		155
Lowest levels		
Illinois	−1.07	24
Kansas	−2.40	21
Michigan	−1.71	23
Texas	−3.07	12
Colorado	−3.23	10
Wisconsin	−2.59	18
Virginia	−3.65	5
Florida	−3.17	11
California	−3.05	13
New Mexico	−3.92	3
Nevada	−3.81	4
Arizona	−4.90	1
Total		145

a. Calculated by least squares regression.
b. Largest decrease is ranked first.

coxon (Mann-Whitney) rank sum test. These conclusions are unaltered when ^{137}Cs is substituted for ^{90}Sr.

It is possible that the adverse effects of radioactive fallout on infant mortality were not felt immediately, but only after a lag of several years. In order to test for this possibility, the rate of change of the infant mortality rate from 1960 to 1970 was calculated for each of the 12 high-fallout states and each of the 12 with low fallout. The rates of change, which were obtained by fitting a least squares linear trend to the natural logarithm of annual observations, were then ranked from 1 to 24, and the ranks for each group of states were summed. The results, presented in Table 10.2, give no support to the view that radioactive fallout affected infant mortality with a lag. With respect to rates of decline of infant mortality, the two groups of states are indistinguishable.

Multivariate Analyses

It is well known that the infant mortality rate varies among states and over time for reasons other than radioactive fallout. It is desirable, therefore, to test for possible effects of fallout while controlling for other determinants of infant mortality. Data for the 48 states in each of 11 years (1960–1970) are pooled, and infant mortality is regressed on the radioactivity measures and other variables across the 528 state-year observations. A list of the variables, summary statistics, and sources is presented in Table 10.3. Ten alternative models are tested.

The dependent variables are total infant mortality, neonatal mortality (death in the first 28 days of life), and post-neonatal mortality (death in the second through twelfth months of life). The dependent variables are specified in logarithms in order to measure the effects of the independent variables on percentage differences in mortality. The independent variables T and $T2$ are time-trend variables designed to measure the impact of technological change and other time-related phenomena. These trends are effectively and efficiently described by allowing for a shift in the rate of change at 1965. The trend from 1960 to 1965 is measured by T, while $T2$ measures the change in that trend after 1965. Thus, the trend 1965–1970 is equal to the sum of the coefficients for T and $T2$. Two other specific in-

Table 10.3 Variables used in multiple regressions

Variable	Unit of measurement	Mean[a]	Standard deviation[a]	Minimum	Maximum	Source
Ln infant mortality	Log of deaths per 1,000 live births	3.155	0.149	2.661	3.728	A
Ln neonatal mortality	Log of deaths per 1,000 live births	2.843	0.115	2.391	3.232	A
Ln post-neonatal mortality	Log of deaths per 1,000 live births	1.822	0.272	0.978	2.789	A
^{90}Sr	pCi/liter	12.773	7.573	1.000	54.000	B
^{137}Cs	pCi/liter	40.967	48.368	0.000	255.000	B
T (1960 = 1; 1970 = 11)	—	5.792	3.186	1.00	11.00	—
$T2$ (1966 = 1; 1970 = 5)	—	1.275	1.757	0.00	5.00	—
%NWBR	Percent	15.887	10.098	0.106	54.178	A
Ln INC	Log of income in $100 per capita in 1970 dollars	3.494	0.214	2.761	3.885	C

Sources: A: National Center for Health Statistics, *Vital Statistics of the U.S., Mortality,* Part A (1960–1970); B: U.S. Department of Health, Education, and Welfare, Public Health Service, Division of Radiological Health, *Radiological Health Data Monthly Reports* (1960–1970); C: Department of Commerce, Bureau of Economic Analysis, *Survey of Current Business* (April 1971, p. 21).

a. Weighted by number of births for each state-year observation.

dependent variables that have figured prominently in previous studies of infant mortality are racial composition and standard of living (Antonovsky and Bernstein, 1977; Brooks, 1975). In order to control for these effects, the percentage of births that are nonwhite and the logarithm of per capita income are included in model 1.

There are undoubtedly other variables that affect infant mortality—including genetic, cultural, and environmental factors as well as differences in medical care—but these are difficult to identify and measure (Grahn and Kratchman, 1963). Because it is impossible to specify a full model, model 2 includes two sets of dummy variables for the nine Census divisions on the assumption that there is geographic variation in the unspecified variables. The first set of dummy variables is designed to capture those unspecified division-specific effects that were present in 1960 (that is, the "fixed" effect). A second set of variables are interaction terms between each division dummy and a time trend to allow for systematic variation in the unspecified division-specific effects over time. Radioactivity is measured by the ^{90}Sr (or ^{137}Cs) in milk averaged over 12 monthly estimates for each year. Each state-year observation is weighted by the number of births.

The regression results are presented in Tables 10.4 and 10.5. In every regression except one (post-neonatal model 2) the coefficient for ^{90}Sr is not significantly different from zero at the 5 percent confidence level, and in that one the direction of effect is negative. We cannot with confidence reject the null hypothesis that the true effect of ^{90}Sr on infant mortality is zero. We can also ask the question, "What are the chances that we are incorrectly accepting the null hypothesis if the true coefficient of ^{90}Sr is large enough to account for the difference between the actual level of infant mortality in 1963–1964 and the level that would have been observed if mortality had continued to decrease after 1955 at the same rate as it did in the period 1945–1955?" This difference is approximately 25 percent. Since the average level of ^{90}Sr in the United Sates in 1963–1964 was a bit under 25 pCi/liter, the ^{90}Sr coefficient would have to be about 0.01 (that is, a 1 percent change in infant mortality per 1 pCi/liter change in ^{90}Sr) if ^{90}Sr were responsible for the "excess mortality" in 1963–1964. Given an observed coefficient of -0.0007 with a standard deviation of 0.0004, it is clear that the chances

Table 10.4 Results of regressions of infant mortality in ^{90}Sr and other variables, pooled cross sections of states, annual observations 1960–1970 (N = 528)

	Total		Neonatal		Post-neonatal	
	Model 1[a]	Model 2[b]	Model 1[a]	Model 2[b]	Model 1[a]	Model 2[b]
R^2	.866	.900	.714	.804	.847	.880
Intercept	3.861	3.630	3.059	2.861	3.725	3.204
	(68.16)	(42.14)	(48.06)	(30.92)	(33.68)	(18.61)
^{90}Sr	−.00069	−.00075	.00068	−.00045	−.00453	−.00133
	(−1.61)	(−1.78)	(1.41)	(−.99)	(−5.41)	(−1.57)
T	−.0019	−.0106	−.0114	−.0200	.0227	.0116
	(−.91)	(−3.97)	(−4.85)	(−7.00)	(5.57)	(2.19)
$T2$	−.0344	−.0344	−.0172	−.0228	−.0810	−.0638
	(−9.18)	(−9.97)	(−4.08)	(−6.15)	(−11.07)	(−9.26)
%$NWBR$	.0085	.0078	.0058	.0049	.0152	.0142
	(30.45)	(24.23)	(18.36)	(14.21)	(27.79)	(22.18)
Ln INC	−.2227	−.1534	−.0654	−.0089	−.6052	−.4420
	(−13.70)	(−6.34)	(−3.58)	(−.34)	(−19.08)	(−9.14)

Note: t-statistics in parentheses: $p < 0.05$ if $|t| > 1.96$; $p < 0.01$ if $|t| > 2.58$; $p < 0.001$ i $|t| > 3.29$. Dependent variables in logarithms.
a. The division dummy variables are excluded.
b. Two sets of division dummy variables are included; see Table 10.5 for their coefficients.

that we are incorrectly accepting the null hypothesis (conditional on the true coefficient being 0.01) are vanishingly small.

When ^{137}Cs is substituted for ^{90}Sr the results are similar, and the coefficients of the other variables are virtually unaltered. Furthermore, tests of eight alternative models reveal that the principal conclusion is insensitive to changes in specification of the time trend, the geographic dummy variables, the period of study, or the timing of the relation between ^{90}Sr and mortality (see Table 10.6).

Discussion

Although the statistical tests do not provide support for the view that infant mortality in the 1960s was significantly affected by radioactive fallout, it must be emphasized that the levels of radioactivity were quite low, and no extrapolation of these results to higher levels is warranted. Similarly, the tests reported here pertain only to infant mortality; no conclusions concerning other possible health effects (such as fetal loss or cancer later in life) are implied. Finally, the conclusion of "no effect" must be qual-

Table 10.5 Regression coefficients of division dummy variables

Geographic division	Total		Neonatal		Post-neonatal	
	Fixed effect	Differential trend	Fixed effect	Differential trend	Fixed effect	Differential trend
New England	−.0089	.0085	.0076	.0116	−.0569	−.0027
	(−.39)	(2.52)	(.31)	(3.19)	(−1.25)	(−.40)
Middle Atlantic	.0014	.0092	.0431	.0108	−.1128	.0040
	(.08)	(3.70)	(2.41)	(4.03)	(−3.39)	(.80)
East North Central	−.0196	.0118	.0110	.0135	−.0930	.0062
	(−1.21)	(4.91)	(.63)	(5.23)	(−2.87)	(1.29)
West North Central	−.0359	.0085	−.0103	.0121	−.0823	−.0050
	(−1.74)	(2.82)	(−.47)	(3.75)	(−2.00)	(−.84)
South Atlantic	.0465	.0040	.0549	.0081	.0439	−.0065
	(2.31)	(1.54)	(2.54)	(2.89)	(1.09)	(−1.26)
East South Central	.0761	.0048	.0950	.0095	.0580	−.0063
	(3.00)	(1.51)	(3.49)	(2.78)	(1.15)	(−1.00)
West South Central	.0450	.0048	.0486	.0104	.0705	−.0105
	(2.16)	(1.69)	(2.17)	(3.42)	(1.69)	(−1.86)
Mountain	.1370	−.0058	.0975	−.0002	.2252	−.0184
	(5.50)	(−1.60)	(3.64)	(−.06)	(4.52)	(−2.53)

Note: Each divisional coefficient shows the difference between that division and the Pacific division. *t*-statistics in parentheses: $p < 0.05$ if $|t| > 1.96$; $p < 0.01$ if $|t| > 2.58$; $p < 0.001$ if $|t| > 3.29$.

Table 10.6 Coefficients of ^{90}Sr, %*NWBR,* and ln *INC* in alternative specifications of ln infant mortality regression

Model	Change from Model 2, Table 10.4	^{90}Sr	% *NWBR*	ln *INC*
3	Quadratic time trend instead of splined linear trends	−.00055 (−1.30)	.0078 (23.90)	−.1494 (−6.09)
4	Region instead of division dummy variables	−.00139 (−3.08)	.0081 (25.69)	−.2259 (−10.66)
5	State instead of division dummy variables	.00055 (1.80)	.0111 (4.04)	.1088 (1.60)
6[a]	Previous year Sr-90 instead of current year	−.00123 (−2.39)	.0078 (23.24)	−.1666 (−6.48)
7[b]	Average of 3 previous years' Sr-90 instead of current year	−.00149 (−2.22)	.0082 (20.65)	−.1828 (−5.93)
8	Pooled cross-section 1960–65 instead of 1960–70	−.00073 (−1.47)	.0076 (18.55)	−.1314 (−4.39)
9[c]	Data base average of 1960–65 instead of pooled cross-section, 1960–70	−.00335 (−2.09)	.0086 (11.08)	−.2697 (−5.76)
10[d]	Year dummies instead of splined linear trends; state instead of division dummy variables	−.00028 (−.46)	.0170 (9.48)	.1916 (2.67)

Note: *t*-statistics in parentheses.
a. 1961–1970.
b. 1963–1970.
c. Division dummy variables excluded.
d. Interaction with time trend excluded.

ified because of possible errors in measurement of radioactivity or possible omission of variables that are correlated with infant mortality and fallout.

The results for the other variables do not suggest major specification errors in the regressions in Table 10.4. The coefficients for racial composition and per capita income, for instance, are statistically significant and consistent with expectations. The coefficient for %*NWBR* indicates that the nonwhite rate is about 80 percent (0.008 × 100) above the white rate after controlling for per capita income and other division-related differences.

Income has a significantly favorable effect on infant mortality, and this effect is much stronger for the post-neonatal than for the neonatal period.

The coefficient for *T2* indicates that there was a marked acceleration in the rate of decrease in infant mortality after 1965 even after controlling for changes in fallout, income, and racial composition. This acceleration was particularly rapid for post-neonatal mortality. The coefficients for *T* show that infant mortality declined relatively slowly in the early 1960s even after controlling for possible effects of radioactive fallout. Several explanations have been proposed for the post-1965 improvement, including more effective contraception, legalized abortion, maternal and child health centers in poverty areas, scientific advances in neonatology, and Medicaid (Eisner et al., 1978). Additional research is necessary in order to sort out the relative importance of these explanations, as well as to explain the slow improvement prior to 1965.

11 | Time Preference and Health

This chapter reports the results of an exploratory effort in a new area: the relationship between intertemporal choice, health behavior, and health status. Intertemporal choice (or time preference) is, of course, a subject much discussed by economists and psychologists (see Maital and Maital, 1978). There is also a large literature on individual behavior (for example, cigarette smoking, diet, exercise) and health status. This study, however, seems to be the first attempt to bring these subjects together and to test empirically for possible interrelations.

In the first section I briefly review some of the considerations that suggest that an investigation of time preference might throw light on health behavior and health status. These include empirical studies of the relation between schooling and health; epidemiological investigations of the health effects of cigarette smoking, diet, exercise, and the like; and theoretical issues concerning investment in human capital, imperfections in capital markets, and optimizing behavior. The second section considers the critical problem of the measurement of time preference and reviews some recent efforts by other investigators to measure time preference in contexts other than health. I then describe a pilot questionnaire given to 500 men and women and present the results of correlation and regression analyses of their replies. The chapter concludes with a discussion of questions raised by this exploratory research.

Background

Empirical Considerations

Cross-sectional studies of the determinants of health status in the United States usually report a strong association between health and years of schooling. This result typically appears regardless of whether health is measured objectively (for example, mortality rates) or subjectively (for example, self-evaluation), and is equally robust in studies of differences across groups (states or cities) or across individuals (household survey data). Simple correlations between health and years of schooling are usually significant in both the statistical and the practical sense. Furthermore, the relation remains strong after controlling for other variables such as income.

Probably the most thorough investigation of this relationship has been carried out by Michael Grossman in "The Correlation between Health and Schooling" (1975). This study of middle-aged men is particularly notable for two reasons. First, a statistically significant effect of schooling on health remains after controlling for a large number of other variables, including family background, health status in high school, income, job satisfaction, and scores on physical and mental tests taken by the men when they were in their early twenties. Second, each of the men had at least a high school diploma; the mean level of schooling was over 15 years. Grossman's finding that the favorable effects of additional schooling persist even at high levels of schooling is in sharp contrast to the relation between income and health, which is positive at low levels of income but seems to be much weaker or nonexistent at average or high levels (Auster, Leveson, and Sarachek, 1969).

While the relationship between schooling and health seems well established, the mechanisms through which schooling affects health are less clear. Grossman has interpreted the empirical results as support for a household production function model; additional years of schooling make the individual a more efficient producer of health. This efficiency may arise through wiser use of medical care or, what is more likely, through differences in cigarette smoking, diet, and other elements of lifestyle.

The view that "the greatest potential for improving the health of the American people . . . is to be found in what people do and don't do to and for themselves" (Fuchs, 1967) has gained widespread acceptance in recent years because of the influence of numerous studies by epidemiologists and social scientists interested in health.[1] These studies report significant differences in health status and life expectancy associated with factors such as cigarette smoking, diet, and exercise. Not only is a statistical correlation well established, but in many instances there is some understanding of the causal mechanisms as well—for example, the role of diet and exercise in the prevention of atherosclerosis. What is not understood at all well is the cause of individual variation in health-related behavior.

From an economic point of view, many of these behaviors have a common characteristic: they involve trade-offs between current costs and future benefits. The costs may be purely psychic, such as the loss of pleasure from passing up a rich dessert or a cigarette. They may involve time (for example, jogging), or they may involve other costs, including financial and nonfinancial resources. The expected benefits typically take the form of reductions in the probability of morbidity and mortality from one or more diseases sometime in the future.

Theoretical Considerations

The acceptance of a current cost for a future benefit constitutes an investment. Becker's development of the theory of investment in human capital (Becker, 1964) and Grossman's application of this theory specifically to health (Grossman, 1972a) provide a convenient framework for thinking about these health behaviors. Suppose individuals differ in their willingness or ability to undertake investments, that is, they have different time preferences. Such differences might help to explain variations in cigarette smoking, diet, and the like. Furthermore, this approach suggests possible links with the health–schooling relationship that has been found by so many investigators.

There are at least two ways in which individual variation in time preference could explain the correlation between schooling and health.[2] First, suppose that differences in time preference are established early in life, are relatively stable, and do affect subsequent behavior.[3] These differences might stem from differences in the education or income of parents, the stability of the family, the values associated with different religions, or from other background characteristics. Given variation in time preference, it would not be surprising to observe that individuals with low rates of time discount would invest in many years of schooling and would also invest in health-enhancing activities. According to this view, schooling has no direct effect on health; the observed correlation is a result of both schooling and health being dependent on time preference.

A second possibility (the two explanations are not mutually exclusive) is that schooling actually affects time preference; those with more schooling are more willing to invest at a lower rate of return.[4] Thus, more schooling could result in better health by increasing investments in health. The empirical portion of this chapter, based on a single cross-section survey, cannot distinguish between these two hypotheses, but we can test for possible relations between schooling and time preference.

Empirical investigation of time preference through survey questions designed to elicit marginal rates of time discount depends critically on capital markets being "imperfect." If capital markets were perfect (that is, if individuals could borrow and lend without limit at a single market rate of interest), marginal rates would be equal for all regardless of time preference. Differences across individuals in time preference might still result in differences in nontradable health-related activities, but these would not be predictable from the replies to interest-rate questions. However, if capital markets are not perfect (an assumption of this chapter), individuals may well have different rates of interest at the margin, and these may be related to health behavior and health status.

Let us imagine a two-period world. Suppose utility in each period depends on consumption of goods (G). Utility in the first period also is a function of some activity C_1 (for simplicity assumed to be free with respect to G) which affects health (and therefore utility) in period two. For example, C_1 might be cigarette smoking:

$$U_1 = U_1(G_1, C_1),$$

$$U_2 = U_2(G_2, H_2), \text{ where } H_2 = H(C_1).$$

A wealth-compensated increase in the rate of interest (r) will, ceteris paribus, alter the allocation of wealth between G_1 and G_2. But if the marginal utility of C_1 depends on the quantity of G_1 (and the marginal utility of H_2 depends on the quantity of G_2), the change in r will also affect C_1 (and H_2). If G_1 and C_1 (and G_2 and H_2) are substitutes, an increase in r will lead to an increase in C_1 and a decrease in H_2. If the relationship is complementary (which seems less plausible to me), the reverse would be true.

It should be emphasized that (given imperfect capital markets) differences across individuals in marginal rates of interest can be the result of differences in underlying preference functions (indifference curves) or differences in opportunities to borrow and lend.[5] In general, it will not be possible to distinguish between these sources empirically, although controlling for family income (as a proxy for "opportunities") may move the analysis somewhat closer to a focus on preference functions per se.

Because time preference is probably only one of many factors affecting the demand for cigarettes, jogging, or other health-related behaviors, we can hardly expect perfect correlation among these activities. Differences in time preference across individuals, however, should result in some positive correlations among these behaviors.

Measurement of Time Preference

In recent years there have been several attempts to measure time preference through household survey techniques. The objectives of the investigators have varied greatly, but the general approach has been similar: the respondent is confronted with a hypothetical situation involving different sums of money at different points in time and is asked to express a preference that will implicitly reveal a rate of time discount.

Thomas and Ward (1979)

Psychologists Ewart A. C. Thomas and Wanda E. Ward were interested in relations between time preference and various psychological measures of temporal orientation[6] and measures of optimism or pessimism. They were also interested in possible effects of time preference on saving and spending behavior. Their sample consisted of 63 college students who were asked 24 open-ended time-preference questions of the following type:

"If offered $100 now or X dollars in six months, what would be the *smallest* amount of money (X dollars) you would accept rather than the immediately available $100?" Some questions gave the future amount and asked the respondent to choose a current value; others gave both amounts and asked for the time period that would make them commensurate. Still others were formulated as payments rather than as receipts, and some were expressed in terms of goods rather than dollar amounts.

Implicit discount rates were found to be negatively correlated with future time orientation and positively correlated with "big spending." The group results were considered satisfactory, but the measurement of time preference was "disappointing" to the authors because of the "high instability of parameter estimates for individual subjects."

West (SRI) (1978)

Economists involved in the Seattle-Denver income maintenance experiment were interested in time preference because the bias introduced by the finite length of the experiment (compared to a national program of indefinite life) would vary depending on the household's rate of time discount (Metcalf, 1974). The families in the experiment (more than 1,500 in each city) were asked a large number and variety of time-preference questions. Some were open-ended, similar to those of Thomas and Ward. Some were "cascades" of the following type: "Suppose you had a choice between a cash bonus of $100 today and $200 a year from now; which would you choose?" If the respondent chooses $200, the question is repeated, with $175 substituted for $200, and so on until the respondent chooses $100. Some cascade questions go up instead of down; some involve payments rather than receipts; and some involve different time periods.

The mean interest rates implicit in the replies of these low-income respondents were typically quite high, but the correlation between questions was typically low (r = about 0.1 or 0.2). The author, Richard W. West, expressed some concern that "the measures are not reliable" (p. 23).

Maital and Maital (1978)

A paper by an economist and a psychologist, Shlomo Maital and Sharona Maital, reviews some of the economic and psychological literature on time preference and reports the results of a survey of 515 Israeli adults. The Maitals' focus is on the role of time preference in the intergenerational transmission of income inequality. They asked one cascade question involving choice between a sum of money now and higher sums one year from now. A similar question in which gift certificates for a week's shopping at a supermarket were substituted for money was asked in an attempt to measure the real as opposed to the nominal implicit rate of interest.

The implicit interest rate was negatively correlated with years of schooling ($r = -0.08$) and with a dummy variable which took a value of 1 if the subject and the subject's father were born in Israel ($r = -0.12$). The nominal rate was negatively correlated with income ($r = -0.14$), but the real rate was not. The authors concluded that the ability to defer gratification is part of the process of socialization and that "after adolescence the propensity to delay gratification is quite stable" (p. 192). This may be correct, but it is not clear that the conclusion follows from their results.

Thaler (1979)

In a questionnaire administered to approximately 75 college students,[7] Richard Thaler posed a large number of open-ended money choices primarily to learn how the implicit interest rate varies with the amount of money involved, the time period, the starting point of the comparison, and whether the choice involves receipt or payment. He found that the implicit rate was lower the larger the amount of money and the longer the time period. Also, choices involving two points both in the future typically invoked a smaller implicit interest rate than choices involving the present versus the future. He concluded that there is a "psychic fixed cost" to waiting, as well as a cost that varies with amount and time.

I included a few questions on health status in the Thaler questionnaire and found a significant negative correlation between health and median implicit interest rate across individuals. This result led me to undertake the larger pilot survey described in the following section.

The Pilot Survey

In November 1979, Stephen Cole and Ann Cole conducted at my request a survey measuring time preference, health status, and health behavior as well as a large number of family background and current socioeconomic variables.[8] Telephone interviews approximately twenty minutes in length were conducted with 508 individuals living in Nassau and Suffolk Counties (on Long Island just east of New York City). Respondents were selected through a random sample of telephone numbers;[9] interviews were completed with 58 percent of the eligible respondents. The characteristics of the respondents conformed closely to census data for the two counties, but the possibility of selection bias remains, especially with respect to some of the family background variables.

The sample was restricted to individuals aged 25–64, and interviewers were instructed to obtain an approximately equal distribution between female and male respondents. The respondents differ from a national sample with respect to religion (55 percent Catholic and 17 percent Jewish), race (3 percent black), and schooling (about one year above the national average). They are also somewhat more affluent and in slightly better health. Allowing for the predominantly suburban middleclass character of the two counties, the distributions of replies on the health, health behavior, family background, and socioeconomic variables conform closely to those obtained in national surveys.

The principal approach to the measurement of time preference was through a series of six questions asking the respondent to choose between a sum of money now and a larger sum at a specific point in the future,[10] for example, "Would you choose $1,500 now or $4,000 in five years?" The amount and the time period varied, as did the interest rate implicit in each question. The lowest implicit rate was 10.1 percent per annum (continuously compounded); the highest was 51.1 percent. This dichotomous-choice type of question was used because it was deemed simpler for the respondent than the open-ended or cascade type questions discussed previously.[11]

In addition to the series of questions dealing with implicit interest rates, a cascade type question with an explicit interest rate (beginning at 6 percent and rising to 50 percent) was asked. The survey also included four attitudinal questions, for example, "Do you agree or disagree with this statement: 'It makes more sense to spend your money now rather than save it for the future'?" In addition, each respondent was asked to choose an expected rate of change of prices for the coming year. The final time-preference questions dealt with the respondent's use of credit during car purchases or through unpaid balances on bank credit cards.

Empirical Results

One of the purposes of the pilot survey was to determine whether respondents would, in a brief telephone interview, give sensible answers to hypothetical money-choice questions when the interest rates implicit in the questions are far from transparent. The data presented in Table 11.1 suggest that many respondents do give sensible replies; some do not. The six implicit-interest-rate questions ask the respondent to choose between taking a smaller prize now or waiting for a larger prize. A priori we expect the fraction of respondents taking the prize now to diminish as the implicit interest rate rises. Table 11.1 shows that this did occur. For the sample as a whole, 76 percent chose "now" for the question with an implicit interest rate of 10.1 percent per annum; only 33 percent did so when the implicit interest rate was 51.1 percent.

Not only do the group results conform to a priori expectations, but almost two-thirds of the respondents gave replies that were internally consistent for each individual. A set of replies was defined as consistent if the respondent never answered "now" to a question with an implicit interest rate that was higher than the rate in another question to which the answer was "wait."[12] The last three columns of Table 11.1 show results for the sample divided into three groups: those with consistent answers, those whose answers would be consistent if one reply

Table 11.1 Mean probability of taking prize now

Question number	Implicit compound interest rate (% per annum)	All respondents (N = 504)	Number of inconsistent answers		
			0 (N = 329)	1 (N = 124)	2 or 3 (N = 51)
30	10.1	.76	.78	.75	.61
32	15.7	.61	.66	.56	.34
28	19.6	.58	.59	.60	.41
29	30.5	.52	.52	.48	.61
33	40.2	.34	.35	.28	.41
31	51.1	.33	.25	.37	.71

were reversed (about one-fourth of the sample), and those whose replies would require two or three reversals in order to achieve consistency (about 10 percent of the sample).[13] The relation between the fraction taking the prize now and the implicit interest rate is much weaker for those respondents with inconsistent answers and much stronger for those with consistent answers. Most of the results reported here are based on analyses limited to those respondents with consistent replies.

Table 11.2 presents the results of regressions in which each question to each individual is treated as an observation. When the regressions are run by OLS, the dependent variable is dichotomous, taking a value of 1 if the reply is "now" and 0 if it is "wait." The right-side variables are the *compound* interest rate implicit in each question, the *simple* implicit interest rate, and the individual's *explicit* interest rate given in reply to the cascade question mentioned in the previous section. We see that the probability that a given individual will reply "now" to a given question falls sharply as the interest rate implicit in the question rises, and rises rapidly as the individual's explicit interest rate rises. These results hold for the entire sample and are particularly strong for those respondents classified as consistent, but do not hold for the other respondents. Logistic regressions estimated by a maximum likelihood procedure give similar results when evaluated at the mean probability of taking "now" (see marginal effects in brackets).

The contrast between the compound interest rate and the simple interest rate coefficients, depending on the consistency class, suggests one possible reason why some respondents give inconsistent replies.[14] The two interest rates are, of course, highly correlated, but not perfectly so. Those giving consistent replies seem to have been influenced by the implicit compound rate, while those with the most inconsistent replies seem to have been influenced primarily by the simple rate. We also see that there is a close connection between the explicit rate and the probability of choosing "now" for the consistent individuals, but not for those whose replies to the implicit-rate questions were inconsistent.

Inasmuch as these results are based on replies to only six questions, they can only be suggestive, not definitive. (It would be desirable to see if the distinction between the compound and simple interest rate holds up in a survey based on a large number

Table 11.2 Regressions of probability of taking prize now on interest rate variables

	All respondents	Number of inconsistent answers		
		0	1	2 or 3
N	2952	1956	719	277
R^2	.106	.158	.082	.026
Intercept	.733	.783	.733	.414
	(.022)	(.026)	(.046)	(.074)
Question compound implicit interest rate (% per annum)	−.0073**	−.0111**	−.0037	.0106*
	(.0012)	(.0014)	(.0024)	(.0040)
	[−.0071]	[−.0126]	[−.0034]	[.0135]
Question simple implicit interest rate (% per annum)	−.0017**	−.0008	−.0032**	−.0042*
	(.0006)	(.0007)	(.0011)	(.0019)
	[−.0020]	[−.0007]	[−.0037]	[−.0053]
Respondent explicit interest rate (% per annum)	.0054**	.0068**	.0020	.0010
	(.0008)	(.0009)	(.0019)	(.0025)
	[.0064]	[.0090]	[.0019]	[.0010]

Note: Regressions based on person-question observations. The OLS regression coefficients are shown first with their standard errors in parentheses below. The marginal effects (at mean probability) from the logistic regressions are in brackets.

*$p < .05$.

**$p < .01$.

of questions.) For this sample, this distinction gives stronger results than do regressions based on Thaler's hypotheses about the effects of length of time or amount of money on the willingness to wait.

Table 11.3 reports the results of regressions similar to those in Table 11.2, but designed to measure the effects of individual characteristics on the probability of the individual choosing "now" in response to the implicit-interest-rate questions. The regressions are limited to respondents with consistent replies and are run separately for females and males because preliminary analysis revealed significant interaction effects for some variables. A brief discussion of the additional variables follows.

AGE: Respondents placed themselves in one of four age categories: 25–34, 35–44, 45–54, or 55–64. The midpoint of each category was used to construct a continuous variable. There was no a priori expectation for this variable. Maital and Maital had found a positive correlation between age and the "real" interest rate ($r = 0.10$), but no relation with the nominal rate.

PARED: Parents' education is the mean of the years of schooling of the respondent's mother and father. The separate schooling variables are highly correlated, and do not yield any significant information when included separately. A priori I expected a negative coefficient for *PARED*, at least prior to inclusion of other variables that are also affected by *PARED* (for example, the respondent's own years of schooling).

LIVPAR: This is a dummy variable taking a value of 1 if the respondent lived with both parents until age 16, and 0 otherwise. Some of the psychological literature suggests that this coefficient should be negative, that is, it should work much the same way as *PARED*.

CATH, JEW: These are dummy variables taking a value of 1 if the respondent is Catholic (or Jewish), and 0 if Protestant or other.

EXINFL: Expected inflation is a continuous variable derived from the respondent's reply to the question about expected price change during the coming year. A positive coefficient is expected when the implicit interest rate is held constant. At any given nominal

Table 11.3 Regressions of probability of taking prize now on socioeconomic variables

	Females (N = 969)[a]					Males (N = 939)[a]				
	(1)	(2)	(3)	(S.E.)	(3L)	(1)	(2)	(3)	(S.E.)	(3L)
Compound implicit interest rate of question (% per annum)	−.011**	−.011**	−.011**	(.001)	[−.014]	−.013**	−.013**	−.013**	(.001)	[−.016]
AGE	.002	.001	.002	(.002)	[.003]	−.003**	−.002*	−.002*	(.001)	[−.002]
PARED	−.003	.007	.013**	(.005)	[.016]	−.031**	−.029**	−.030**	(.006)	[−.037]
LIVPAR	.066	.091*	.105**	(.042)	[.138]	.061	.049	.058	(.048)	[.065]
CATH	−.046	−.057	−.078*	(.033)	[−.089]	−.033	−.017	−.018	(.038)	[−.006]
JEW	−.222**	−.164**	−.137**	(.046)	[−.197]	−.064	−.081	−.086	(.045)	[−.110]
EXINFL	.015**	.013**	.013**	(.003)	[.017]	.004	.004	.005	(.003)	[.003]
≤12YRS	—	.116***	.087*	(.036)	[.111]	—	.129**	.142**	(.042)	[.170]
≥16YRS	—	−.134**	−.138**	(.040)	[−.161]	—	.164**	.161**	(.039)	[.218]
ADJINC	—	—	−.016**	(.003)	[−.019]	—	—	.004	(.003)	[.004]
Intercept	.647	.566	.648	(.125)	—	1.257	1.115	1.063	(.129)	—
R^2	.155	.186	.210	—	—	.176	.192	.194	—	—

Note: Regressions based on person-question observations. The coefficients from the OLS regressions are in columns 1–3. The marginal effects (at mean probability) from the logistic regressions are in column 3L.
a. Consistent respondents only.
*$p < .05$.
**$p < .01$.

rate, the respondent should be less willing to wait if prices are expected to rise rapidly because the implicit "real" rate of interest is lower.

≤ *12YRS* and ≥ *16YRS:* These are dummy variables for the respondent's own years of schooling. The omitted class is those with 13 to 15 years of schooling. A positive coefficient is expected for ≤ *12YRS* and a negative one for ≥ *16YRS*, for reasons discussed in the first section of this chapter.

ADJINC: Adjusted family income is a continuous variable derived as follows. The respondent placed total family income in one of the following categories: under \$15,000, \$15,000 to \$25,000, \$25,000 to \$35,000, or over \$35,000. Values of 10, 20, 30, and 40 were assigned to each category. Sixty of the respondents did not answer the income question, but an income category was assigned to them on the basis of their reply to a social class question and a regression of income on social class. Total family income was divided by adult equivalents to create adjusted family income. "Adult equivalents" is the weighted sum of the number of adults and the number of children in the household with the following weights: respondent = 1; each additional adult = 0.8; first child = 0.5; second child = 0.4; each additional child = 0.3. A negative coefficient was expected for *ADJINC* both because of a possible effect of income on time preference, and an effect of time preference on income.[15]

Three alternative OLS specifications (for each sex) allow us to look first only at the background variables (controlling for the implicit interest rate and expected inflation), then at the effect of schooling (which is probably affected by the family background variables and may be a route through which they affect time preference), and finally at the effect of family income. The regressions were also estimated in logistic form by maximum likelihood; the results are similar to those for OLS. The coefficients from the logistic version of the third specification, converted to marginal effects at the mean probability of taking "now," are shown in column (3L) of Table 11.3.

In the first specification, *AGE* and *PARED* are statistically significant for males in the expected direction, while *JEW* is highly significant for females. A coefficient of −0.22 indicates that, other things being equal, a Jewish female respondent has 0.22 lower probability of answering "now" than does a Protestant or other female. The sign of the *LIVPAR* coefficient is opposite to that expected, perhaps because of sample selection bias. It may be that most persons with divorced parents do have high rates of time discount, but those who "make it" to a middle-class suburban community are probably atypical and may have low rates of time discount.

The schooling variables behave as expected for females and are highly significant. For males, the ≤ *12YRS* coefficient is as expected, but the ≥ *16YRS* coefficient has the wrong sign and is statistically significant. It is not obvious why men with 16 years of schooling or more should be, ceteris paribus, more eager to take the prize now than men with 13 to 15 years; possibly the former have better opportunities to invest the money.

The income variable works as expected for females and is significant; it has the wrong sign for males but is not significant. In the fullest specification, *LIVPAR* and *PARED* are statistically significant for females with signs opposite to that expected. Some of the background and socioeconomic variables are highly correlated with one another (see Table 11.4 for the zero-order correlation matrix), and multicollinearity may explain some of the perverse results. *EXINFL* is statistically significant in the expected direction and has approximately the same effect as the nominal implicit interest rate on the probability of taking the prize now.

The model underlying the regressions reported in Table 11.3 treats time preference (as reflected in the choice between "now" and "wait") as dependent on years of schooling. As previously

Table 11.4 Zero-order correlations among selected variables

	SCHOOL	HSRANK	PARED	LIVPAR	ADJINC	IMPINT	EXINFL
SCHOOL	—	.47	.37	.21	.25	−.23	−.05
HSRANK	.33	—	.21	.09	.15	−.11	−.03
PARED	.30	.19	—	.02	.29	−.07	.01
LIVPAR	.20	.10	.15	—	.07	.02	.02
ADJINC	.27	.09	.14	−.04	—	−.23	.01
IMPINT	−.03	.03	−.21	.02	−.02	—	.19
EXINFL	.18	−.01	.03	−.05	−.06	.03	—

Note: Females: upper right triangle; males: lower left triangle. $r \geq |\,0.21\,|$ $p < 0.01$; $r \geq |\,0.17\,|$ $p < 0.05$.

discussed, some writers believe that differences in time preference are established early in life and are stable; they would treat years of schooling as dependent on time preference. Table 11.5 presents the results of regressions in which number of years of schooling is regressed on time preference and other variables. The new variables are as follows.

IMPINT: An implicit interest rate is calculated for each respondent who gave consistent answers to the six implicit-interest-rate questions. Those respondents who answered "now" to some questions and "wait" to others were assigned a rate equal to the mean of the highest implicit rate to which they answered "now" and the lowest to which they answered "wait."[16] Those respondents who always chose "wait" were assigned a rate of 5 percent and those who always chose "now" were assigned 60 percent. The higher the respondent's *IMPINT*, the lower should be the years of schooling. The variable *EXINFL* should work in the opposite direction.

HSRANK: The respondent's scholastic performance in high school was inferred from replies to the question: When you were in high school were you (percentage of sample in each category shown in parentheses):

(1) an excellent student (10%)
(2) an above-average student (28%)
(3) an average student (57%)
(4) a below-average student (5%).

Grade averages of 95, 85, 75, and 65 were assigned to the four categories respectively, and the variable is treated as a continuous variable. A positive coefficient is expected.

HSHLTH: Health in high school was treated as a dummy variable taking a value of 1 if the respondent recalled his or her health as being "better than most of the other kids" (26 percent), and 0 if it was "about average" (70 percent) or "worse than most of the other kids" (4 percent). A positive coefficient is also expected for this variable.

The results of these regressions again give weak support for the view that there is a relation between time preference and schooling, but leave open the question of the direction of the causality. In the first specification the coefficient of *IMPINT* is highly significant for females, and is still significant when the family-background variables are introduced. *EXINFL* has the

Table 11.5 Regression of years of schooling on implicit interest rate and other variables

	Females (N = 162)[a]				Males (N = 157)[a]			
	(1)	(2)	(3)	(S.E.)	(1)	(2)	(3)	(S.E.)
AGE	−.066**	−.035**	−.038*	(.016)	−.045*	−.035	−.043*	(.017)
IMPINT	−.024***	−.019*	−.014	(.008)	−.004	.003	−.000	(.009)
EXINFL	−.036	−.032	−.031	(.029)	.104*	.106*	.107**	(.040)
PARED	—	.223**	.150**	(.056)	—	.137	.091	(.074)
LIVPAR	—	1.252*	1.025*	(.456)	—	1.398*	1.299*	(.568)
CATH	—	.082	−.143	(.357)	—	−1.346**	−1.157*	(.460)
JEW	—	1.276*	1.077*	(.488)	—	.899	.730	(.550)
HSRANK	—	—	.120**	(.021)	—	—	.089**	(.027)
HSHLTH	—	—	.130	(.367)	—	—	.109	(.403)
Intercept	17.367	12.116	3.562	(1.951)	15.277	12.505	6.426	(2.351)
R^2	.128	.274	.411	—	.072	.273	.324	—

a. Consistent respondents only.
*$p < .05$.
**$p < .01$.

wrong sign and is not significant. For males the reverse is true: *EXINFL* is significant with the expected sign, but *IMPINT* shows no effect.

The background variables work as expected, with *PARED* and *LIVPAR* both raising years of schooling. *HSRANK* has a very strong effect, but the causality may be partly the reverse of that assumed in this regression, that is, individuals who plan to go on to college may exert more effort to do well in high school. *HSHLTH* shows practically no effect on years of schooling. In general, this variable has very low correlations with other socioeconomic or health variables, suggesting that it may be poorly measured.

One of the purposes of the pilot survey was to determine the correlation among alternative measures of time preference. These correlation coefficients, shown in Table 11.6, indicate a weak but statistically significant correlation between the implicit and explicit interest rates and between the implicit rate and replies to the two simple attitudinal questions ("spend now" and "don't worry"). The other two attitudinal questions, which are more complex because they introduce considerations such as life insurance and the education of children, do not correlate well with either the implicit or explicit rates, although they are correlated with each other. The fact that the credit card debit and car loan dummy variables are not significantly correlated with the interest rate variables would be disturbing, but given the timing of the pilot survey, there may be an easy explanation: the interest rates on these loans were legally restricted to unrealistically low levels, given the high interest rates prevailing at that time and given the high rates revealed by the respondents in replies to the implicit-rate questions.

Explanations aside, the low correlations across time-preference questions must be a source of some concern. They suggest the need for further refinement in the survey techniques and the need to understand better how the specific context of a decision affects intertemporal choice.

Investment in Health

Do differences in time preference affect investments in health? Some crude measures of these investments were obtained by asking the respondents about their cigarette smoking, dental visits, exercise, weight (as a proxy for diet), and seat belt usage.

Table 11.6 Correlation coefficients[a] among time preference variables (N = 329)[b]

	Implicit interest	Explicit interest	Don't sacrifice	Spend now	No life insurance	Don't worry	Credit card debit	Use car loan
Implicit interest	—	.23**	.00	.23**	-.06	.14*	.09	.06
Explicit interest	.23**	—	.02	.11	-.04	.08	-.02	.00
Don't sacrifice[c]	-.01	.03	—	.08	.25**	.09	.07	.12*
Spend now[d]	.23**	.11*	.09*	—	.03	.11	.11	.04
No life insurance[e]	-.06	-.04	.26**	.02	—	-.06	-.07	-.01
Don't worry[f]	.14**	.08	.09*	.10*	-.05	—	.08	.09
Credit card debit	.09	-.03	.07	.11*	-.08	.09*	—	.21**
Use car loan	.06	.00	.13*	.04	-.01	.10*	.19**	—

a. Upper right triangle shows simple correlations; lower left triangle shows partial correlations controlling for age and sex.
b. Only respondents with consistent answers to implicit interest rate questions.
c. Disagree with statement in question 35.
d. Agree with statement in question 36.
e. Disagree with statement in question 37.
f. Agree with statement in question 38.
*p<.05.
**p<.01.

Replies to questions about these behaviors were converted to continuous variables as follows.

		Assigned value	% of sample
SMOKE	Question: Do you currently smoke cigarettes?		
	Replies:		
	(1) No.	0	64
	(2) Yes, less than a pack a day.	10	12
	(3) Yes, about a pack a day.	20	14
	(4) Yes, more than a pack a day.	30	10
OVWT	Question: Would you say that you are currently . . .		
	Replies:		
	(1) underweight.	0	5
	(2) about the right weight.	0	39
	(3) about 5–10 pounds overweight.	7.5	35
	(4) about 11–20 pounds overweight.	15	12
	(5) more than 20 pounds overweight.	30	9
DENTDEL	Question: When did you have your last dental checkup?		
	Replies:		
	(1) Within the last year.	0.5	72
	(2) About one or two years ago.	1.5	19
	(3) About three to five years ago.	4.0	5
	(4) More than five years ago.	8.0	4
EXER	Question: How often do you exercise for 30 minutes or more?		
	Replies:		
	(1) Never.	0	40
	(2) Once a month or less.	1	9
	(3) Several times a month.	2.5	9
	(4) About once a week.	4	10
	(5) Two or three times a week.	10	16
	(6) More than three times a week.	18	16

		Assigned value	% of sample
STBELT	Question: When you are in a car, how often do you use seat belts?		
	Replies:		
	(1) All the time.	1.00	21
	(2) Most of the time.	0.75	7
	(3) Some of the time.	0.30	13
	(4) Rarely or never.	0.05	59

The correlation between favorable health behaviors is positive for every possible pair (reversing signs where appropriate), but the coefficients are quite low and only some are statistically significant (see Table 11.7). The correlations with seat belt usage suggest that individual differences with respect to health in general may be more important than differences in time preference. Moreover, the generally low correlations underscore the fact that even if there is a common factor at work across behaviors, there are also other factors that are specific to particular behaviors. The low coefficients may also be attributable to the rough approximations used to measure the variables.

In order to test for possible effects of time preference, the health behavior variables were regressed on *IMPINT, EXINFL,* and several other variables. The results for cigarette smoking are reported in Table 11.8. They confirm the expectation that cigarette smoking increases with higher *IMPINT,* and decreases with higher *EXINFL,* but the size of the effect of *IMPINT* is quite small. We also see an effect of schooling on cigarette smoking as expected; the difference between the coefficients

Table 11.7 Correlations coefficients[a] among health-related behavior variables (N = 508)

	SMOKE	OVWT	DENTDEL	EXER	STBELT
SMOKE	—	.01	.06	−.08	−.12**
OVWT	.01	—	.06	−.18**	−.12**
DENTDEL	.05	.06	—	−.01	−.07
EXER	−.08*	−.17**	−.01	—	.09*
STBELT	−.12**	−.12**	−.08*	.09*	—

a. Upper right triangle shows simple correlations; lower left triangle shows partial correlations, controlling for age and sex.
*$p<.05$.
**$p<.01$.

Table 11.8 Regression of number of cigarettes smoked per day on socioeconomic variables

	Females (N = 162)[a]				Males (N = 157)[a]			
	(1)	(2)	(3)	(S.E.)	(1)	(2)	(3)	(S.E.)
AGE	-.041	-.075	-.081	(.076)	.018	.037	.025	(.080)
IMPINT	.072*	.074*	.063	(.036)	.092*	.098*	.091*	(.043)
EXINFL	-.280*	-.297*	-.292*	(.136)	-.263	-.275	-.155	(.186)
PARED	—	-.376	-.313	(.268)	—	.234	.403	(.337)
LIVPAR	—	.117	-.049	(2.139)	—	-2.887	-1.326	(2.664)
CATH	—	-2.325	-2.604	(1.658)	—	-.617	-1.647	(2.136)
JEW	—	.092	1.012	(2.300)	—	-1.224	-.758	(2.537)
≤ 12YRS	—	—	-2.089	(1.814)	—	—	5.325*	(2.315)
≥ 16YRS	—	—	-5.568**	(2.045)	—	—	-.853	(2.207)
Intercept	8.606	15.284	17.595	(6.097)	5.759	5.577	1.102	(7.018)
R^2	.043	.067	.110		.043	.054	.108	
Dependent variable mean	—	—	—	6.42	—	—	—	6.82
Dependent variable standard deviation	—	—	—	9.43	—	—	—	10.68

a. Only respondents with consistent answers to implicit-interest-rate questions.
*p<.05.
**p<.01.

Table 11.9 Regressions of health status[a] on time preference, schooling, and age

	Females					Males				
	IMPINT	EXINFL	SCHOOL	AGE	R_2	IMPINT	EXINFL	SCHOOL	AGE	R_2
*ln*HLTH										
(1)	-.003	-.004	—	-.015*	.045	-.003	.018	—	-.021**	.084
	(.003)	(.012)		(.006)		(.003)	(.015)		(.006)	
(2)	—	—	.059*	-.010	.069	—	—	.059*	-.020**	.106
			(.025)	(.006)				(.027)	(.006)	
(3)	-.002	-.001	.054*	-.011	.072	-.003	.013	.054	-.020**	.115
	(.003)	(.011)	(.026)	(.006)		(.004)	(.016)	(.028)	(.006)	
MNEXHLTH										
(1)	-.001	.001	—	-.007**	.062	-.002*	.001	—	-.011**	.208
	(.001)	(.005)		(.002)		(.001)	(.005)		(.002)	
(2)	—	—	.013	-.006**	.071	—	—	.009	-.011**	.189
			(.010)	(.002)				(.008)	(.002)	
(3)	-.000	.002	.013	-.006**	.072	-.002*	.001	.009	-.011**	.214
	(.001)	(.005)	(.010)	(.002)		(.001)	(.005)	(.008)	(.002)	

a. For definitions and measurement of health status variables, see text.
*$p<.05$.
**$p<.01$.

for $\leq 12YRS$ and $\geq 16YRS$ is statistically significant for males. The overall explanatory power of the regression is low; most of the variation in cigarette smoking is not explained by these variables, and the addition of $ADJINC$ was of little value.

Regressions for the other health behaviors were even less satisfactory. The total explanatory power was low, and $IMPINT$ was not statistically significant except for $EXER$ for males, where the sign was the opposite of that expected.

Health Status

In the first section of this chapter, questions were raised about whether differences in time preference could help explain health status or throw light on the relation between health status and schooling. Table 11.9 reports the results of regressions addressed to these questions. The top section of the table uses as the dependent variable $ln\ HLTH$, the same variable used by Grossman (1975) in "The Correlation between Health and Schooling." It is obtained by taking the logarithms of values given to replies to the question: In general, would you consider your health to be:

	Assigned value	% of sample
(1) Excellent	1.0	43
(2) Good	9.8	45
(3) Fair	26.4	9
(4) Poor	86.7	3

Grossman obtained these values from a regression of work-loss weeks due to illness on self-evaluation of health status.[17]

The results support Grossman's finding of a strong effect of schooling on health, and it appears that the effect is equally strong for females and males.[18] The coefficients for $IMPINT$ have the expected negative sign, but are not statistically significant. When time preference and schooling are entered simultaneously, the latter clearly dominates the former. When $ADJINC$ is added to the regression, its coefficient is not significant, and the other results are unchanged.

Three other sets of health status questions were asked in addition to the subjective self-evaluation. One used a checklist of symptoms and diagnoses; a second requested information on utilization of hospitals, drugs, and physicians' services; and the third asked about the respondent's ability to walk or jog a mile. These measures are significantly correlated with each other and with self-evaluation of health status, even after controlling for age and sex (partial correlation coefficients are typically about 0.20). A composite health status variable *MNEXHLTH* was calculated from the four measures by assigning a value of 0.25 to respondents for each of the following:

(1) Self-evaluation excellent (44%)
(2) Zero symptoms (47%)
(3) Very low medical care utilization[19] (64%)
(4) Able to jog a mile (61%)

This "mean proportion of excellent health measures" is the dependent variable in the regressions reported in the bottom section of Table 11.9. They indicate a stronger effect for time preference and a relatively weaker effect for schooling.[20] *IMPINT* actually achieves statistical significance for males. It appears that the choice of health status measure makes a difference.

Unresolved Questions

This exploratory study leaves unresolved many empirical and theoretical questions concerning time preference, health behavior, and health status. The attempt to measure implicit interest rates through a series of six dichotomous choices between "money now" and "money in the future" produced answers that are clearly not all "noise," but neither are they completely satisfactory. About one-third of the respondents had at least one inconsistent reply. Moreover, one-half of those who were consistent answered all the questions the same way (either all "now" or all "wait"). An extension of the range of the implicit interest rates might yield more information about this group. An increase in the number of questions would be desirable for many reasons, but the Coles believe that six is about all the respondents will tolerate as part of the total telephone interview.

At a time of sharply rising prices, the measurement of "real" versus "nominal" interest rates presents a major problem which is solved only partially by including a question on expected inflation. The *EXINFL* variable usually works as expected—opposite to *IMPINT*—but the coefficients are not always equal, and sometimes the signs are inconsistent.

The mean implicit interest rate in this survey of 30 percent per annum is substantially lower than the rates reported in surveys by other investigators. This rate is still high, however, compared to current borrowing and lending rates, and high compared to the mean response to the explicit-interest-rate question (14 percent). What accounts for the difference? Also, although the implicit and explicit rates are significantly correlated ($r = 0.23$ for the two-thirds of the sample with consistent replies), why isn't the correlation higher?

The pilot survey confirms our a priori expectation of a correlation between schooling and time preference, but other types of data are needed if we are to learn something about the direction of the causality. The effect of time preference on health behavior and on health status is usually in the expected direction, but is not always statistically significant, and even when it is statistically significant the size of the effect is frequently small. This may be partly a result of errors in the measurement of time preference, but it may also indicate weaknesses in the specification of the model. For instance, the assumption that investment behavior is affected only by time preference is probably unrealistic. Investments typically involve uncertainty as well as time preference because future values of any variable, whether the price of a stock or the state of health, cannot be known with certainty. Thus, individual attitudes toward risk will also affect investment behavior. The uncertainty element is probably particularly large in the case of such investments in health as giving up cigarettes, eliminating fatty foods, jogging, and the like. Even the best information available indicates only the *average* expected benefit from such health investments; the return to any individual is highly uncertain. Only a minority of cigarette smokers will actually contract lung cancer, while giving up cigarette smoking does not provide a guarantee against the disease. Therefore, individual differences with respect to uncertainty can also affect health investment and health status.

Psychologists Kahneman and Tversky, in their highly original and provocative work on prospect theory (1979), have suggested that most individuals prefer certain to uncertain *gains*, but prefer uncertainty to certainty with respect to *losses*. For example, most individuals, when offered a choice between (A) a certain gain of $500 or (B) an equal chance to win $1,000 or nothing, will choose A. The same individuals, when offered a choice between (A) a certain loss of $500 or (B) an equal chance to lose $1,000 or nothing, will choose B.

Such asymmetry in risk aversion, if applicable to health-related behavior, could be important. Consider a person who is contemplating giving up some current pleasurable activity or undertaking an unpleasant one in return for the chance of an improvement in health status sometime in the future. The immediate action involves a loss with a high degree of certainty, but the future gain is quite uncertain for the individual even though it may be highly predictable, on average, for a large population. Thus, the stronger the individual's asymmetry with respect to uncertainty (as described by Kahneman and Tversky), the less likely will he be to undertake the health-enhancing action. This conclusion is unaltered if one reverses the framing of the decision and thinks of the current activity, such as cigarette smoking, as a "gain" (where certainty is preferred) and the possibility of ill health in the future as the "loss." Thus, individual differences in risk aversion may confound attempts to measure time preference or to analyze the effects of time preference on health.

This survey and the analyses reported here also highlight problems of measurement of health status and health investment. When health is measured by subjective self-evaluation, the results are different from those obtained when a composite health measure based on self-evaluation, medical care utilization, symptoms, and physical ability is used. Problems in the measurement of health investment surface when we examine a variable such as exercise; it seems that exercise is undertaken for many reasons other than to improve health, and these other reasons may swamp an effect of time preference. Perhaps more detailed questions concerning the type and intensity of exercise would help.

I conclude this report of exploratory research on a note of cautious optimism. Crude but useful measures of time preference, health investment, and health status can be obtained, even through very inexpensive telephone interviews. Time preference *is* related to schooling, and also shows some relation to health investment and health status. However, none of the relationships found in these data are particularly strong.

Whether improvements in survey design, more accurate measurement of variables, and better specification of models will produce more significant results remains to be determined.

Appendix: Time Preference Questions

A. Implicit interest rate

Given your present circumstances, suppose you won a tax-free prize at a local bank and were offered a choice between two prizes. I am going to read off pairs of choices, and for each pair you tell me which prize you would choose.

28.	1 = $1,500 now, or	DON'T [3 = don't know	
	2 = $4,000 in 5 years	READ [9 = refuse	28
29.	1 = $1,000 now, or	DON'T [3 = don't know	
	2 = $2,500 in 3 years	READ [9 = refuse	29
30.	1 = $4,000 now, or	DON'T [3 = don't know	
	2 = $6,000 in 4 years	READ [9 = refuse	30
31.	1 = $750 now, or	DON'T [3 = don't know	
	2 = $1,250 in 1 year	READ [9 = refuse	31
32.	1 = $2,500 now, or	DON'T [3 = don't know	
	2 = $4,000 in 3 years	READ [9 = refuse	32
33.	1 = $500 now, or	DON'T [3 = don't know	
	2 = $2,500 in 4 years	READ [9 = refuse	33

B. Explicit interest rate

34. Suppose you won a tax-free prize of $10,000 at a local bank. You then had a choice between getting the money now or leaving it in the bank for one year. How much interest would the bank have to pay you in order for you to agree to leave the money in the bank? [CASCADE—STOP READING WHEN CHOICE MENTIONED]

1 = 6%	7 = 50%	
2 = 8%	8 = take the	
3 = 10%	money	
4 = 15%	now	
5 = 20%	DON'T [9 = don't know	
6 = 30%	READ or refuse	34

C. Attitudinal questions

Do you agree or disagree with the following statements?
(Categories for Questions 35 to 38)

1 = agree	DON'T [3 = don't know
2 = disagree	READ [9 = refuse

35. Parents should make financial sacrifices in order to save money for their children's education.

_____
35

36. It makes more sense to spend your money now rather than saving it for the future.

_____
36

37. A working man should have life insurance equivalent to at least three times his annual income even if paying for this insurance means he would have to live on a tight budget.

_____
37

38. Most people spend too much time worrying about the future and not enough time enjoying themselves today.

_____
38

D. Expected inflation

39. In general, during the coming year do you expect prices to:

1 = decrease
2 = stay about the same
3 = increase by about 5 percent
4 = increase by about 10 percent
5 = increase by about 15 percent
6 = increase by about 20 percent
7 = increase by about 30 percent or more

DON'T [8 = don't know
READ [9 = refuse

_____
39

E. Use of credit

54. At the end of each month do you usually pay the balance on all your outstanding credit cards, or do you have a debit balance on which you must pay interest?

1 = pay all balances   DON'T [9 = don't know
2 = have debit balance   READ   or refuse
3 = have no credit cards

_____
54

55. When you or your spouse buy a car, do you pay cash or take a car loan?

1 = pay cash   DON'T [9 = refuse
2 = take a car loan   READ
3 = have done both in
      the past
4 = never buy cars

_____
55

Schooling and Health: The Cigarette Connection

One of the strongest generalizations to emerge from empirical research on health in the United States is a positive correlation between years of schooling and health status. At one time this relationship was viewed as a "class" or "socioeconomic status" effect and was thought to be significantly influenced by a positive relation between schooling and income and a positive effect of income on health (Antonovsky, 1967). Numerous studies by economists during the past decade, however, have revealed a large, statistically significant relationship between health and years of schooling after controlling for differences in income.[1] The central question now is: Is increased schooling a causal factor for better health, or are both schooling and health differences manifestations of some other underlying third variable?

In a detailed exploration of the subject, Grossman (1975) hypothesized that additional years of schooling make an individual a more efficient producer of his own health. Schooling could increase knowledge about health effects of behavior and medical-care options, change preferences, or train a person to better process and act upon information. Or perhaps schooling increases the individual's ability to develop strategies of self-control (Thaler and Shefrin, 1981). On the other hand, the schooling–health correlation may result from the action of some underlying differences among individuals that affect both schooling and health behaviors, such as family socialization,

Written with Phillip Farrell.

mental ability, or internal rate of time preference. One attempt to test for schooling effects in the use of, and outcomes from, in-hospital surgical operations had essentially negative results (Garrison, 1981). Education was not systematically related to the stage of the disease at the time of surgery, qualifications of the surgeon, length of hospital stay, or even outcome of the surgery (controlling for the initially better general health of those with more schooling).

This chapter examines the possibility that schooling affects health through an effect on cigarette smoking—an important determinant of health status. It is well known that cigarette smoking and years of schooling are negatively correlated, at least at high school levels or above. In a 1975 national probability survey, the proportion of high school graduates who smoked was more than 50 percent higher than that of college graduates (U.S. Department of Health, Education, and Welfare, 1976). A negative relation between smoking and health is also well established. Among males with life insurance, the gross difference in life expectancy at age 35 between nonsmokers and those who smoke a pack a day is approximately six years (Harris, 1981). Even within a relatively homogeneous population, such as regular participants in the Kaiser-Permanente Multiphasic Health checkups, the age-sex-race-adjusted death rate for cigarette smokers is double that of nonsmokers (Friedman et al., 1981).

Our research strategy is to examine the smoking behavior of different cohorts of men and women before and after they have completed their formal schooling. If additional years of schooling have an effect, this will show up in a change in behavior. We first describe the source and nature of our sample of retrospective smoking histories, define the variables, and explain the method of analysis. We also examine the possibility of a bias toward underreporting of smoking behaviors in the survey and present evidence that such bias is insignificant. Next we present and interpret the results of the data analysis. Our principal finding is that the amount of formal schooling a person will eventually achieve predicts his smoking behavior *before* the schooling is actually realized, and that realizing the additional years of schooling has no marginal effect on smoking behavior. We reject the hypothesis that schooling differences are causal to smoking differences in favor of the existence of one or more underlying third variables that are determinants of both schooling and smoking behaviors. Our second finding is that the strong negative correlation between schooling and smoking developed only after the spread of information that smoking was a serious health hazard. This implies that the mechanism behind the schooling–smoking relation may also give rise to the schooling–health relationship. Finally, we speculate on the nature of the third variable behind the schooling–smoking correlation and present some evidence that casts doubt on either the social-class or the mental-ability hypothesis.

Data and Methods

The Sample

The data used in this study are drawn from 2,504 personal interviews conducted in the fall of 1979 by the Stanford Heart Disease Prevention Program (SHDPP) among residents aged 12 to 75 years in randomly selected households in four small California cities: Modesto, Monterey, Salinas, and San Luis Obispo. All cities are located in predominantly agricultural areas; their populations range between 30,000 and 130,000 (in 1975). The interviews were conducted as part of a health education experiment designed to test the effectiveness of techniques for altering smoking, exercise, and dietary behaviors in order to reduce risk of heart disease (Maccoby and Solomon, 1981).

The relations between schooling and health and between schooling and smoking status in this sample are similar to those reported in national surveys. Health status, as measured by days of normal activity limited by illness, health care utilization, and personal satisfaction with health, shows systematic improvement with increased schooling. The proportion smoking cigarettes on a daily basis declines with years of schooling (except at the very lowest levels of schooling). Men are more likely to smoke than women, and the proportion smoking is higher at age 24 than at age 17.

For the regression analyses that follow, a subset of 1,183 survey respondents was selected consisting of white, non-Hispanic men and women who were not students at the time of the survey, who had completed 12 to 18 years of schooling, and who were at least 24 years old; 45 percent were men and 55 percent women. Nonwhites and Hispanics (about 17 percent of the survey respondents) were excluded because the sample size was inadequate to explore interactions among ethnicity, schooling, and smoking. Persons still in school or under age 24 were excluded in order to focus on those who had had ample opportunity to reveal their decisions about schooling and initiation of smoking. More than 90 percent of the "ever regular smokers" in the SHDPP survey began smoking by age 24. Using a higher cut-off age (to capture a higher percentage of all possible smokers) would remove from the study too many of the younger cohorts who have been most exposed to information about the health consequences of smoking.

To test the hypothesis of a causal relationship between schooling and smoking, we observed the smoking behavior of our sample of individuals at age 17, when they all had approximately the same amount of schooling, and at age 24, when they had completed differing amounts of schooling. Assuming uninterrupted attendance in school from age 6 onward, those with more than 18 years of schooling were excluded so that everyone in our sample (including those who reached age 24 in 1979) could be observed after the completion of schooling. Persons with less than 12 years of schooling were excluded so that the entire sample would still be in school at age 17. This lower schooling limit was selected as a compromise between including persons with a wide range of schooling achievement and observing them all while still in school at an age when a significant proportion of all eventual smokers had already begun to smoke.

With this sample we can study the effects of additional years of schooling (beyond 12) on smoking behavior; we cannot explicitly investigate the effects of differences in the quality or type of schooling, although the effects should be similar since differences in quality of schooling are a particular dimension of quantity of education, other things being equal.

The Variables

Respondents to the SHDPP 1979 survey were asked if they had ever smoked cigarettes on a daily basis. Those who responded affirmatively are classified as "ever regular smokers." Ever regular smokers were also asked at what age they began smoking and whether they had smoked in the past week. Those who had smoked in the past week are considered "current regular smokers"; those who had not are considered "former regular smokers." Former regular smokers were asked how long ago they stopped smoking. The answers to these questions were used to construct retrospective histories of smoking status.[2]

Education was recorded in the SHDPP 1979 survey as number of years of formal schooling completed. Education was tried in the analyses in both continuous and categorical forms with similar results. Family background characteristics, such as cultural traditions (including religion), income, and whether or not the parents smoked, are possibly important influences on whether a person begins to smoke. Unfortunately, the only such background characteristic included in the 1979 SHDPP survey was the father's years of completed schooling.[3] The absence of other background variables may be less of a problem in this relatively homogeneous sample than in a national sample.

Cohorts were defined according to historical periods of possibly different smoking behavior. The critical years were believed to be entry into World War II (1942), the first appearance in the popular press of articles linking smoking to lung cancer (ca. 1953),[4] and the publication of the first Surgeon General's Report on Smoking and Health (U.S. Department of Health, Education, and Welfare, 1964). Survey respondents were assigned to the cohort that included the calendar year when they were 17 years of age. The four cohorts defined by these three important years were roughly equal in size in these data.

Possible Bias in Variables

Potential systematic bias in the measurement of smoking status is an important concern, especially if bias is correlated with education. The most obvious potential source of bias when survey results are used is the possibility that respondents lie about their smoking status or history in order to avoid perceived social stigma or disapproval. Fortunately, the SHDPP survey tested for the presence of two smoking by-products: carbon monoxide in expired air samples and thiocyanate in blood samples. These tests establish the veracity of self-reported current smoking behavior and, by extension, previous smoking behavior (since the motivation to lie—social stigma—would be less strong for previous smoking than for current smoking). All of the female self-reported nonsmokers (including former smokers) and 97.5 percent of the male ones had levels of smoking by-products well below "threshold levels" used to classify typical smokers (8 ppm CO and 100 micromoles/liter thiocyanate; see Vogt et al., 1977). For self-reported nonsmokers, mean levels of these by-products (and thus the probability of lying) decreased with increased years of schooling, though only the differences in CO levels were statistically significant.[5] If present at all, systematic bias due to "lying" is thus very minor and works in the direction of reducing, not increasing, the observed strength of the schooling–smoking relation.

Another potential source of bias is differential survivorship of smokers and nonsmokers. The direction and size of bias depend on the absolute difference in mortality, the true proportion who were smokers at different levels of schooling, and possible effects on death rates of interactions between smoking and education. We have attempted to estimate the potential bias assuming mortality rates for smokers that were double those of nonsmokers, and concluded that even for our oldest cohort the effect is small unless the interaction between smoking and education was very large.[6] Most important of all, considering the purposes of this study, the effect on the comparison between the schooling–smoking relation at ages 17 and 24 is negligible.

The Model

Our analysis is designed to test two questions: whether the schooling–smoking relation developed as a result of the spread of information about adverse health effects of smoking (that is, whether it is health-motivated); and whether the relation is only observable after schooling differences are realized (that is, whether schooling differences are causal to smoking differences). Our model must therefore permit estimation of the schooling–smoking relation separately by cohort and at ages before and after the schooling is actually realized. The model must also take into account the fact that the observation of individual smoking behavior is dichotomous, not continuous. It is also desirable to control for other influences in the decision to smoke. Clearly, men and women have been influenced by different societal attitudes and expectations toward smoking in the last half-century (Harris, 1980). Our model will therefore estimate the smoking–schooling relation separately by sex. The only other background control variable available in this sample is father's education, which will be included in the model.

To meet these needs, we divide the sample into subsets defined by sex and cohort, and then estimate the parameters of the logistic function[7]

$$P_a = 1/(1 + e^{-\beta X}),$$

where P_a is the probability of smoking at age a (17 or 24), X is the vector of independent variables consisting of intercept, own years of schooling completed and father's years of schooling completed, and β is the vector of estimated parameters. Observed proportions of smokers correspond closely to proportions predicted by these regressions, indicating the appropriateness of this functional form.

Results

Table 12.1 reports the results of maximum-likelihood logit regressions in which the probability of smoking is a function of years of own schooling and years of father's schooling, separately estimated by sex and cohort. Identical regressions were estimated for the probability of smoking at age 17 and age 24 with schooling measured in both cases as the number of years the individual would eventually complete (by 1979). This specification permits a test of whether the schooling–smoking relation observed in this sample was established before or after the additional years of schooling were obtained. The schooling coefficients by cohort allow a test of whether the effect was associated with the news of adverse health effects from smoking.

The most striking result is the absence of any significant increase in the size of the schooling coefficient between the ages of 17 and 24.[8] The negative relation between completed schooling and smoking is generally as strong at age 17 as it is at age 24 for all cohorts; for women, the relationship is even stronger at age 17 than at age 24 for the two most recent cohorts. At age 17, however, the individuals were all still in the same school grade (approximately). The relative differences in the probability of smoking that are observed at age 24 between persons with differing years of schooling are already present at age 17, before the schooling is obtained. The additional schooling cannot be the cause of the differential smoking behavior, since the realization of the schooling does not have any marginal effect on the size of the schooling coefficient.

The second important result is that the differences in smoking

Table 12.1 Maximum-likelihood logit regression results for probability of smoking at age 17 and age 24, by sex and age cohort:[a] white men and women aged 24 to 75 years, with 12 to 18 years of completed schooling

Variable	Men				Women			
	1921–41	1942–52	1953–63	1964–72	1921–41	1942–52	1953–63	1964–72
				Smoking at age 17				
Years of schooling	−0.098	−0.141	−0.487[c]	−0.317[c]	0.026	−0.130	−0.305[b]	−0.454
	(0.123)	(0.110)	(0.131)	(0.100)	(0.127)	(0.152)	(0.136)	(0.122)
Father's years of schooling	−0.065	0.115	0.033	−0.083	0.012	0.059	0.122	−0.040
	(0.057)	(0.068)	(0.066)	(0.051)	(0.074)	(0.073)	(0.068)	(0.057)
Intercept	0.851	0.217	5.984[c]	4.614[c]	−2.664	−0.736	1.407	5.556[c]
	(1.618)	(1.528)	(1.728)	(1.362)	(1.690)	(1.947)	(1.630)	(1.546)
N	130	98	120	178	189	130	143	195
$\bar{P}$	0.262	0.327	0.375	0.287	0.101	0.131	0.210	0.246
				Smoking at age 24				
Years of schooling	−0.078	−0.154	−0.490[c]	−0.352[c]	−0.108	−0.160	−0.098	−0.305[c]
	(0.104)	(0.101)	(0.125)	(0.090)	(0.084)	(0.100)	(0.091)	(0.094)
Father's years of schooling	−0.012	0.103	0.090	−0.092	0.098[b]	0.021	−0.020	0.004
	(0.049)	(0.066)	(0.063)	(0.049)	(0.049)	(0.051)	(0.051)	(0.049)
Intercept	1.766	1.349	6.541[c]	6.065[c]	−0.011	1.589	1.521	3.706[c]
	(1.366)	(1.444)	(1.681)	(1.290)	(1.087)	(1.307)	(1.193)	(1.209)
N	130	98	120	178	189	130	143	195
$\bar{P}$	0.646	0.520	0.617	0.455	0.365	0.408	0.483	0.379

Note: Asymptotic standard errors of coefficients in parentheses.
a. Cohort defined by calendar year when respondent became 17 years old.
b. Significant at $p<0.05$.
c. Significant at $p<0.01$.

by years of schooling appear to be motivated, at least in part, by health concerns. This can be seen in the variation in the schooling coefficients by cohort, which shows how the schooling–smoking relation has changed over time. This variation is important because before 1953 there was little public discussion linking cigarettes to bad health, and before 1964 there was little explicit public antismoking policy.

The regression results in Table 12.1 show that schooling has a sharply different relation to smoking in the periods before and after the health consequences of smoking became a major public concern, rather than a gradually changing relation over time. Though all but one are negative, the schooling coefficients for the two pre-1953 cohorts for all sex/age smoking combinations are small; none are significantly different from zero ($p > 0.10$ for all). On the other hand, all the post-1953 cohort coefficients are strongly negative and significantly different from zero (at $p < 0.01$), except for the 1953–1963 cohort for women, where the coefficient at age 17 is less significant (different from zero at $p < 0.05$) and the coefficient at age 24 is still quite small and insignificant.

The only significant differences in schooling coefficients among cohorts are between the pre-1953 and post-1953 cohorts, not within either of these two groupings ($p > 0.10$ for all within-group tests). For men at both ages, post-1953 cohort coefficients are significantly different from the pre-1953 cohort coefficients (at $p < 0.05$). For women, the only strongly significant difference ($p < 0.05$) is between the 1964–1972 cohort and the pre-1953 cohorts at age 17. The results for women show a weaker relation between the schooling coefficient and the spread of information about health effects of smoking than do the results for men. The "pure schooling" correlation for women may be contaminated more than for men by correlations between schooling and social class and between social class and propensity to smoke (Harris, 1980).

The coefficients for father's schooling by cohort in Table 12.1 are small, and all but one are statistically insignificant. Nor do we find any systematic pattern of variation in the coefficients by cohort. Even if own schooling is left out of the regression or father's schooling is restricted to have the same coefficient across all cohorts, the father's schooling coefficient remains weak. Father's schooling may perform poorly in these regressions because of correlation with several potentially conflicting influences on smoking, such as social class, own education, and family income.

The intercept coefficients in Table 12.1 show the partial effect of cohort, holding the effect of interactions between schooling and cohort at zero. To obtain the mean effect of cohort holding schooling constant at some nonzero level, one must sum the simple intercept coefficient and the effect of the schooling coefficient evaluated at the specified level of schooling. We evaluated the intercohort effects with schooling held constant at the mean value of the whole sample (rather than zero) to judge the overall time trend in smoking behavior for the average person.

At mean schooling levels, the partial effect of cohort for men is increased smoking in successively younger cohorts up to the 1953–1963 cohort for both ages (except for a dip at age 24 in the 1942–1952 cohort), followed by a sharp decline in smoking in the 1964–1972 cohort. For women, smoking increases in successive cohorts right through the 1964–1972 cohort at age 17; at age 24, smoking increases through the 1953–1963 cohort and then drops sharply in the 1964–1972 cohort. None of these cohort-to-cohort changes are statistically significant (at $p < 0.05$), however, except the decrease in smoking among 24-year-old men in the 1964–1972 cohort. This overall trend in smoking corresponds to that found in other surveys (Harris, 1979).

One way to illuminate the differences in the schooling–smoking relation by cohort, age, and sex is to examine the predicted probabilities of smoking implied by the regression results. Table 12.2 shows those predictions for the end values and midpoint of years of schooling, for each cohort/age/sex combination. These predicted probabilities clearly show the dramatic change in the schooling–smoking relation between the pre- and post-"health concern" cohorts. The strong negative relation between schooling and smoking came about primarily from decreases in smoking by the highly educated; smoking probabilities for those with only 12 years of schooling are generally as high or higher in the post-"health concern" cohorts as in the pre-"health concern" cohorts. Table 12.2 also reaffirms that the schooling–smoking relationship observed at age 24, after schooling was completed, could be accounted for by equally strong differences in smoking probabilities among the same individuals at age 17, before they had obtained differential amounts of schooling.

Table 12.2 Predicted probability of smoking at ages 17 and 24, by sex, cohort, and years of completed schooling:[a] white men and women aged 24–75 years, with 12 to 18 years of completed schooling

Cohort[b]	Age 17			Age 24		
	12 years schooling	15 years schooling	18 years schooling	12 years schooling	15 years schooling	18 years schooling
			Men			
1921–41	0.26	0.21	0.17	0.67	0.61	0.56
1942–52	0.44	0.34	0.25	0.65	0.54	0.43
1953–63	0.62	0.28	0.08	0.84	0.54	0.21
1964–72	0.48	0.26	0.12	0.70	0.44	0.22
			Women			
1921–41	0.10	0.10	0.11	0.44	0.36	0.29
1942–52	0.16	0.11	0.08	0.47	0.36	0.26
1953–63	0.28	0.14	0.06	0.53	0.46	0.39
1964–72	0.42	0.16	0.05	0.52	0.30	0.15

a. Based on maximum-likelihood logit regressions of probability of smoking reported in Table 12.1. Probabilities are evaluated at mean father's schooling.

b. Defined by calendar year when age 17.

Discussion

The data examined in this study reject the hypothesis that additional years of schooling play a significant causal role in the schooling–smoking correlation.[9] There are apparently one or more "third variables" that affect both smoking and years of schooling. These data do, however, support the hypothesis that the schooling–smoking relation—and, by implication, the effect of any underlying third variable—is related to considerations of the health consequences of smoking.

What is the third variable that leads to differences in both schooling and smoking? The data do not support the view that differences in social class are the underlying cause. First, the effect of father's schooling is very weak and is not statistically significant even in regressions that omit the individual's own schooling. Second, "class" effects should presumably have been present for the older cohorts as well as the more recent ones, but no significant relation between schooling and smoking emerges until the post-1953 cohorts.

Mental ability is another possible third variable. Those individuals who complete additional schooling are presumably more intelligent. The incidence of smoking among high school students has also been negatively correlated with academic performance, which itself is a correlate of mental ability (Borland and Rudolph, 1975). Thus, even though all the subjects in our sample have the same number of years of schooling at age 17, those of greater mental ability may more rapidly absorb and act upon information about the harmful effects of smoking, as well as obtain more additional schooling. If the schooling–smoking correlation were primarily due to superior mental ability, however, one might expect that it would become weaker over time as knowledge about the harmful effects of smoking became more widely diffused. The analysis by cohort provides no significant evidence of such weakening over time.

In Chapter 11 I suggested that both schooling and smoking behavior are related to individual differences in time discount, that is, willingness and ability to incur current costs for future benefits. Schooling has long been recognized as a form of investment; decisions about cigarette smoking have a similar character. Assuming imperfect capital markets, so that no single marginal rate of time discount would prevail for all persons in all domains, differences in time discount could explain the observed correlation between schooling and smoking. The data in this study are consistent with this hypothesis, but cannot test it.

Cigarette smoking is undoubtedly an important intervening variable in the correlation between schooling and health. If, as this study suggests, additional years of schooling are not causally related to smoking, identification of the third variable that affects both may provide a key to understanding the schooling–health relation.

HEALTH POLICY IV

**From Bismarck
to Woodcock**

Almost a century ago Prince Otto Eduard Leopold von Bismarck, the principal creator and first chancellor of the new German nation-state, introduced compulsory national health insurance to the Western world. Since then, nation after nation has followed his lead until today almost every developed country has a full-blown national health insurance plan. Some significant benchmarks along the way have been the Russian system (introduced by Lenin after the Bolshevik Revolution), the British National Health Service initiated by Beveridge and Bevan in 1945, and the Canadian federal-provincial plans (hospital care in the late 1950s, physicians' services in the late 1960s). In nearly all cases these plans built on previous systems of medical organization and finance that reflected particular national traditions, values, and circumstances (Abel-Smith, 1964).

In some health plans, such as those in the communist countries, the government has direct responsibility for providing services. In others, the production of medical care is still at least partially in the private sector, but the payment for care is through taxes or compulsory insurance premiums which are really earmarked taxes. Even in the United States, the last major holdout against the worldwide trend, government funds pay directly for almost half of all health care expenditures and pay indirectly for an appreciable additional share through tax exemptions and allowances.[1] Moreover, most observers believe that it is only a question of *when* Congress will enact national health insurance, not *if* it will.

Almost as obvious (to many economists) as the rise of public subsidy of health insurance is the "irrational" aspect of such programs. Health insurance, in effect, reduces the price the consumer faces at the time of purchase of medical care and therefore induces excessive demand. Because the direct cost to the consumer is less than the true cost to society of providing that care, he tends to overconsume medical care relative to other goods and services. This misallocation of resources results in a significant "welfare loss," which Martin Feldstein (1973) has estimated at a minimum of $5 billion per annum in the United States.

Not only does society seem to be irrationally bent on encouraging people to overuse medical care, but in the free market for health insurance, people also tend to buy the "wrong" kind. Most economists agree that, to the extent that health insurance serves a useful purpose, it is to protect consumers against large, unexpected bills for medical care. All insurance policies are actuarily "unfair," that is, they carry a load factor for administrative costs, but if consumers are risk-averse, it is worthwhile for them to pay these costs in order to protect themselves against unpredictable (for the individual) large losses. It follows, therefore, that consumers should prefer major medical (catastrophe) insurance, that is, plans with substantial deductibles or copayment provisions for moderate expenses but ample coverage for very large expenses. Instead, we observe a strong preference for "first-dollar" or shallow coverage. Of the privately held hospital insurance policies in the United States, the number covering the first day of hospitalization is several times greater than the number covering long-term stays.

Another apparent irrationality with respect to health insurance was alleged by Milton Friedman in a *Newsweek* column in April 1975. He noted that Leonard Woodcock, president of the United Automobile Workers union (UAW), is leading the drive for universal comprehensive national health insurance despite the fact that such a measure is "against the interest of . . . members of his own union, and even of the officials of that union . . . The UAW is a strong union and its members are among the highest paid industrial workers. If they wish to receive part of their pay in the form of medical care, they can afford, and hence can get, a larger amount than the average citizen. But in a governmental program, they are simply average citizens. In addition, a union or company plan would be far more responsive to their demands and needs than a universal national plan, so that they would get more per dollar spent" (Friedman, 1975). Friedman says that Woodcock is an "intelligent man," and therefore finds his behavior a "major puzzle."

From Bismarck to Woodcock, it seems that economists are drowning in a sea of irrationality. But other economists warn us against jumping to the irrationality conclusion. In particular, George Stigler has taught us to look beyond the surface appearance of political actions in search of their actual consequences and of the interests that they serve. He writes, "It seems unfruitful . . . to conclude from the studies of the effects of various policies that those policies which did not achieve their announced goals, or had perverse effects . . . are simply mistakes of the society" (Stigler, 1975). In short, when confronted with some consistent and widespread behavior that we cannot explain, we should not blithely assume that it is attributable to lack of information or bad judgment. We should be wary of what might be called the "fallacy of misplaced ignorance." It may be that the behavior we observe is more consistent with the self-interest of particular individuals or groups than it first appears.

It is to George Stigler (1958b) that we are also indebted for the "survivor principle," one of his many contributions to the study of industrial organization. The basic notion is simple: if we want to learn something about the relative efficiency of differently sized firms in an industry, Stigler tells us to look at that industry over time and notice which size classes seem to flourish and which do not. Can the "survivor principle" be applied to institutions as well? If so, national health insurance seems to pass with flying colors. No country that has tried it has abandoned it, and those that have tried it partially usually expand it. It may not be unreasonable to infer, therefore, that national health insurance does serve some *general* interests; that is, there may be some welfare gains lying below the surface that more than offset the losses so apparent to many economists. The following sections explore some of the special or general benefits that might explain the widespread pursuit of national health insurance.

Implicit National Health Insurance

Some of the observed behavior would seem less irrational if we assume that the United States already has *implicit* national health insurance, especially for catastrophic illness. If it is true that most uninsured people who need care can get it one way or another—through government hospitals, philanthropy, or bad debts—then it may be rational for people to buy only shallow coverage, or indeed, not to buy any insurance at all. To suggest that there is implicit insurance in the United States covering nearly everyone is not at all to suggest that there is equal access to equal quality care. We know that so-called free care may often have some stigma attached to it, may be less pleasant and less prompt, and may fail in other ways as well. But it cannot be denied that a good deal of medical care is delivered every year in the United States to persons who do not have explicit insurance or the money to pay for it.

Those individuals without explicit insurance are essentially free riders. Those who do carry extensive insurance, such as the automobile workers, in effect pay twice—once through the premiums for their own insurance and again through taxes or inflated costs to cover care for those without explicit insurance. If this is a significant factor, it could be perfectly rational for the automobile workers to support *universal compulsory* insurance. Why society provides implicit or (in most countries) explicit coverage for all remains to be explained.

An Attempt to Control Providers

Another reason why the UAW leaders and others may favor a single national health plan is the hope of gaining some control over the providers of medical care—the hospitals and the physicians. In recent years one of the major frustrations faced by the auto workers and other groups with extensive insurance coverage is the rapid escalation in the price of medical care. They may believe that only a single-source national health insurance plan will be in a position to control provider behavior and stop the escalation in costs. Moreover, there is strong evidence that they are not alone in this view. One of the puzzles for economists has been to explain the traditional opposition of the medical profession to legislation which, at least in the short run, increases the demand for their services. This opposition probably stems in part from the belief that national health insurance would ultimately result in an increase in government control over providers.

Tax Advantages

Why do people buy shallow coverage—where the administrative load is high and the risk element relatively small? One reason is that when the premium is paid by the employer, the implicit income is free of tax. Even health insurance premiums paid by the individual are partially deductible from taxable income. If the tax laws allowed employers to provide tax-free "food insurance," we would undoubtedly see a sharp increase in that type of fringe benefit. But again the explanation is not very satisfactory. Why do the tax laws encourage the purchase of medical care but not food, clothing, or other necessities? In an attempt to answer this question, we should consider some of the characteristics of medical care and health insurance that are different from conventional commodities.

Externalities

One explanation for the popularity of national health insurance that has great appeal for economists at the theoretical level is that there are substantial external benefits associated with the consumption of medical care. If this were true, then governmental subsidy of care need not be irrational; indeed it might be irrational not to provide that subsidy. The best example of potential externalities is the prevention or treatment of communicable diseases such as tuberculosis. In earlier times these diseases constituted a very significant portion of overall health problems, but they are much less important today. Furthermore, if a concern with externalities were the chief motivation, it would be logical and feasible to subsidize those services (for example, venereal disease clinics) that are clearly addressed to the communicable diseases. However, even economists who are strong advocates of national health insurance, such as Lester Thurow, do not rely on the externality argument. Thurow (1974) writes, "Once a society gets beyond public health measures and communicable diseases, medical care does not generate externalities."

Mark Pauly (1971) has called attention to one special kind of externality that probably is operative: it involves the satisfaction people get from knowing that someone else who is sick is getting medical attention. This satisfaction could be purchased by voluntary philanthropy, but the total amount so purchased is likely to be less than socially optimal because each individual's giving tends to be based on his or her private satisfaction, ignoring the effects on others. Thus the solution may be compulsory philanthropy, that is, tax-supported programs.

A Matter of "Life or Death"

Another explanation for national health insurance that has great appeal at the theoretical level but carries less conviction empirically is that "the market should not determine life or death." This theme is advanced by Arthur Okun in his book *Equality and Efficiency: The Big Tradeoff* (1975) and is a basic tenet of those who argue that "health care is a right." There is considerable logic in the argument that society may be unwilling to accept the consequences of an unequal distribution of income for certain kinds of allocation decisions, such as who serves in the army during wartime, who gets police protection, and who faces other life-threatening situations. It may be easier and more efficient to control such allocations directly than to try to redistribute money income (possibly only temporarily) to achieve the desired allocation.

Although this explanation has a certain theoretical appeal, one problem with it is that the vast majority of health services do not remotely approach a "life or death" situation. Moreover, the ability of medical care to make any significant contribution to life expectancy came long after Bismarck and Lenin advocated national health insurance. Even today, when some medical care is very effective, it is possible that housing, nutrition, and occupation have more influence on life expectancy than does medical care, yet we allow inequality in the distribution of income to determine allocation decisions in those areas. According to Peter Townsend (1974), there is no evidence that the British National Health Service has reduced class differences in infant mortality, maternal mortality, or overall life expectancy. If equalizing life expectancy were society's goal, it is not at all clear that heavy emphasis on national health insurance would be an optimal strategy.

The emphasis on medical care rather than on other programs that might affect life expectancy is sometimes defended by the statement that the former is more feasible. Although diet or exercise or occupation may have more effect on life expectancy than does medical care, it may be technically simpler to alter people's consumption of medical care than to alter their diet, amount of exercise, or occupation. It has also been argued that it is politically more feasible to push medical care rather than alternative strategies. The distinction between technical and political feasibility is not, of course, clear-cut because the former depends in part on what we are willing to do in the way of permitting government to intrude on personal decisions—a political question. However, to the extent that the popularity of national health insurance is said to be attributable to its political feasibility, we have really not explained much. Its political popularity is precisely the question we started with.

The Growth of Egalitarianism

Life expectancy aside, one way of interpreting the growth of national health insurance is an expression of the desire for greater equality in society. British economists John Jewkes and Sylvia Jewkes (1963) have written, "The driving force behind the creation of the National Health Service was not the search for efficiency or for profitable social investment. It was something quite different: it was a surging national desire to share something equally." An American economist, C. M. Lindsay, has developed a theoretical model that analyzes alternative methods for satisfying the demand for equality of access to medical care. Among other things, he shows that if this demand for equality is widespread, there are externalities similar to those discussed by Pauly in connection with philanthropy. Thus a free-market approach will result in less equality than people really demand. He also shows that the British National Health Service can perhaps best be understood as an attempt to satisfy this demand for equality. He concludes, "The politician's sensitive ear may read the preferences of his constituents better than the econometrician with his computer" (Lindsay, 1969).

Why the demand for equality has grown over time and why it should find expression in medical care more than in other goods and services are not easy questions to answer. Is there really more altruism in society now than before? Were Bismarck and Lenin the most altruistic political leaders of their time? Is it simply the case that equality is a normal "good," that is, we buy more of it when our income rises? If this is the explanation, what are the implications for equality in a no-growth economy?

Perhaps there has been no real increase in altruism at all. Perhaps what we observe is a response to an increase in the ability of the less well-off to make life miserable for the well-off through strikes, violence, and other social disruptions. In this view, health insurance is part of an effort to buy domestic stability. It may be that industrialization and urbanization make us all more interdependent, thus increasing the power of the "have-nots" to force redistributions of one kind or another. Or perhaps there has been a decline in the willingness of the "haves" to use force to preserve the status quo.

Such speculations, if they contain some validity, would explain a general increase in egalitarian legislation, but they would not help much in explaining why this legislation has focused heavily on medical care. Indeed, is it not curious that society should choose to emphasize equality in access to a service that makes little difference at the margin in life expectancy or to economic or political position and power? A cynic might argue that it is not curious at all, since it is precisely because medical care does not make much difference that those with power are willing to share it more equally with those with less. Indeed, one might argue that the more a society has significant, enduring class distinctions, the more it needs the symbolic equality of national health insurance to blunt pressures for changes that alter fundamental class or power relationships.

One egalitarian goal that has always had considerable acceptance in the United States is equality of opportunity. Thus, a popular argument in favor of national health insurance is that it would help to equalize access to medical care for children. Some recent theoretical work on the economics of the family, however, calls into question the effectiveness of such programs. Gary Becker (1976) has argued that the thrust of programs aimed at increasing investment in disadvantaged children can be blunted by parents who may decrease their own allocation of time and money to their children as investment by the state increases. The increase in the welfare of the children, therefore, may be no greater than if a cash subsidy equal to the cost of the program were given directly to the parents. The ability of the "head" to reallocate family resources may not, however, be as unconstrained as Becker's model assumes. There may be legal or social constraints, or there may be a desire on the part of the head to maintain the child's obedience, respect, or affection. Thus the importance of the reallocation effect is an empirical question that we know virtually nothing about at present.

Paternalism

An argument advanced by Thurow (1974, p. 193) in favor of transfers in kind—such as national health insurance—is that some individuals are not competent to make their own decisions.[2] He writes, "Increasingly we are coming to recognize that the world is not neatly divided into the competent and the incompetent. There is a continuum of individuals ranging from those who are competent to make any and all decisions to those who are incompetent to make any and all decisions." Thurow argues that if society desires to raise each family up to some minimum level of *real* welfare, it may be more efficient to do it through in-kind transfers than through cash grants. Even if we agree with this general argument, it does not follow as a matter of logic that subsidizing medical care brings us closer to a social optimum. It may be the case, for instance, that the "less able" managers tend to *overvalue* medical care relative to other goods and services, in which case Thurow should want to constrain their utilization rather than encourage it.

More generally, there is the question of whether government will, on average, make "better" decisions than individuals. As Arrow (1973) has stated in a slightly different context, "If many individuals, given proper information, refuse to fasten their seat belts or insist on smoking themselves into lung cancer or drinking themselves into incompetence, there is no reason to suppose they will be any more sensible in their capacity as democratic voters." Two arguments have been suggested to blunt Arrow's critique. The first is that the less able are less likely to vote; therefore the electoral process produces decisions that reflect the judgment of the more able members of society. Second, it has been suggested that there is considerable scope for discretionary behavior by elected representatives; they do not simply follow the dictates of their constituents (Breton, 1974). It may be that their judgment is generally better than that of the average citizen.

An Offset to an "Unjust Tax"

Suppose the United States were defeated by an enemy in war and had to pay an annual tribute to the enemy of $100 billion.[3] Suppose further that the enemy collected this tribute by a tax of a variable amount on American citizens chosen at random. The U. S. government might decide that this tribute tax was unjust and that it would be more equitable for the federal government to pay the tribute from revenues raised by normal methods of taxation. If the enemy insisted on collecting the tribute from individual citizens on a random basis, the government could choose to reimburse those paying the tribute.

Some observers believe there is a close parallel between the tribute example and expenditures for medical care. They see ill health and the consumption of medical care as largely beyond the control of the individual citizen—the cost is like an unjust tax—and the purpose of national health insurance is to prevent medical expenditures from unjustly changing the distribution of income. There is, of course, the question of whether, or how much, individuals can influence and control the amount of their medical expenditures. Putting that to one side, however, and assuming that the analogy is a good one, there are still some questions that arise.

One might ask why the government has to intervene to protect people against the tribute tax. Why couldn't citizens in their private lives buy insurance against being taxed for tribute? The total cost and the probabilities are known; therefore private insurance companies could easily set appropriate premiums. One answer might be that this is also inequitable to the extent that some people can afford the insurance more easily than others. The government could easily remedy this, however, by some modest changes in the distribution of income. Another problem, of course, is that some people might not buy the insurance. They would be "free riders" because if they were hit with a big tribute tax they would be unable to pay, and others would have to pay in their place. Furthermore, they would be wiped out financially, so that society would have to support their families.

To be sure, the government could both redistribute income to take care of the premium and make insurance compulsory, but that becomes almost indistinguishable from a national insurance plan. The only difference then would be whether there is a single organization, the government, underwriting the insurance, or whether there are several private insurance companies.

In the tribute tax example we have assumed that the probability of loss would be identical across the population, but this is clearly not true for health insurance. One argument advanced in support of national health insurance is that it does not require higher-risk individuals to pay higher premiums. A counter-argument is that individuals do have some discretion concerning behavior that affects health and concerning the utilization of medical care for given health conditions. National health insurance, it is alleged, distorts that behavior. A related argument is that medical care will always have to be rationed in some way, and that national health insurance requires the introduction of rationing devices other than price and income. These devices carry their own potential for inequity and inefficiency.

The Decline of the Family

Illness is as old as mankind, and while frequently in the past and not infrequently today, there is little that can be done to change the course of disease, there is much that can be done to provide care, sympathy, and support. Traditionally most of these functions were provided within the family. The family was both the mechanism for *insuring* against the consequences of disease and disability, and the locus of the *production* of care. The only rival to the family in this respect until modern times was the church, a subject to be considered in the following section.

With industrialization and urbanization, the provision of insurance and of care tended to move out of the family and into the market. Thus, much of the observed increase in medical care's share of total economic acitivity is an accounting illusion. It is the result of a shift in the production of care from the home, where it is not considered part of national output, to hospitals, nursing homes, and the like, where it is counted as part of the GNP. Unlike the production of bread, however, which also moved from the family to the market (and stayed there), medical care, or at least medical insurance, increasingly became a function of the state.

One possible explanation is that the state is more efficient because there are significant economies of scale. With respect to the *production* of medical care, the economies of scale argument can fairly safely be rejected. Except for some exotic tertiary procedures, the economies of scale in the production of physicians' services and hospital services are exhausted at the local or small region level. For the insurance function itself, however, there may be significant economies of scale. Definitive studies are not available, but the proposition that a single national health insurance plan would be cheaper to administer than multiple plans cannot be rejected out of hand (LeClair, 1975).[4] To be sure, a single plan would presumably reduce consumer satisfaction to the extent that the coverage of the plan would represent a compromise among the variety of plans that different individuals and groups might prefer.

The relationship between the declining importance of the family and the growing importance of the state is complex. Not only can the latter be viewed as a consequence of the former, but the causality can also run the other way. Every time the state assumes an additional function, such as health insurance, child care, or benefits for the elderly, the need for close family ties becomes weaker. Geographic mobility probably plays a significant role in this two-way relationship: one of the reasons why people rely more on the state and less on their family is that frequently the family is geographically dispersed. The other side of the coin is that once the state assumes responsibilities that formerly resided with the family, individuals feel freer to move away from the family, both literally and figuratively.

It has often been alleged that intrafamily dependency relationships are inhibiting and destructive to individual fulfillment. Whether a dependency relationship with the state will prove less burdensome remains to be seen. There is also the question of whether the efficient provision of impersonal "caring" is feasible.

The Decline of Religion

In traditional societies when the family was unable to meet the needs of the sick, organized religion frequently took over. Indeed, practically all of the early hospitals in Europe were built and staffed by the church and served primarily the poor. The development of strong religious ties, with tithes or contributions that are frequently indistinguishable from modern taxes, can be viewed as an alternative mechanism for dealing with the philanthropic externalities discussed previously. Moreover, at a time when technical medical care was so ineffective, religion offered a particular kind of symbolic equality—in the next world if not in this one. Thus the decline of organized religion, along with the weakening of the family, may have created a vacuum which the state is called upon to fill.

The "Political" Role

When refugees from the Soviet Union were interviewed in Western Europe after World War II, they invariably praised the West and disparaged life in Russia—with one notable exception: they said they sorely missed the comprehensive health insurance provided by the Soviet state (Field, 1967). It may be that one of the most effective ways of increasing allegiance to the state is through national health insurance. This was undoubtedly a prime motive for Bismarck as he tried to weld the diverse German principalities into a nation. It is also alleged that he saw national health insurance as an instrument to reduce or blur the tension and conflicts between social classes.

We live at a time when many of the traditional symbols and institutions that held a nation together have been weakened or have fallen into disrepute. A more sophisticated public requires more sophisticated symbols, and national health insurance may fit the role particularly well.

Why Is the United States Last?

One rough test of the various explanations that have been proposed is to see if they help us understand why the United States is the last major developed country without national health insurance. Several reasons for the lag can be suggested. First, there is a long tradition in the United States of distrust of government. This country was largely settled by immigrants who had had unfavorable experiences with governments in Europe and who had learned to fear government rather than looking to it for support and protection. Second, it is important to note the heterogeneity of our population compared to some of the more homogeneous populations of Europe. We are certainly not a single "people" the way, say, the Japanese are. Brian Abel-Smith (1964) has noted, for instance, that the American poor were often Negroes or new immigrants with whose needs the older white settlers did not readily identify.

The distrust of government and the heterogeneity of the population probably account for the much better developed nongovernmental voluntary institutions in the United States. Close observers of the American scene ever since de Tocqueville have commented on the profusion of private nonprofit organizations to deal with problems which in other countries might be considered the province of government. These organizations can be viewed as devices for internalizing the philanthropic externalities discussed earlier in this chapter, but the organizations are frequently limited to individuals of similar ethnic background, religion, region, occupation, or other shared characteristic.

Another possible reason for the difference in attitudes between the United States and Europe is the greater equality of opportunity in this country. In the beginning this was based mostly on free or cheap land, and later on widespread public education. Moreover, the historic class barriers have been weaker here than in countries with a strong feudal heritage. To cite one obvious example, consider the family backgrounds of university faculties in Sweden and the United States. Sweden is often hailed as the outstanding example of a democratic welfare state, but the faculty members at the leading universities generally come from upper-class backgrounds. By contrast, the faculties at Harvard, Chicago, Stanford, and other leading American universities include many men and women who were born in modest circumstances. With greater equality of opportunity goes a stronger conviction that the distribution of income is related to effort and ability. Those who succeed in the system have much less sense of noblesse oblige than do the upper classes in Europe, many of whom owe their position to the accident of birth. In the United States, even those who have not succeeded or only partially succeeded seem more willing to acquiesce in the results.

Summing Up

The primary purpose of this inquiry has been to attempt to explain the popularity of national health insurance around the world. My answer at this point is that probably no single explanation will suffice. National health insurance means different things to different people. It always has. Daniel Hirschfield (1970), commenting on the campaign for national health insurance in the United States at the time of World War I, wrote: "Some saw health insurance primarily as an educational and public health measure, while others argued that it was an economic device to precipitate a needed reorganization of medical practice . . . Some saw it as a device to save money for all concerned, while others felt sure that it would increase expenditures significantly."

Externalities, egalitarianism, the decline of the family and traditional religion, the need for national symbols—all these may play a part. In democratic countries with homogeneous populations, people seem to want to take care of one another through programs such as national health insurance, as members of the same family do, although not to the same degree. In autocratic countries with heterogeneous populations, national health insurance is often imposed from above, partly as a device for strengthening national unity. The relative importance of different factors undoubtedly varies from country to country and time to time, but the fact that national health insurance can be viewed as serving so many diverse interests and needs is probably the best answer to why Bismarck and Woodcock are not such strange bedfellows after all.

Economics, Health, and Postindustrial Society

Two hundred years ago the industrial revolution was figuratively and literally beginning to pick up steam. In a few Western countries agricultural advances, which came faster than population growth, enabled some men and women to escape from grinding poverty. Life for most, however, was still "nasty, brutish, and short." Infant mortality rates of 200 or 300 per 1,000 births were the rule, and life expectancy in Western Europe was not very different from what it had been under the Romans. The great majority of men and women worked on farms, producing barely enough to feed themselves plus a small surplus for the relatively few workers engaged in the production of other goods and services. Widows and orphans, the sick, the elderly, and the destitute relied primarily on family and church for help in their time of need.

Agriculture continued to dominate employment for another century; as recently as 1877, half the United States labor force was still engaged in farming. Then, very quickly—in less than 30 minutes if we think of recorded history as a "day"—most of the countries of Western Europe and North America became industrialized. But the process of economic development did not stop with industrialization. As Colin Clark noted so accurately in 1960: "The most important concomitant of economic progress is the movement of labor from agriculture to manufacture, and from manufacture to commerce and services." By 1957 the United States had become the world's first "service economy"—that is, the first nation in which more than half of the labor force was engaged in producing services rather than goods.

Today, many Western societies can be described as "postindustrial" (Bell, 1973). Such societies are characterized by a variety of special features—affluence, urbanization, infant mortality rates of 10 to 15 per 1,000, high female labor force participation, low fertility, decreased importance of the family and traditional religions, increased importance of the state, long life expectancy, and, of course, a substantial change in the locus of economic activity. The hospital, the classroom, and the shopping center have replaced the coal mine, the steel mill, and the assembly line as the major work sites of modern society. "Industrial man" has been succeeded by "postindustrial person," but the import of this transformation for society has not yet been fully analyzed.

In this chapter I shall focus on one of the largest and fastest-growing industries in postindustrial society—medical care—and on a range of problems specifically related to medicine and health. I will use the discipline of economics to provide some insights concerning these problems, and will also attempt to use the health field to illuminate more general problems of postindustrial society. In this last respect I wish to ally myself with H. Scott Gordon, who wrote in 1971: "I have never regarded economics as a discipline that is inherently narrow." At the same time, I am aware of the limits of economics—both those limits that stem from shortcomings in current theoretical and empirical knowledge and those limits that are inherent in any science of man. For instance, it should be clear that economics alone does not, indeed should not, tell us whether it is better to devote resources to extending the life of an 80-year-old man with terminal cancer or to reducing the risk of birth defects in a population of newborns. What economics does do is to help us arrange the relevant information in a systematic way and make explicit the choices that individuals and society face. Therein lies much of its unpopularity. Economics has earned the label "the dismal science" because it constantly reminds us that we have been turned out of the Garden of Eden. Many people prefer to pretend that choices do not have to be made; many like to believe that they are not being made at present.

This chapter will not offer that kind of comfort or reassurance; neither will it supply simple answers to the major policy issues of the day. It is, rather, an attempt on my part to report some key findings from more than a decade of research in health economics, and to offer some generalizations from these findings. I am aware that such generalizations, based on only one aspect of society, must necessarily be speculative.

The Determinants of Health

In this section I will review some major results concerning the determinants of health, especially the roles played by medical care, income, and education. We will see that changes in health are much more dependent on nonmedical factors than on the quantity of medical care. Nevertheless, medical care has become one of the largest industries in modern society, and I will discuss some of the reasons for this rapid growth.

Medical Care

One of the first things economics does is to sensitize us to the distinction between *inputs* and *outputs*—that is, in the present context, to the difference between *medical care* and *health*. This perspective can be found in the wise observations of René Dubos and has been ably articulated in Canada by Marc Lalonde (Dubos, 1959; Lalonde, 1974). It remained for economists, however, to develop the matter systematically and quantitatively in multivariate analyses that examine the effect on health of medical inputs, income, education, and other variables.

The basic finding is the following: when the state of medical science and other health-determining variables are held constant, the marginal contribution of medical care to health is very small in modern nations. Those who advocate ever more physicians, nurses, hospitals, and the like are either mistaken or have in mind objectives other than the improvement of the health of the population. The earliest studies that reported this conclusion were greeted with skepticism in some quarters because the analyses typically relied on mortality as the measure of health. It was suggested that mortality is a rather crude index of health, and that more sophisticated measures would reveal the favorable effects of greater numbers of physicians, nurses, and hospital beds. A Rand study, however, based on six sensitive indicators of ill health (elevated cholesterol levels, varicose veins, high blood pressure, abnormal chest x-ray, abnormal electrocardiogram, and an unfavorable periodontal index) provides striking confirmation of the results based on mortality (Newhouse and Friedlander, 1980). Variations in the amount of health resources available across 39 metropolitan areas of the United States had no systematic effect on these health measures taken alone or in linear combination.

Examples of the distinction between medical care and health can be drawn from many countries other than the United States. In Great Britain, for instance, the National Health Service (NHS) has undoubtedly served to reduce class differences in access to medical care, but the traditionally large class differentials in infant mortality and life expectancy are no smaller after three decades of the NHS. Moreover, despite free access to medical care, time lost from work because of sickness has actually increased greatly in Britain in recent decades. The number of sick days depends on many factors in addition to health, but these data hardly support the notion that there has been a large payoff from the NHS in that area (Townsend, 1974). The discrepancy between health and medical care is even sharper in the Soviet Union. In recent years there apparently has been a deterioration in health as measured either by infant mortality or life expectancy, even though the Soviet medical care system is said to have expanded (Davis and Feshbach, 1978).

There are several reasons why an increase in medical resources, given a reasonable quantity as a base, does not have much effect on health. First, if physicians are scarce, they tend to concentrate on those patients for whom their attention is likely to make the most difference. As doctors become more plentiful, they naturally tend to spend more time on patients less in need of attention. Second, patients also alter their behavior depending on how easy or difficult it is to get to see a physician. When physicians are more numerous, patients tend to seek attention for more trivial conditions. Third, many of the most effective interventions, such as vaccinations or treatment of bacterial infections, require only modest amounts of resources. Quite often, one "shot" goes a long way. On the other hand, the long-term benefits of some of the most expensive procedures, such as open-heart surgery or organ transplants, are still in doubt. Fourth, there is the problem of "iatrogenic disease"—illness that arises as a result of medical care. Because medical and surgical interventions are more powerful than ever before, they carry with them greater risk. Sometimes too much care, or the wrong care, can be more deleterious to health than no care at all. Finally, it is abundantly clear that factors other than medical care (genes, environment, life-style) play crucial roles in many of the most important health problems.

Income and Inequality

For most of man's history, income has been the primary determinant of health and life expectancy—the major explanation for differences in health among nations and among groups within a nation. A strong income effect is still observed in the less developed nations, but in the United States the relation between income and life expectancy has tended to disappear. This is true when health is measured by mortality, or by indicators such as high blood pressure, varicose veins, elevated cholesterol levels, and abnormal x-rays or cardiograms, or by subjective evaluation of health status. Other things being equal, there is no longer a clearly discernible effect of income on health except at the deepest levels of poverty. I regard the disappearance of the income effect as an important aspect of postindustrial society, but the fact is not widely known, and the implications are rarely discussed. To realize one such implication, consider how attitudes toward economic growth might differ depending on whether further growth was or was not expected to reduce mortality.

The favorable effect of economic growth and technological change on *average* life expectancy is well known. Less appreciated is the extent to which growth has also reduced *inequality* in life expectancy across individuals and groups. The principal reason for the reduction is that general economic growth, even if unaccompanied by any reduction in income inequality, has more favorable effects on the health of the very poor than on those who have already reached a level of living well above subsistence. A second reason is that many effective medical discoveries of the past half-century, such as antibiotics, have been relatively low in cost and widely available.

Consider the following statistics taken from U. S. life tables for the white population. At the turn of this century, given the age-specific death rates then prevailing, one-fourth of a newborn cohort of males would die before the age of 23. On the other hand, one-fourth could expect to live beyond the age of

72. In other words, the variation in life expectancy was great. One simple measure of variation is the interquartile ratio—that is, the difference between the age of death at the third quartile and at the first quartile divided by the median age at death. For white males in 1900, this variation was 86 percent [(72 − 23) ÷ 57], but by 1975 it had fallen to 26 percent. This large reduction is attributable in part to drastic declines in infant and child mortality, but even if one looks at years of life remaining at age 20, the interquartile ratio fell from 59 percent to 35 percent between 1900 and 1975. White females experienced a similar decline in variation in life expectancy. Furthermore, nearly all of the decline occurred before the advent of Medicare and Medicaid.

Not only has the distribution of life expectancy become much more nearly equal within the white population, but the difference between white and nonwhite life expectancy has also been reduced substantially in this century. In 1900 life expectancy for whites was 47 percent higher than for nonwhites, while in 1975 the differential was only 8 percent. The overall reduction in inequality of life expectancy bears a strong relationship to reduction in inequality by income class. In 1900 those with short life expectancy were disproportionately from the lower half of the income distribution. Now, with the correlation between income and life expectancy much weaker, we can say that with respect to the most precious good of all, life itself, the United States is approaching an egalitarian distribution.

Education

Despite the general trend toward equality in life expectancy, there is one factor—education—that consistently appears as a significant correlate of good health. The same research by health economists that reveals the small marginal contributions of medical care and of income to health reports a strong positive relation between health and years of schooling. In the United States, regardless of the way health is measured (for example, mortality, morbidity, symptoms, or subjective evaluation), and regardless of the unit of observation (for example, individuals, city or state averages), number of years of schooling usually emerges as the most powerful correlate of good health. Michael Grossman, an economist who has done extensive research on this question, has tended to interpret this relationship as evidence that schooling increases the individual's efficiency in producing health, although he recognizes that some causality may run from better health to more schooling (Grossman, 1975). The way in which schooling contributes to efficiency in producing health has never been made explicit, but Grossman has speculated that persons with more education might choose healthier diets, be more aware of health risks, obtain healthier occupations, and use medical care more wisely.

I accept the "efficiency" hypothesis, but I think that it explains only a part of the correlation. One reason for my skepticism is that Grossman did not find any favorable effect of IQ on health, holding constant schooling and other variables. If more years of schooling increase efficiency in producing health, it seems that a higher IQ ought to work in the same direction. Furthermore, recent research on surgical utilization casts doubt on the proposition that better-educated individuals use medical care differently from the less educated. While the probability of surgery is much lower for the highly educated than for the rest of the U. S. population, a study by Louis Garrison (1978) shows that the highly educated who do undergo surgery enter the hospital at the same stage of disease as do the less educated. He also finds that the better-educated patients choose the same kinds of physicians, have about the same length of stay, and—apart from the fact that their general health is a little better than average—have about the same outcomes from surgery. Thus, at least in the context of in-hospital surgery, there is little support for the "efficiency" effect in the use of medical care.

The most plausible explanation for the lower surgery rates of the highly educated is that they have less need for surgery, that is, they are in better health. The question remains, why? One explanation that I favor is that both schooling and health are manifestations of differences among individuals in their willingness and/or ability to invest in human capital. Both schooling and health-related activities involve incurring current costs for the sake of future benefits, and it seems quite clear that individuals differ in the "rate of return" that will induce them (or their parents) to undertake such investments. There are numerous possible reasons for such differences. For instance, some individuals have much better access to capital than do others. And even holding access to capital constant, individuals differ in their skills of self-control and in their ability to visualize the future.

Recent preliminary research gives modest support for this view. A colleague and I surveyed a group of young adults to ascertain their rate of time discount, measured by the extra money they would require to wait for a money award in the future rather than collecting a smaller sum in the present. My colleague was interested in the pattern of the rates, that is, how they changed with length of time involved, size of the award, and so on. I added a few questions about the respondents' health and then looked at the relation between health and discount rate across individuals. I found a strong, statistically significant negative correlation between the rate of discount and the subjective assessment of health. For the 25 percent of the sample with the lowest discount rates, the probability of being in excellent health was 63 percent; for the quarter with the highest rates, the probability was only 32 percent.

Some recent statistics from England seem to provide additional support for my view of the correlation between health and schooling. A study of cigarette smoking revealed that among men in social class I (highly educated), the proportion who smoked fell almost by half between 1958 and 1975. In contrast, among men in social class V (poorly educated), the proportion scarcely changed. It seems unlikely that this difference in behavior occurs primarily because the men in class V have not heard about the dangers of smoking or do not understand the implications for health; it is more likely that they are unwilling (or unable) to give up a present pleasure for a distant and uncertain benefit. I suspect that if one compared these two groups of men with regard to other aspects of behavior that involve explicit or implicit rates of time discount (such as saving or buying on credit), one would find similar differences.

Progress in Medical Science

A discussion of the determinants of health should give some consideration to the effects of progress in medical science. Economics not only cautions us to distinguish between inputs and outputs but also calls attention to the distinction between the marginal product of an additional unit of input, holding constant the production function, and the shift of that function through technological progress. In the first instance, we ask what would be the effects on health of an increase in the quantity of physicians, nurses, and hospitals, assuming no change in the way care is delivered. In the second, we ask what would be the effects on health of an advance in medical science, assuming no change in the quantity of physicians, nurses, and hospitals.

With respect to the latter question, it seems to me that the "medical care doesn't matter" argument is overstated by some writers. To be sure, medical progress was slow until well into the twentieth century, but from about 1935 to about 1955, a period that marked the introduction of anti-infectious drugs, major improvements in health were recorded in all industrial nations. The decreases in mortality were far greater than could be attributed to general economic advance, increases in the *quantity* of medical care, or similar changes. The only reasonable explanation, in my view, is that advances in medical knowledge changed the structural relations governing the production of health. In a study of changes in infant mortality in 15 Western nations between 1937 and 1965, for instance, I estimated that the change in structure accounted for at least half of the large decline in infant mortality over that period (Fuchs, 1974b).

The application of medical and public health knowledge also improved health in the less developed countries, and at un-precedented speed. In a sample of 16 less developed countries studied by demographer Samuel H. Preston, life expectancy was only 39 years in 1940, but rose to 60 years by 1970 (Preston, 1980). He and I estimated that about two-thirds of the increase was attributable to better health technology and similar struc-tural changes and only one-third to a rise in per capita income. By contrast, in the United States the same change in life expec-tancy—from 39 to 60 years—required three-quarters of a cen-tury, from 1855 to 1930, because health technology was de-veloping so slowly at that time.

It remains true that advances in medical science do not come at a steady or predictable pace. During the 1960s many "break-throughs" were hailed, and expenditures for medical care rose appreciably, but the favorable consequences for health were quite limited. In recent years, however, U. S. death rates, es-pecially from heart disease, have decreased rapidly. For men and women at most ages, the probability of death from arte-riosclerotic heart disease in 1975 was 20 to 25 percent lower than in 1968. Analysts who are technologically inclined attribute most of this large decrease to better control of hypertension, special coronary care units in hospitals, open-heart surgery, and similar medical innovations. Other observers are more prone to credit changes in diet, smoking, exercise, and other aspects of personal behavior. We do not know the true explanation; I suspect that there is some validity to both points of view.

The Growth of Medical Care

Although the pace of medical advance has been highly uneven, the growth of expenditures for medical care has been unrelenting. For at least the past three decades (and probably for much longer), the share of gross national product (GNP) devoted to medical care has steadily increased in the United States and many other countries. Today, in every postindustrial society, health care absorbs a substantial portion of the nation's resources; in several, the share devoted to health is rapidly approaching 10 percent. In the remainder of this section I will consider several possible explanations for the rapid growth of health care as an industry.

Income and productivity. One popular, but I believe exaggerated, explanation for the relative growth of service employment is the growth of per capita income. With respect to health care, higher income is clearly not a *direct* causal factor. Precise estimates of the income elasticity of the demand for health care differ, but almost all investigators agree that is is well below unity—that is, people behave as if health care is a "necessity." It follows, therefore, that the direct effect of a rise in per capita income should be a *decrease* in health care's share of real GNP. Some services other than health may be considered as "luxuries," that is, they have income elasticities greater than one, but it is interesting to note that according to the U. S. national income accounts there has been only a small increase in the service sector's share of gross product measured in *constant* dollars (Fuchs, 1978a). To be specific, during the past 30 years, while service employment was growing from 46 percent to 61 percent of total employment, the share of real output (1972 dollars) originating in the service sector changed only from 51 percent to 56 percent. If services had the high income elasticity of demand that is often ascribed to them, the growth of service output would surely have been more rapid.

The differential trends in employment and real output are the result of a relatively slow growth of output per worker in services. In this respect, health care has been no exception. Labor input per patient, especially in hospitals, has grown at an extremely rapid rate. In 1976 there were 304 full-time equivalent employees per 100 patients in the U. S. short-term hospitals, compared with 178 per 100 patients in 1950. Taken at face value, these data suggest that there has been a *decrease* in productivity, but this is highly problematic. The character of hospital activity has changed greatly since 1950. Each patient now has many more laboratory and x-ray tests; more complex surgery is performed; and new treatment approaches, such as intensive care units, have proliferated. I use the word "activity" rather than "output" deliberately, because we are far from knowing how much this increased activity has resulted in better health. Some changes in medical technology, such as the anti-infectious drugs mentioned previously, have clearly raised productivity enormously, but the only thing we know with certainty about some of the other technological changes is that they have greatly raised expenditures.

One reason for the difficulty of measuring productivity in medical care is that the consumer is an integral part of the production process. Health depends not only on how efficiently the physicians and nurses work, but also on what the patient does. Similar problems arise in attempts to measure change in real output and productivity in education, social services, police protection, entertainment, and many other service industries. As more and more of the work force becomes employed in industries whose output cannot be accurately measured, the "real" GNP will become increasingly unreliable as a measure of the welfare of society. We will probably be forced to abandon faith in a single summary index for measuring long-term changes or for international comparisons. Instead, welfare comparisons will be sought through mortality and morbidity indexes, crime rates, reading ability, and other more direct indicators of well-being.

Medical technology. The rapid growth of medical technology—the vast expansion in the character and scope of interventions that physicians can undertake—has been a major factor in the growth of health expenditures in recent decades. Familiar examples include renal dialysis, open-heart surgery, organ transplants, and high-energy cancer treatments. These innovations, attributable in large part to the investment in medical research of the past quarter-century, may or may not make major contributions to improved health, but relative ineffectiveness does not deter their use.

In the past I have referred to the proclivity of physicians to employ new technologies simply because they exist as the "technological imperative" (Fuchs, 1968). Recent economic research, however, provides a different explanation for the emphasis on expensive treatments that yield little in terms of lives saved, while preventive activities with high potential yield per dollar of expenditures are denied resources. Such behavior may be fully consistent with consumer sovereignty (that is, willingness to pay) even in a population with uniform incomes and preferences. The reason is that the amount most people are willing to pay for a given reduction in the probability of death is positively related to the *level* of the probability. Thus, a person facing almost certain death would usually be willing to pay a great deal for even a small increase in the chance of survival; that same person, facing a low probability of death, would not pay nearly as much for the same increase in survival probability. If one infers the "value of life" from the amount the person is willing to pay for the change in the probability of survival, it is clear that the value of life varies for the same individual, depending on the circumstances.

Imagine a cancer treatment program that costs $1 million per life saved, and another program to lower the probability of getting cancer that costs only $500,000 per life saved. People might be more willing to pay for the *treatment,* if sick, than to pay for the *prevention,* if well. This behavior is not necessarily irrational, nor need it be the result of some "death-denying" psychological quirk. We do not think it odd that a thirsty man will pay a large amount for a small drink of water if there is very little available, but is not willing to pay much for a drink when water is plentiful and he is not particularly thirsty.

The medical profession has been frequently criticized for failing to allocate resources so as to maximize the number of lives saved, but some of this criticism may be unjustified—at least in the sense that the emphasis on heroic efforts in life-threatening situations at the expense of preventive measures may be a reasonable response to consumer preferences. If we seek a health care system that does what people want it to do (regardless of whether that preference is expressed in the market or through political processes), we should expect considerable inequality at the margin in costs per life saved. To the extent that we deem this an undesirable outcome, the way to guard against it is to rule out the *possibility* of relatively high-cost interventions. If the intervention is unknown, society may, in some sense, be better off. For instance, suppose the very expensive cancer treatment did not exist; people might be more likely to avail themselves of the cancer prevention program. Perhaps even more to the point, suppose a project to develop a cancer treatment with the characteristics described above was being considered. It could be socially advantageous *not* to support the research, even though, once completed, the results would be used.

Government, family, and religion. The growth of government, the decline in importance of the family, and the weakening of traditional religion are three closely related factors that I believe have also contributed substantially to the growth of the health care industry. The growing importance of government will be discussed in detail in the next section. At this point I want to call attention to the fact that subsidization of health care by government induces additional demand. Nearly all health economists believe that the *price* elasticity of demand for care is smaller than one, but no one believes that it is zero. It follows, therefore, that a reduction in the price of care to the patient through public (or private) insurance increases the quantity demanded. To get some idea of the possible magnitude of this effect, let us assume that the total price (including money, time, and psychic costs) of care has been reduced by one-half as a result of government intervention, and let us also assume that the price elasticity of demand is −0.5. If nothing else changed, the increase in quantity demanded would be two-fifths. A decline in price of three-fourths with an elasticity of −0.28 would produce approximately the same change.[1] These examples suggest that the government's effect on price has probably been a major factor in increased utilization.

The effects of the decline of the family and of traditional religion are more difficult to quantify, but I offer a few examples to convey the flavor of the argument. Consider nursing homes, which are by far the fastest-growing component of the health care sector in the United States; their share of total spending climbed from less than 2 percent in 1960 to almost 8 percent in 1977. Nursing home expenditures now exceed spending for drugs or for dentists' services; the only larger categories are hospitals and physicians' services. But what is a nursing home and what services does it provide? I would argue that it provides very little that was not provided in the past at home by the family. Indeed, in some cases it does not provide as much. To be sure, the growth of nursing homes is attributable in part to growth in the relative number of the elderly. But more important, in my opinion, is the growth in female labor force participation and the mobility of the population. Elderly widows comprise the bulk of the nursing home population, and there has been a tremendous increase in the percentage of widows age 65 and over who live alone. In 1950 that figure was 25 percent; in 1976 it was 65 percent. True enough, rising income makes living alone possible and helps pay for nursing home care; however, a considerable amount of what we think of as an *increase* in health care is not an increase at all, but rather a substitute for care that was formerly provided within the family.

The same may be said about the growth of child care and many other services. Contrary to the assumption underlying the national income accounts, these services do not represent a completely new addition to the nation's output; they are in part simply a transfer from home production to the exchange economy. The rise of female labor force participation and the growth of service employment are bound together in a nexus of mutual reinforcement. Each is both cause and consequence of the other.

Not only does purchased medical care in part take the place of the family, but I believe that it is also frequently a modern substitute for religion. This is most obvious in the case of mental illness, and the similarity between psychiatry and religion has been frequently discussed. It needs to be emphasized, however, that many visits to physicians who are not psychiatrists are undertaken for reasons other than specific diagnostic or therapeutic intervention. The patient may be seeking sympathy, or reassurance, or help in facing death (his own or that of someone close to him). The patient may want to unburden himself to an authority figure who will keep his secrets confidential. There may be a desire to find someone to assume responsibility for a difficult decision, or there may be a need for validation of a course of action already decided upon. The ability to state "The doctor says I should (or shouldn't) do this" often is worth a great deal.

In an earlier day, priests, ministers, and rabbis met many of these demands. For some people they still do, but today many find a white coat more reassuring than a black one, a medical center more impressive than a cathedral. One striking change is in the customary site of death. In an earlier day dying was usually a private affair, attended by family and friends, and legitimized by priest or shaman or witch doctor. Today, in most Western nations, more than half of all deaths occur in hospitals. The physician is now our chief ambassador to death.

The analogy I have drawn between medical care and religion may be regarded as disparagement of care by those who share Marx's opinion of religion as the "opium of the people." But it is well to remember that in the very same passage Marx also called religion the "heart of a heartless world . . . the spirit of spiritless conditions." Despite the many criticisms that can be raised about medicine today—its high cost, its preoccupation with technology, its fragmentation into specialties and subspecialties—the truth is that for many people it is the "heart of a heartless world . . . the spirit of spiritless conditions."

The Growth of Government

The extension of the scope of government in the health field, like the extension of government in many other aspects of postindustrial society, is too obvious to require elaboration. I shall, therefore, move immediately to a consideration of possible explanations. One likely reason is the ever-increasing complexity of modern life. Consumers are now faced with a bewildering array of goods and services, and they feel a great need for information about them. There can be significant economies of scale in the provision of information about the quality of beef, the purity of drugs, and the safety of airlines; thus it may be more efficient to have a single agency, the government, provide that information.

Many observers also believe that urbanization and the growth of population and income have increased the importance of *externalities,* so that there is legitimate scope for the government to do more than simply provide information. An externality in health exists if Brown's consumption or other actions have favorable (or unfavorable) effects on Smith's health, but these effects are not reflected in the prices Brown faces and there is no feasible way for Brown and Smith to make a private arrangement that would cause Brown to take these effects into account. Familiar examples in this category include vaccinations (positive externality) and air pollution (negative externality). When externalities exist, the solution most economists prefer is to use subsidies or taxes to bring private costs (or benefits) into line with social costs (or benefits). Direct regulation that compels or forbids certain activities outright should generally be avoided unless the costs of administering the subsidies or taxes are unreasonably high.

A special kind of externality discussed by Calabresi and Bobbitt (1978) in their book *Tragic Choices* concerns society's unwillingness to "see" some of its members (typically the very poor) take unusual risks or pursue degrading activities. An example is the inhibition of the sale of kidneys or other organs by living donors. Calabresi and Bobbitt refer to society's unwillingness to countenance behavior that is an "affront to values" as a "moralism." Is it really "moral," however, to force an already disadvantaged person to be more disadvantaged by denying him the opportunity to do something which he thinks it is to his advantage to do? It seems to me that inhibitions of this character might more accurately be described as "aestheticisms"; that is, they are really matters of taste. The importance of taste and social conventions in these matters is nicely illustrated by the fact that society readily permits individuals to work in coal mines and to pursue other activities that are far more dangerous to health than is the absence of one kidney.

Or consider public policy with respect to abortions. At one time most governments forbade them. More recently we have seen governments encourage abortion through subsidies. Someday governments may compel an abortion rather than allow the birth of a horribly deformed child, either because the public does not want to have to support the child, or simply because it upsets people to see or hear about such a child. In each case the majority in society uses government to influence the behavior of others, always in the name of "morality," but probably because such behavior affects the majority through tangible or psychological externalities. One can speculate that such psychological externalities have grown in importance with urbanization, affluence, and, especially, more rapid, widespread, and vivid communications.

A pure libertarian, confronted with these alternative governmental policies toward abortion, would say: "A plague on *all* your houses." The libertarian position is that the government should not forbid abortions, should not subsidize them, should not compel them—in short, should do nothing to interfere with the right of the individual to do as he or she pleases—unless the action harms someone else. Ah, there's the rub. What constitutes harm? The libertarian would not allow murder, robbery, or rape. Many libertarians would go along with economically sound measures to deal with air pollution. But what if I find abortion, or prostitutes soliciting on the street, more offensive than air pollution, and most voters feel as I do? The distinction between physiological and psychological harm is rather fragile; the head is connected to the body, and we know that there are important interchanges between the psyche and the soma. This discussion illustrates the importance of widely shared values for the smooth functioning of a democratic society. As Tawney (1926) has written: "The condition of effective action in a complex civilization is cooperation. And the condition of cooperation is agreement, both to ends to which effort should be applied, and the criteria by which its success is to be judged."

In postindustrial society, governments clearly go far beyond providing information or dealing with obvious externalities. In the United States, especially, the government, in the name of health and safety, now undertakes detailed regulation and control of thousands of products and activities. One possible reason for the proliferation of government interventions is that they serve as a form of "precommitment" concerning certain kinds of behavior. In other words, Smith may vote for laws that force persons in Brown's circumstances to behave in ways contrary to Brown's preference in order to precommit himself (Smith) if his circumstances should change to those of Brown. Smith, then, might think that if he were to become poor he would be tempted to sell a kidney. He might therefore now vote to make such sales illegal in order to prevent himself from ever taking such action.

I believe that health insurance can in part be regarded as a form of precommitment; the insured is precommitting himself or herself to disregard price in making decisions about the utilization of care. Economists have had a great deal of difficulty explaining the popularity of "first dollar" coverage in health insurance policies. It is easy to see why risk-averse individuals might want to insure against large medical bills, but why would they want to bear the administrative costs and the excess utilization costs associated with insurance for small bills that they could pay out of their normal income? One possible answer is that they do not want money costs to influence their decisions about the utilization of care. *Compulsory* health insurance can be viewed as precommitment to buy insurance regardless of changes in income or other circumstances.

Conventional economic analysis regards precommitment as irrational; why should anyone ever want to gratuitously restrict his options? Economist Richard Thaler has suggested an answer: precommitment may be a rational strategy for dealing with problems of self-control (Shefrin and Thaler, 1977). Such problems can arise when there is tension between alternative behaviors that have very different implications for our welfare in the short and long run. For instance, in the short run I may get pleasure from smoking or from spending, but I also know that in the long run I will suffer from the effects of smoking or from a lack of savings. Thus I may precommit myself by taking a job where smoking is prohibited, and I may join a Christmas Club. The financial field offers numerous examples of precommitment strategies, including front-end loaded life insurance policies and mutual fund plans, passbook loans, and prepayment of real estate taxes to banks. Even installment buying has a precommitment aspect, as evidenced by the many consumers who pay high consumer loan interest rates while maintaining low-yielding savings accounts.

Government regulation may also be a strategy to reduce the opportunity to make decisions that turn out badly. Consider airline safety. Instead of the current practice of setting a single standard of safety, the government could merely provide information about the safety standards adhered to by different airlines and let individuals choose among airlines on the basis of safety, price, and so on. There are costs associated with making airlines safer; one could imagine consumers being offered a choice between a high price/high safety airline and a low price/low safety line. Conventional economics tells us that the larger the range of choice, the greater is consumer welfare. But many (perhaps most) people would not like to make this kind of choice; they prefer to have the Federal Aviation Authority set a single minimum "safe" standard that all scheduled airlines must meet. In doing so, people seek to minimize the regret or guilt that they might experience if there is a crash.

There has been some discussion in economics about the "costs" of decision making, but these costs have generally been assumed to be experienced in the process of *making* the decision, that is, acquiring the information and taking time to think about alternatives. Having the government set a single safety standard clearly reduces those costs. The point at issue here, however, is that there are psychic costs associated with having *made* a decision that turns out badly, and individuals may very well opt for government regulations that preclude such decisions.

The growth of government can also be viewed as a substitute for family or church as the principal institution assisting individuals who experience economic or social misfortune. Private insurance could conceivably do the same job, but problems of "free riders" (those who do not buy insurance and then need help anyway), adverse selection (the tendency for the poorer risks to buy the insurance), or excessive sales and administrative costs may make universal, compulsory programs the more sensible way to proceed. Moreover, a principal thrust of many government programs is to combine insurance with *redistribution*. Indeed, I believe that an unrelenting pressure for a more egalitarian society is one of the most important explanations for the growth of government in health and other areas.

The conditions of modern life seem to compel a more equal sharing of material goods and political power. In *Equality and Efficiency: The Big Tradeoff*, Arthur Okun (1975) assumes that this sharing occurs because people have a "preference" for equality. Perhaps some do, but it is also possible that many who have power and goods would rather not share them; their ability to maintain inequality, however, may vary with circumstances. It seems to me that, the more affluent and the more complex a society becomes, the more it depends on the willing, cooperative, conscientious efforts of the people who work in that society and the more difficult it is to obtain satisfactory effort through the use of force.

When the main task at hand consisted of hauling large blocks of stone from the river to the pyramid, it was a relatively simple matter to rope a dozen slaves together and use a whip and the threat of starvation to secure compliance. In feudal societies, the predominantly agricultural work force was kept in line despite huge inequalities in income through force, the need for protection, the limited mobility of the poor, and through the promise of heaven and the threat of hell. But when a nation's workers are airplane mechanics, teachers, and operating-room nurses, for example, it is clear that such techniques will not do. A few dissatisfied air traffic controllers can change the pace of a continent. Even such low-paid work as the changing of tires in a tire store involves considerable potential for danger and disruption. It would be very expensive to check every bolt on every wheel, but the management lives in fear that a few carelessly tightened bolts will allow a wheel to fall off and result in a million-dollar damage suit against the company. Furthermore, in the affluent postindustrial society virtually all persons live above a subsistence level—and will be maintained at above subsistence whether they work or not.

The problem of getting everyone to "go along" is compounded by the declining force of religion, nationalism, and other traditional control structures. Calls to serve "God and country" do not meet with as enthusiastic a response as they once did, whether that service is military or some onerous and not particularly rewarding civilian task. A weakening of hierarchical structures is evident wherever we look—in the family, in the church, in the school, in the workplace. Romantics of the Right yearn for a return to the "good old days," but such yearning is not likely to avail much against economic growth and technological change. As Norman Macrae (1976) has so aptly noted in *America's Third Century:* "It is pointless to say . . . that society must therefore return to being ruled by the old conventions, religious restrictions, craven obedience to the convenience of the boss at work. Individuals will not accept these restrictions now they see that wealth and the birth control pill and transport technology make them no longer necessary."

The preoccupation with equality, or the *appearance* of equality, is evident in many discussions about health. With respect to the British National Health Service, for instance, economists John Jewkes and Sylvia Jewkes (1963) have argued that it was created primarily in pursuit of the goal of equality. As noted in the previous section, the results of the NHS seem consistent with that view.

Or think of the buckets of ink that have been spilled over regional inequality in the physician/population ratio in Canada, the United States, and most other countries. In the United States, at least, this interminable discussion has proceeded without any evidence that health is adversely affected by a low physician/population ratio. Indeed, in the United States one cannot even show that the number of physician visits per capita is significantly lower in areas that have been identified as "medically underserved." Moreover, the oft-heard argument that an overall increase in the number of physicians will result in a reduction in regional inequality seems to be without empirical foundation.

The more one examines this issue, the more puzzling it appears. Nearly everyone says that regional inequality in physician supply is bad, but no one quite explains why. Nearly everyone says that it should be reduced, but not much is done about reducing it. For a long time in California, the state's political leaders voiced loud complaints about how difficult it was to get physicians to settle in rural areas, while at the same time setting fee schedules for Medi-Cal (Medicaid) patients that reimbursed rural physicians at a lower rate than their urban counterparts. In my view, national health insurance and other governmental interventions in health are best viewed as political acts undertaken for political and social objectives that are minimally related to the health of the population. This seems to be an inescapable conclusion from the evidence now available.

Theories of the Right and Left

The discussion of the proper role of government in society is central to the debate between the ideologues of the Right and the Left, a debate that seems to me to capture a degree of attention far in excess of the merits of the theories propounded by either side. The positions of the arch-conservatives and the radicals are usually clear-cut and often provocative. In my judgment, however, they are ultimately unsatisfactory either as analyses of how we have come to our present position or as prescriptions for where we ought to go from here. I shall try to illustrate my proposition with references to health and medical care, but I believe the same critique is valid in a more general framework.

I begin with the Right, and I admit at the outset that some of its favorite themes seem to have considerable value. For one thing, it is the Right that regularly reminds us of the efficiency of a *decentralized* price system as a mechanism for allocating scarce resources. Frankly, it is a shame that we need to be reminded of this; surely, theory and experience combine to teach us that the alternative (some sort of centralized control) will usually be much less efficient. Second, we should be indebted to the Right for reminding us, in the words of a Milton Friedman lecture title, of "the fragility of freedom." Accustomed as we are to freedom of speech, press, religion, and more, we are too prone to take them for granted—to imagine that they are the normal and expected state of affairs—rather than, as any comprehensive view of past or contemporary societies reveals, a precious exception. When conservatives insist that there are important complementarities between property rights and human rights, we ignore them at our peril.

So much for their good points; where does the Right go wrong? One big problem is that the Right, with the notable exception of Joseph Schumpeter (1942), seems to lack any plausible view of the historical development of society. This is nicely illustrated if one looks at the Right's analysis of the growth of national health insurance around the world. How does the Right deal with such a phenomenon? The first response (and often the last) is to castigate it as one more deplorable trend toward socialism. When pressed for an explanation of the trend, the Right offers two types of theories. First, there is the "people are stupid" explanation: the same people who are supposedly so knowledgeable when running businesses or choosing occupations or spending money are presumed foolish, irrational, or worse when they must make choices about government policy. This is not very convincing. If there is some widespread behavior that we do not understand, we should not automatically attribute it to the other fellow's ignorance or irrationality.

Not all conservatives subscribe to the "people are stupid" theory. A substantial number try to explain the growth of national health insurance and similar (in their view) misguided legislation as the triumph of special interests over the general public interest. Their research strategy is to identify the special groups that gain from policies that seem to result in a general welfare loss (and many economists believe national health insurance fits that category because it encourages excessive utilization). A second task is to figure out how the special groups are able to assert and maintain their interest over that of the majority. Sometimes this strategy is useful, but with respect to the growth of national health insurance, it has not been notably successful. Indeed, in the United States, one special interest group that has benefited greatly from Medicare and Medicaid has been the physicians, and they were in the forefront of the groups that opposed such legislation.

What the Right apparently cannot accept—but neither can it refute—is the hypothesis that national health insurance comes to developed countries not out of ignorance, not out of irrationality, not at the behest of narrowly defined special interest groups, but because most of the people want it, because it meets certain needs better than alternative forms of organization. That these needs are often political, social, and psychological rather than physiological is one of the principal themes of this chapter.

Another problem with the Right is its failure to apply its own economic reasoning to institutions and to goals. For instance, granted that the market is an efficient institution for allocating most goods and services, the extension of the market mechanism to all aspects of human society at the expense of other institutions such as the family may well run into diminishing returns. For the market to be most effective, it needs complementary inputs from other institutions, just as capital needs labor and land.

Or consider the Right's preoccupation with the goal of freedom. It is easy to agree that certain basic freedoms of thought and expression are essential to a good society, but it is more difficult to accept George Stigler's position that freedom should always dominate other goals. He writes (1958a; italics mine): "The supreme goal of the Western world is the development of the individual: the creation for the individual of a *maximum* area of personal freedom, and with this a corresponding area of personal responsibility." It seems odd to me that an economist would want to maximize personal freedom or any other single goal rather than to find an optimum balance among various goals. Surely the law of decreasing marginal utility must apply to freedom as well as to other goals, and one suspects that there is increasing marginal disutility to the personal responsibility that Stigler notes is a corollary of freedom. It is reasonable to suppose that there is some *combination* of freedom and responsibility that is optimal, although that optimum probably varies among individuals depending on their ability to benefit from freedom and to handle responsibility.

Let us turn now to the Left, and let us again begin on a positive note. We should be grateful to the Left for two reasons. First, it reminds us that a decentralized price system is not *always* the best way to allocate scarce resources. There are things such as externalities and transaction costs that may mean that some allocation problems are better handled by institutions other than the market. More important, the Left at its best makes a contribution by keeping before us a vision of a just society. Like the prophets of old, it scolds, it warns, it preaches. And so it should. The Left reaffirms in secular form the ancient cry for justice. The big problem with the Left is not its inability to identify important problems; it is its analysis of the causes and its proposed solutions that must give one pause. Who among us would not like to see a world free of war, poverty, racism, sexism, and ignorance? Or, to narrow it down to the field of health, who among us does not think that health is better than illness, life better than death? But to state worthwhile goals is one thing; to have some good ideas about how to reach them is another.

Consider leftist critiques of health and medical care. First, there is the naive reformist position, typified by, say, John Kenneth Galbraith (1958). According to this view, the problem is one of insufficient public funds: if only we had more hospitals, more physicians, more medical schools, and so on, the problem would be solved. This at a time when, in the United States, there is excess hospital capacity in every major metropolitan area, when general surgeons are carrying what they themselves agree is only 40 percent of a reasonable work load (and there is widespread suspicion that many of the operations should not be performed), and when iatrogenic illness (arising out of the medical care process itself) is a major problem! That so many on the Left can still believe so many shibboleths is a tribute to the triumph of ideology over analysis.

There is another type of leftist critique, however, which is slightly more sophisticated and far more radical. Far from simply prescribing "more medical care," these leftist critics argue that the "system" is at fault. The trouble, we are told, is that providers are oriented to profits rather than to health; that if only we made the system more "democratic," placed public health at top priority, put physicians on salaries, and so on, all would be well. Would it? Right now in the United States about 95 percent of the hospital industry is in the hands of nonprofit organizations, either public or private, yet the escalation in costs in these hospitals has been tremendous, and the emphasis on complex, esoteric technology great. When we look at other systems with other forms of organization and reimbursement, such as in England or Russia, do we see more emphasis on preventive medicine, more action on environmental health problems, more consumer control of the medical care process? The answer is overwhelmingly negative. Indeed, even in China and Cuba, which have done some fine things in delivering simple but effective medical care to the general population, a basic health problem like cigarette smoking is left virtually untouched. Some say this is because certain communist leaders are avid smokers, or because tobacco is an important crop. Whatever the reason, it is a strange way for these governments to fulfill their self-proclaimed responsibility for the health of the people.

Because the Left is so eager to attribute the problems of the world to capitalism, it ignores some basic observations about human behavior. Most of the health problems that it identifies existed before capitalism and persist in noncapitalist countries. Many problems arise from the conflict between health and other goals, rather than from the evil or selfish intent of physicians. Personal behavior and genetic endowment are far more important to health than is medical care—whatever the system. Even when medical care is relevant, health is rarely something one person can *give* to another. It comes, if at all, from the efforts of physician and patient working together, often in the face of uncertainty and fear.

One of the strongest generalizations warranted by a comparative study of medical care in modern nations is the inability of planning agencies, insurance funds, hospital boards, and other lay authorities to completely control the medical profession. In country after country, the introduction of national health insurance was marked by significant concessions to physicians with respect to methods and levels of reimbursement, procedures for reviewing the quantity and quality of care, geographic and specialty choice, and control over allied (competing?) professions.

What is the problem? In part, the power of physicians derives from their ability to withhold what is sometimes an essential service. A strike by physicians may not be as threatening as one by coal miners in winter, or bartenders on New Year's Eve, but it is not negligible. Emigration by physicians is a more distant, but probably more effective, threat against unacceptable pressure. Because medical skills are more easily transferred from one country to another than are those of most other professions, and because physicians earn a high income, their return from migration is large relative to costs.

In my opinion, more subtle factors are also at work. The effectiveness of medical care depends in considerable measure on a bond of mutual confidence between physician and patient. Too much external control can break that bond. Moreover, physicians, like priests or magicians, can fill their roles effectively only if they are set apart from the common run of mankind. A medical profession that was completely subservient to lay authority would be, in several respects, a less effective profession. This is not to say that fee-for-service reimbursement never leads to overutilization, or that licensure laws are completely in the public interest, or that present institutional arrangements are ideal. It is to say that many of the most difficult problems of health and medical care transcend particular forms of economic and political organization—a conclusion that the Left leaves out.

Concluding Remarks

What speculative generalizations can be drawn from a broad economic study of health and medical care in modern society? First, I am impressed by the widespread confusion between process and product, the tendency to identify medical care with health, even though the connection is a fairly limited one. I wonder if that same confusion does not exist in other aspects of society, for example, schooling vis-à-vis wisdom, litigation vis-à-vis justice, or police activity vis-à-vis public safety? In the case of medical care and national health insurance, it seems clear to me that institutions often serve purposes other than those that are explicitly articulated. From the health insurance of Bismarck's administration to the Professional Standards Review Organizations of Nixon's, we can see sharp differences between the stated and the actual intent of health legislation.

The growth of big government in modern society stands as a major challenge for social analysis. My reading of its role in health and medical care leads me to emphasize two factors: the decline of other institutions and the pressure for a more egalitarian society. It seems clear to me that the success of the market system in the Western world was attributable in no small measure to the existence of strong nonmarket institutions such as the family and religion. The fruits of the market system—science, technology, urbanization, affluence—are undermining these institutions, which were the foundations of the social order. Human beings need more than an abundance of material goods. They need a sense of purpose in life, secure relationships with other human beings, something or someone to believe in. With the decline of the family and of religion, the inability of the market system to meet such needs becomes obvious, and the state rushes in to fill the vacuum. But it does so imperfectly because it is so large and so impersonal.

The affluence and complexity of modern life also contribute to the pressure for more equality, and government is now the chief institution for undertaking redistributive functions. This is not to suggest that the pressure for equality is always met quickly and fully. On the contrary, much legislation is designed to give symbolic recognition of the ideal of equality, but does not involve significant redistribution. This is not necessarily to be condemned; a preoccupation with equality and the neglect of other goals can be socially harmful. It is useful to recall Lord Acton's comment on the French Revolution (1907): "The finest opportunity ever given to the world was thrown away because the passion for equality made vain the hope of freedom."

For all its weakness, the family is probably still the greatest single barrier to equality in postindustrial society. As long as mothers and fathers pass on to their offspring their own particular genetic endowment, their own special heritage and values, attempts to achieve complete equality will be frustrated. At some point we shall have to ask whether that last increment of equality is worth the loss of so valuable an institution as the family—one that can stand as a refuge from impersonal markets and authoritarian government.

Government also grows because the majority frequently sees no feasible alternative for dealing with the complexity and interdependence of modern life. Thus, it seems to me that the fulminations of the Right against the ever-increasing role of government are often misdirected. The constant assertions that this or that regulation or subsidy is irrational and inefficient often fall on deaf ears, because the majority does not see it that way. As I have tried to show with illustrations from health, some individual governmental interventions can perhaps be justified economically—because of economies of scale, or because of externalities (tangible or psychological), or as precommitment strategies, or as techniques for shifting responsibility, or as redistributive mechanisms introduced to buy social tranquillity. The point that I think needs emphasis is that the cumulative impact of the growth of government is to weaken (and ultimately destroy) other useful institutions, such as the market, family, and private associations of a religious, fraternal, and philanthropic character. Thus we should be wary of the constant expansion of government, and especially centralized government, not only because any particular proposed expansion is "inefficient"—it may well pass a comprehensive cost-benefit test for a majority of the population—but because there are other goals besides efficiency.

For me the key word is *balance,* both in the goals that we set and in the institutions that we nourish in order to pursue these goals. I value freedom *and* justice *and* efficiency, and economics tells me that I may have to give up a little of one goal to ensure the partial achievement of others. Moreover, I believe the best way to seek multiple goals is through a multiplicity of institutions—the market, government, the family, and others. No single institution is superior for all goals. Moreover, diversification, be it of institutions, genes, or security holdings, is the best assurance of stability and survival in the face of an uncertain future. Above all, we must avoid concentration of power. In the spirit of the lowered aspirations of our time, I conclude that, although diffusion of power may keep us from reaching Utopia, it also limits the harm that may befall us.

Recent years have witnessed numerous battles for control within and between health care institutions and professions. These battles are likely to intensify in the years ahead because of mounting economic pressures as well as changes in the social and technological framework within which physicians, hospital administrators, and other health professionals must function.

The economic pressures will be felt first by physicians because there is likely to be a drastic slowdown in the rate of growth of real health care expenditures per physician. These expenditures grew at 3.6 percent per annum between 1950 and 1980, but during the 1980s the rate of increase will probably be under 2.6 percent per annum and may be as low as 1.6 percent per annum (Fuchs, 1981a). The principal reasons for the slowdown are: (1) slow growth of the economy as a whole; (2) rapid growth in the number of physicians; and (3) a slowdown in the rate at which the health care sector increases its share of the gross national product.

The economy is likely to grow more slowly because of lagging productivity and because the labor force will not expand as rapidly as it did during the decades when female labor force participation was zooming and the baby boom of the 1950s was reaching working age. With respect to the number of physicians, there has been some discussion recently about reducing the size of medical school classes, but in most instances this is still just talk. It is no easier to turn off the education pipeline of physicians than it is to turn it on; thus a rapid increase in the number of practicing physicians by 1990 seems almost inevitable.

To be sure, even if the economy as a whole slows down and the number of physicians inreases, health care expenditures per physician could still grow rapidly if the health care sector acquires more and more resources from the rest of the economy. This could happen—if some highly effective, highly expensive new technologies appear—but it seems to me unlikely that it will. Resistance to rapid expansion of government spending for health care is already very great, both in the form of the public's reluctance to pay higher taxes and also in the increased competition within government from other agencies fighting for their share of public funds. Private health care spending is also being watched more carefully, with growing numbers of business firms becoming more conscious of health care costs and other groups in the community asking what they can do to hold down the rate of growth of health expenditures.

Suppose health care expenditures per physician do increase more slowly. Why should that matter? It will matter critically for physicians, because it is these expenditures that determine what they can do for their patients in terms of hospitalization, tests, drugs, and other elements of care. Equally important, these expenditures determine the physician's own income. Once this becomes apparent I believe that physicians, in their own self-interest, will give more thought to how they can influence the overall rate of growth of health care expenditures and, in particular, how they can hold down the nonphysician portion of these expenditures. Given a limit on total health care spending, physicians' incomes will depend heavily on their success in slowing the rate of growth of spending for hospitals, drugs, and similar items.

Thus, not out of ideology, not as a consequence of exhortations from economists or politicians, but rather in pursuit of their own self-interest, physicians will be attracted to modes of medical practice that are conducive to holding down the growth of expenditures. Many physicians are already practicing in such modes—prepaid group practices, independent practice associations, primary care networks—and many others will join in the future. Furthermore, new kinds of organizations and new modes of practice will develop to compete with those that are already in place.

The key feature of all these modes is physician-centered control of, and responsibility for, the *total* health care bill. It is the total bill that really matters to the taxpayer, to the patient, and to the insurance carrier. And, in the end, it will be the total health care bill that is going to matter to physicians in terms of preserving and enhancing their earning power. I believe that it is inevitable that the American medical care delivery system is going to become more *organized* and more *competitive* as a consequence of these forces.

The intensification of competition has been forecast, hailed, and decried by many observers. Competition, of course, can take many different forms. One form has been outlined (and deplored) by Dr. Arnold S. Relman, editor of *The New England Journal of Medicine*, in a stimulating article entitled "The New Medical-Industrial Complex" (1980). Relman discusses the rise of for-profit institutions in the health field, especially in hospitals, and particularly the large chains of hospitals. He also discusses nursing homes, clinical laboratories, kidney dialysis centers, and home health services—all of which operate under a for-profit structure. Relman expresses great concern about this development, charging the for-profit settings with overutilization of care, fragmentation of delivery, overemphasis on medical technology, and "cream skimming"—the practice of treating only the healthiest patients. Relman is also worried about what he terms the "undue influence" on health policy that might be exerted by these for-profit companies and about the ethical problems that the profit motive presents to physicians.

Dr. Relman rendered a great service in publishing this article, but I believe that the facts of the case lead to a somewhat different set of inferences. It seems to me that the important distinctions are not between the for-profit and the nonprofit modes, but along other lines—lines that will shape the emerging battles for control of health care.

The most significant battleline emerging is that between practicing physicians and management. By that I mean the inevitable clash between a fiercely independent profession and a management structure that seeks to gain firmer control over what doctors do. Traditionally, health care has been controlled by physicians, sociologist Elliot Friedson called it "professional dominance." Any analyst who looks at health care from the outside is always in awe of the extent to which, until recently, physicians have controlled the medical enterprise.

That control rests on many things. It originated in the mystery and in the fears that are associated with illness and dying. It is fed by technology. And it is supplemented by government regulation and by licensing, which is a grant of monopoly power that restricts the practice of medicine to physicians. This control is being eroded, however, by the development of large institutions that require vesting significant power in the hands of management if the institution is to function successfully.

The erosion occurs in nonprofit and for-profit institutions alike, but the latter are newer, larger, and seem more threatening to physicians. Consider the Hospital Corporation of America (HCA), which owns or manages some 350 hospitals throughout the United States and has its fingers in a large number of other health care enterprises. HCA reported the following results for the first *quarter* of 1982: revenues totaled $874 million, up 60 percent from the same period of 1981; net income increased 55 percent to $48 million; and earnings per share increased 32 percent. The national scope of HCA's growth is impressive, too. The 1982 first-quarter report stated: "Growth through acquisitions continued during the first three months of 1982 with the addition of several general and one psychiatric hospital with a total of 900 beds. The newly acquired hospitals are located in Florida, Georgia, Kentucky, North Carolina, South Carolina, Tennessee, and Texas. HCA's management of hospitals owned by others also increased during the quarter, with new agreements signed in Arizona, Maine, Mississippi, New Mexico, Pennsylvania, South Carolina, and Texas."

HCA is the largest of its kind, but it is not unique. There are many similar organizations that reflect the emergence of a new era in American medicine. Why is the power of management growing? Why are larger institutions becoming more important? Three main ingredients are involved.The first is the need for capital to finance growth. As medical technology grows more complex, capital requirements for practicing medicine, both in and out of the hospital, grow exponentially. Larger organizations have better, quicker access to capital markets and can finance the technologically intensive medical care of the 1980s on more favorable terms.

A second reason is the growth of government regulation and bureaucracy. Larger organizations have more effective mechanisms for dealing with bureaucratic phenomena: they have the contacts in government, and they employ the counterparts to the reimbursement specialists and the regulators that staff the government agencies. A recent conversation with a physician who practices in a small town in Arizona illustrates this point. He told me that the hospital where he admits patients recently entered into a management contract with one of the large for-profit hospital corporations. When I asked him what this management corporation did for him, he responded, "It's very simple. When there's a problem getting reimbursement from Medicare, when the reimbursements are coming in slowly or there are difficulties of one kind or another, they can deal with it. The management company has a team of experts, some of whom previously worked for the reimbursing agency. They know how to push the buttons, they know whom to call, and they keep the process flowing. When problems of accreditation come up, they know how to get the approvals through, they know how to do the paperwork. In other words, they are good at things that do not have much to do with patient care or efficiency, but rather with the regulatory framework."

The third reason for the growth of management is what I would call a need for the true skills of management—the ability to organize complex technology, bringing together different people from different professions to deliver service as a team. Every large organization, for-profit or nonprofit, needs these skills. Physicians, on the whole, do not like this trend toward larger, management-dominated enterprises; most would prefer to maintain physician dominance over health care. But it simply will not be possible for physicians to dominate medicine in the future as they have in the past. I hope that physicians and management will work out compromises, will understand the legitimate functions and the legitimate concerns of each, and rather than engaging in bloody battle, will develop a unified and comprehensive approach that better meets the needs of patients and society.

Control of medicine, as far as I can see, will never again belong completely to physicians. If this is the case, physicians should decide what parts of the system are most important to them, what parts they would prefer to control in the future. They should look around to determine where doctors have been particularly successful in working out viable arrangements with management. A good example of successful accommodation—where physicians have remained in charge of what is important to them—is the Mayo Clinic in Rochester, Minnesota. A visitor to Mayo cannot help but be impressed by the extent to which the organization has worked out the necessary compromises between the practicing physicians and management. To an outsider, the organization seems to work smoothly. Significant power and authority are vested in management, but they are shared with the practicing physicians. Perhaps the most interesting dimension of this situation is revealed by an exchange I had with one of my students. I was making the point in a lecture that Mayo had struck these compromises between its physicians and the management when a physician in my class, who had done a residency at Mayo, stopped me and said: "Professor Fuchs, you have that one all wrong. The physicians at Mayo perceive that they still have the power." I smiled and responded, "Thank you. That's just the point I am making."

Mayo is a $250-million-a-year operation, and it runs smoothly, efficiently, and profitably. It is not possible for a $250-million-a-year operation to be run smoothly, efficiently, and profitably by practicing physicians. But if the physicians perceive that they still have the power, that is great. It is great because it demonstrates that Mayo physicians still believe they command what is important to them; they do not feel that someone is trying to tell them how to practice medicine. I hope other organizations will be as successful as this one in working out compromises and avoiding this battle.

There is another battle emerging that superficially seems to be related to the for-profit/nonprofit distinction, but really reflects a larger set of issues. This battle pits *university* physicians and hospitals against *community* physicians and hospitals. The university medical centers are facing very difficult times. Biomedical research funds are flat or falling; medical education support is dwindling, and the university medical centers are looking increasingly to patient care to shore up their revenues. At the same time, these centers dread the notion of having to compete for patients in a tight economic environment. In many cases their concern is well justified. When it comes to delivering bread-and-butter care, the chances are that the community physicians and community hospitals can render this care less expensively.

On the other hand, the community hospitals and their affiliated physicians also feel threatened. They see these gleaming medical centers, big and powerful, and they see the famous specialists, and they wonder how the medical centers will use their power, and whether it will be at the expense of the community physicians and hospitals.

The conflict is exacerbated by the proliferation of tertiary types of medical care—activities at the frontier of medicine— which should be performed primarily in medical centers but which increasingly are being undertaken in community settings. This proliferation frequently is bad economics and bad medicine. Eventually, this conflict is going to produce a need for better understanding, a need for compromise, a need to realize the legitimate concerns of each part of the health care enterprise. I am particularly concerned, for example, about what will happen to medical research. Without research, without advancing the state of knowledge, medicine will begin to run up against blank walls. There is only a limited amount of improvement in health that can be purchased by increasing the number of physicians or by adding hospital beds. The great advances have always come from figuring out better and newer ways of preventing or treating disease. Somehow there have to be enough funds generated in the medical centers to support research and to employ faculty who are actively engaged in research.

Society would benefit from the evolution of a medical care system where academic centers concentrated on research, teaching, and tertiary care, and did only as much primary and secondary care as was necessary for them to carry out their principal missions. At the same time, complex tertiary care should be limited primarily to regional medical centers because such centers can provide the specialized services more efficiently, offer higher-quality care, and carry out the research that should accompany all innovations in medicine.

In the preceding discussion of two emerging battles for control of health care, government has not been one of the chief contestants. This may come as a surprise, since the battle for control of health care is often depicted as one of medicine against government. However, this simply is not the case, at least in these two battles. Medicine currently has a little respite from the hot and heavy breath of government. Unfortunately, the medical profession is not using this breathing space as creatively and as constructively as it might. For a time in the late 1970s, physicians were running scared, largely in fear of a government takeover of medical care. When the proregulation forces were in power, organized medicine was more willing to talk about competition, more willing to consider major changes in the system. After the 1980 election, the reaction among medical leaders was, "Let's go back to business as usual." This is a shame, because even though the regulatory threat went away for a time, medicine should not think that it has disappeared forever. It could come back quickly and heavily. Indeed, a case could be made that it already has, in the form of Medicare and Medicaid budget cuts. Medical leaders should use this breathing space to demonstrate real leadership, to make unnecessary the imposition of centralized controls and tighter regulation later in this decade.

There is one other battle that may emerge in the years ahead. The likelihood of struggle on this issue is less certain than for the two already discussed, but there is enough of a possibility to merit some consideration. This battle will pit physicians against physicians, and the basis for it was nicely delineated by Dr. Benson Roe in an article entitled, "The UCR Boondoggle: A Death Knell for Private Practice?" (1981). Roe, an experienced California surgeon, made one central point that every physician is aware of: there is a serious imbalance in the fees physicians receive for different types of work. When a new medical procedure comes along, it is usually reimbursed at a high relative fee. According to Roe, the high fee is justified at first because there is a tremendous amount of cost, effort, and risk involved in the early stages of developing a new procedure. Roe, a cardiac surgeon, describes what was involved in doing those early operations. A high relative fee was justified. But then what happens? The procedure becomes routine, or certainly more routine than it was. The volume grows enormously, unit costs decline, but unlike almost any other industry with this pattern of development, the fee remains relatively high. At some point any physician doing that procedure on a reasonably full-time basis earns a fortune. Of course, not all do because the high fees attract more physicians than are needed to perform the procedure, and they cannot all maintain full work loads.

Sometimes these specialists do not even have half-workloads or one-third workloads, so they do not derive huge incomes, but the cost to the patient and to the taxpayer and, indeed, to society from these disproportionately high fees remains. A few words should be added to complete the picture. Many physicians work hard practicing high-quality care that is *not* procedure-oriented and that does not generate high relative fees. They put in long hours in return for moderate incomes. At some point, the competitive squeeze I discussed earlier could result in confrontations between the different kinds of physicians; that is, there may be a battle within medicine itself between specialists who command large fees for the technology-driven medicine they practice and generalists who render high-quality care that is not procedure-oriented. Again, government would be largely a bystander in this battle, unless it uses the battle among physicians to strenghen its own control over all of them.

In other countries that have had major changes in health legislation, such as the United Kingdom and Canada, one of the techniques that the politicians employed was to turn physicians against each other. The government can create splits within the medical community, play off one type of physician against another, and give one a better deal than the other. It will be important, therefore, for physicians to be attentive to this potential battle within the profession and try to deal constructively with it before it destroys them.

In conclusion, physicians face the likelihood of several unpleasant, unrewarding battles for control of health care. No matter how they are resolved, the next ten years are not likely to be as pleasant as the last thirty. Things are going to be different. A realistic approach for physicians, one that they often recommend to patients, is "Learn to live with it."

Once physicians and other health care specialists understand the reasons for conflict and change, their best hope is to work out appropriate compromises. Let practicing physicians concentrate on treating patients and let management concentrate on managing. Let academic physicians in medical centers concentrate on teaching, research, and tertiary care with only as much primary and secondary patient care as is necessary to perform these functions well, and let community physicians concentrate on less intensive forms of care. Unless the necessary compromises are struck, American medicine will be consumed by conflict in the years to come, and patients and society will be the major sufferers.

Though Much Is Taken

Less than one score years ago this nation brought forth a new system of financing health care for the elderly—Medicare. This system, conceived as part of a broad thrust toward a "Great Society" and dedicated to the proposition that high-quality medical care should be freely available to all persons age 65 and over, is now the subject of intense reexamination. It is altogether fitting and proper that this be done. The rapid rate of growth of health care expenditures, the growing resistance to further increases in governmental taxes or deficits, and the changing circumstances of the elderly make this an appropriate time to ask (and attempt to answer) basic questions about the economic and social forces that affect this age group and this program.

Projections of Medicare outlays and revenues indicate very large future deficits in the hospital insurance trust fund and the supplementary medical insurance trust fund. A wide range of possible solutions to this problem have been proposed, including modification of benefits, changes in methods of reimbursement, and discovery of new sources of funds. This chapter attempts to place the Medicare issue in a broad context by identifying major economic and social trends that concern the elderly and briefly considering the causes and consequences of these trends. I do not discuss Medicare directly, but the questions raised and the data presented will, I hope, contribute to the formulation of improved public policies regarding health care for the elderly.

I begin by supposing that a policymaker with a strong interest in the elderly had disappeared in 1950 and had only recently returned. What would he or she most need to know about the elderly with respect to their current situation and the changes of recent decades? In my judgment there are six areas that are of critical importance: the number of elderly; their health status; use of medical care; labor force participation; income; and their living arrangements. I shall discuss the most dramatic changes in these areas during the past three decades, indicate how current policies may have contributed to these changes, and suggest the need for reconsideration of those policies.

The Number of Elderly

Almost every article and book about the elderly begins by noting that the percentage of the population over age 65 has grown appreciably over time. Why is there so much interest in this percentage? First, it is assumed that most men and women aged 65 and over are not at work; therefore, part of the working generation's output must be transferred to the elderly through Social Security payments, private pension plans, direct provision of services, or other means. The higher the percentage of elderly, the greater is the amount that must be transferred. Second, it is assumed that health deteriorates with age, and that the consumption of medical care increases. Furthermore, it is argued that even though the decline in labor income, the deterioration in health, and the increased use of medical care are, for the most part, foreseeable, many elderly cannot or do not adequately provide for old age by saving or by acquiring a health insurance policy when young that would protect them later in life. (Imperfections in insurance markets, problems of adverse selection, and high administrative and sales costs are said to contribute to this outcome.) Finally, the rise in the number of elderly increases their political power. This increase, coming at a time when economic resources are often allocated through the ballot box rather than the marketplace, raises the possibility of bitter political conflict between the elderly and other groups in society.

The definition of old age—that is, the age of eligibility for retirement and Medicare benefits—is a critical variable in the development of viable programs for the elderly. Consider, for instance, a hypothetical population in which the birth rate equals the death rate and everyone dies at 80 years of age. If every man and woman works from ages 20 to 65 and then retires, the ratio of workers to retirees will be three to one. If, however, the retirement age is 70, there will be five workers for every retiree, thus permitting a substantial increase in benefits or decrease in taxes, or both.

It is conventional to define the elderly with reference to the number of years since birth, but this is largely a concession to administrative convenience rather than the logical result of a closely reasoned argument. Individuals "age" at very different rates, and, in theory at least, the elderly could be defined in terms of years until death, for example, those men and women who will die within some specified time. For instance, we could look at the proportion of the population that will die within one year (the crude death rate). According to this measure, the proportion has *decreased* since 1950. To be sure, it does not make much sense to define infants, children, and young adults as "elderly," even if they are close to death. But a count of persons aged 65 and over who will die within the next several years is informative because much of the interest in the elderly revolves around their need for medical care and other special services. From a different perspective, a count of persons aged 65 and over who are not in the labor force is revealing because it shows the portion of the population that must live on transfer payments, income from capital, or dissaving.

These alternative views of who is old yield different trends in the relative importance of the elderly, as may be seen in Table 16.1. The first row shows the familiar increase in the proportion of the population aged 65 and over, from 8.2 percent in 1950 to 11.3 percent in 1980. The second row, however, shows that if we define the elderly as persons aged 65 and over who will die within five years, this number as a percentage of the total population has increased relatively slowly since 1950 and has hardly grown at all since 1965. Sharp declines in age-specific death rates at ages 65 and above have offset the effect of the increase shown in the first row. On the other hand, if we define the elderly as persons aged 65 and over who are out of the labor force (row 3), that proportion has grown even more rapidly than the percentage over age 65.

Table 16.1 The "elderly" as a proportion of the total population: Alternative definitions

Definition	1950 (%)	1965 (%)	1980 (%)
Age 65 and over	8.2	9.5	11.3
Age 65 and over and within 5 years of death[a]	2.6	3.0	3.1
Age 65 and over and not in the labor force	6.2	7.9	10.0

Sources: U.S. Bureau of the Census, *Current Population Reports*, series P-25, no. 310, June 1965, table 1; no. 519, April 1974, table 2; no. 917, July 1982, table 2 (Washington). U.S. Bureau of the Census, *Historical Statistics of the United States, Colonial Times to 1970* (Washington, 1975), pt. 1, series B189-192. U.S. Bureau of the Census, *Statistical Abstract of the United States, 1982–83* (Washington, 1982), table 109. Employment and Training Administration, *Employment and Training Report of the President, 1981* (Washington, 1981), table A-2.

a. Estimated by author.

Health Status

One of the big surprises of recent years has been the sharp reduction in age-specific mortality of older persons. Between 1965 and 1980 life expectancy at age 65 jumped from 14.6 to 16.4 years. This was a much bigger increase than was expected, based on extrapolation of either the 1935–1965 or 1950–1965 trends (see Table 16.2). The improvement is attributable primarily to a decrease in the risk of death from heart disease or cerebrovascular disorders (strokes), as may be seen in Table 16.3. Why death rates from these causes have plummeted is not well understood. Analysts who are technologically inclined attribute most of the reduction to better control of hypertension, special coronary care units in hospitals, open-heart surgery, and similar medical innovations. Other observers credit changes in diet, smoking, exercise, and other aspects of personal behavior. We do not know the true explanation; there is probably some validity to both points of view.

Are people escaping fatal heart attacks and strokes only to spend more years in poor health? This question is difficult to study because measures of morbidity and disability lack the objectivity of mortality statistics, but in my judgment the answer is no. Restricted-activity days and bed-disability days per hundred persons aged 65 and over were about the same in 1980 as in 1965 (U.S. Bureau of the Census, 1982, p. 119). The percentage of persons reporting activity limitations due to chronic

Table 16.2 Life expectancy at age 65, selected years 1935 to 2000

	1935	1950	1965	1980	2000
Actual	12.5	13.9	14.6	16.4	—
Predicted from 1935–1950 trend	—	—	15.5	—	—
Predicted from 1935–1965 trend	—	—	—	15.8	—
Predicted from 1950–1965 trend	—	—	—	15.3	—
Predicted from 1935–1980 trend	—	—	—	—	18.5
Predicted from 1950–1980 trend	—	—	—	—	18.3
Predicted from 1965–1980 trend	—	—	—	—	19.1

Sources: National Center for Health Statistics, *Health, United States, 1982* (Washington, December 1982), table 10. National Center for Health Statistics, *Vital Statistics of the United States, 1965* (Washington, 1967), Mortality, pt. A, table 5-4. U.S. Bureau of the Census, *Historical Statistics of the United States, Colonial Times to 1970* (Washington, 1975), pt. 1, series A-133. L. Dublin, *Health Progress 1936–1945: A Supplement to Twenty-Five Years of Health Progress* (New York: Metropolitan Life Insurance Company, 1948), table 6. U.S. Bureau of the Census, *Statistical Abstract of the United States 1982–83* (Washington, 1982), p. 71.

conditions rose somewhat from 1970 to 1980, but it is doubtful that this is the result of greater morbidity. For instance, the percentage of elderly persons reporting hypertension without heart involvement rose from 6.4 to 13.1 (U.S. Bureau of the Census, 1982, p. 121), but it is unlikely that hypertension actually increased. Indeed, direct measures of blood pressure among

Table 16.3 Age-specific death rates from heart and cerebrovascular diseases and other causes, 1965 and 1980

Age	Cause	Deaths per 100,000		Change, 1965 to 1980 (percent per annum)
		1965	1980	
65–74	Heart and cerebrovascular diseases	2,057	1,433	−2.4
	Other causes	1,606	1,535	−0.3
75–84	Heart and cerebrovascular diseases	5,261	4,065	−1.7
	Other causes	3,098	3,113	0.0
85 and over	Heart and cerebrovascular diseases	13,256	9,229	−2.4
	Other causes	6,813	5,261	−1.7

Source: National Center for Health Statistics, *Health, United States, 1982* (Washington, December 1982), tables 9, 16, 19.

the elderly over the same period show declines in average levels and a large decline in the percentage of the population aged 65 to 74 with systolic pressure of 160 or more or diastolic pressure of 95 or more (National Center for Health Statistics, 1981, 1982a). Taking all the available mortality and morbidity data into account, I conclude that the health status of the elderly at any given age has improved in recent decades, and that this improvement is primarily the result of lowered incidence or severity of heart disease and cerebrovascular disease.

Death rates from all other causes at ages 65 to 84 were virtually the same in 1980 as in 1965. This relative stability presents a major puzzle, since during those years Medicare substantially improved access to health care for the elderly, especially the poor. Moreover, there were many significant medical advances including new drugs, improved surgical procedures, and enhanced diagnostic techniques. It is difficult to believe that these achievements had no beneficial effect. Age-adjusted death rates from malignant neoplasms (cancer) actually rose between 1965 and 1980 among the elderly, possibly as a result of increases several decades ago in cigarette smoking and environmental hazards. It is encouraging to note that cancer mortality has declined for males aged 35 to 44; perhaps similar declines will begin to show up at older ages as the cohorts with fewer cigarette smokers reach that point in the life cycle.

Will life expectancy at older ages continue to increase at a rapid rate? Some experts say no, arguing that there is a biologically determined average limit for the species of about 85 years (Fries, 1980). Other observers contend that recent large declines in the death rate for the 85-and-over group is evidence against the existence of that limit (Schneider and Brody, 1983). Both groups agree that additional declines in mortality at ages 65 to 84 are possible or even likely; it would, therefore, be prudent to consider the possibility of such declines in planning future programs for the elderly.

Health Care Utilization

The role of additional medical care in improving the health of the elderly is a matter of some dispute. What is beyond dispute is the increased consumption of medical services by the elderly. Between 1965 and 1981 there was a large increase in health expenditures at all age levels, but the *share* accounted for by persons aged 65 and over jumped from 23.8 percent to 32.7 percent. This shift has helped to fan the Medicare financial crisis; it is important, therefore, to examine it in some detail. Two factors are responsible for this increased consumption, and they have been about equal in importance: first, the *number* of elderly grew more rapidly than the rest of the population; second, the change in *per capita* health expenditures by the elderly outpaced the rate for persons under age 65 (see column 1 of Table 16.4). The relative importance of these factors was not the same among the subperiods, however, as may be seen in columns 2–4. Not surprisingly, per capita expenditures among the elderly rose rapidly in the years immediately after the enactment of Medicare (1965–1970). From 1970 to 1976, per capita expenditures rose at about the same rate for both age groups; divergent trends in population accounted for nearly all of the differential change in expenditures. During the period 1976–1981, however, a large differential in the growth of per capita expenditures again emerged. This gap, combined with a continuing difference in population trends, resulted in a total differential change in expenditures of 3.8 percent per annum. This was larger than the difference between the elderly and the rest of the population in the five years immediately following the introduction of Medicare!

The last eight rows of Table 16.4 provide additional detail regarding the surge of spending on the elderly. We see that there was a very sharp *deceleration* in public spending on persons under age 65, while the trend increased slightly for the elderly. Private spending, on the other hand, held steady for persons under 65 and accelerated sharply for those over that age. Expenditures for physicians' services experienced the most rapid increase among the elderly.

What accounts for these divergent trends? One possibility is that increasing competition among physicians for patients led more of them to concentrate on the older men and women in their practice. Another possibility is that the new medical and surgical interventions have been particularly applicable to older persons. These speculations indicate why it is so difficult to predict expenditures on medical care, either in the aggregate or for particular age groups or particular types of service. Sudden advances in medical technology—new drugs, new diagnostic

Table 16.4 Rates of change of health care expenditures, by age, 1965–1981 (percent per annum)

Age group		1965–81 (1)	1965–70 (2)	1970–76 (3)	1976–81 (4)
Real[a] *health care*	65+	8.0	9.2	6.9	8.2
expenditures	<65	5.3	6.6	5.0	4.4
	Differential	2.7	2.6	1.9	3.8
Population	65+	2.2	1.7	2.4	2.4
	<65	0.9	1.0	0.9	0.9
	Differential	1.3	0.7	1.5	1.5
Real[a] *health care*					
expenditures	65+	5.8	7.5	4.5	5.8
per capita	<65	4.3	5.6	4.1	3.5
	Differential	1.5	1.9	0.4	2.3
Public	65+	10.5	21.8	5.3	5.7
	<65	7.2	11.3	6.9	3.5
Private	65+	1.6	−4.3	3.0	6.2
	<65	3.5	4.1	3.1	3.5
Physicians	65+	5.5	5.3	4.2	7.5
	<65	4.1	5.3	3.4	3.9
Hospitals	65+	6.8	9.4	5.4	6.2
	<65	5.8	8.3	5.3	4.0

Sources: U.S. Bureau of the Census, *Current Population Reports,* series P-25, no. 519, April 1974, able 2; no. 917, July 1982, table 2 (Washington). Council of Economic Advisers, *Economic Report of he President, 1982* (Washington, 1982), table B-3. C. R. Fisher, Differences by Age Groups in Health Care Spending, *Health Care Financing Review* 1 (4), 1980, pp. 65–90, table A. Provisional data from he Health Care Financing Administration.
a. Adjusted for inflation by the gross national product deflator.

techniques, new surgical procedures—can dramatically alter utilization. In addition, modifications in insurance coverage, in reimbursement methods, or in the number of physicians can alter the balance of demand and supply, thus inducing changes in the way physicians treat patients and the way patients use physicians. Whatever the cause, the upsurge in per capita expenditures of the elderly is a major factor in the prospective deficits in Medicare.

Does Utilization Rise with Age?

Analysts interested in projecting future health care utilization by the elderly have frequently noted that the age distribution

Table 16.5 Reimbursement per Medicare enrollee by age and sex, 1976 (in dollars)

	Actual			Adjusted for survival status		
Age group	All (1)	Men (2)	Women (3)	All (4)	Men (5)	Women (6)
67–68	518	578	471	624	654	595
69–70	555	613	511	649	667	630
71–72	603	674	551	679	704	660
73–74	657	717	613	712	713	705
75–79	736	793	699	732	716	742
80–84	818	854	798	717	679	741
85 +	866	937	832	595	594	595

Source: Health Care Financing Administration, Office of Research and Demonstrations, *Health Care Financing Program Statistics* (Baltimore, August 1982), Medicare Summary, Use and Reimbursement by Person, 1976–1978, pp. 53, 61. Adjusted expenditures calculated by author.

within the group aged 65-and-over is shifting toward the older ages, and that utilization (as reflected by Medicare reimbursements) rises steadily with age (see the first three columns of Table 16.5). Under the assumption that the cross-sectional age-spending relationship holds constant over time, the effect of the change in age distribution is estimated by applying the cross-sectional data on age-specific expenditures to the change in the age distribution.

Although this procedure is widely used, implicitly if not explicitly, it is incorrect. To the extent that the change in the age distribution is the result of rising life expectancy (that is, falling age-specific death rates), the cross-sectional differences in expenditures by age *overestimate* the changes that would result from an aging population. Health care spending among the elderly is not so much a function of time since birth as it is a function of time to death. The principal reason why expenditures rise with age in cross section (among persons aged 65 and over) is that the proportion of persons near death increases with age. Expenditures are particularly large in the last year of life and, to a lesser extent, in the next to last year. Among Medicare enrollees in 1976, the average reimbursement for those in their last year of life was 6.6 times (and in their next to last year 2.3 times) as large as for those who survived at least two years (Lubitz and Prihoda, 1982). As age-specific death rates fall over time, there will be fewer people in the last year of life in any age category, and this will tend to reduce age-specific health care expenditures.

Age-sex–specific expenditures adjusted for age-sex differences in death rates can be calculated by a method analogous to the indirect method of calculating age-sex–adjusted death rates. Suppose that each person's expenditures depended only on his survival status, for example, last year of life, next to last year, or "survivor." We can estimate a "predicted" expenditure for each age-sex group by multiplying the proportion in each survival status by the all-group average expenditure for each survival status and summing across the three statuses. The higher the death rate of the group, the higher would be its predicted expenditures. The ratio of actual to predicted expenditures for a group tells us whether expenditures are relatively high or low after adjusting for its death rate. This ratio multiplied by the average expenditure for all groups yields the adjusted expenditure for the group.[1]

As may be seen in the last three columns of Table 16.5 and in Figure 16.1, adjustment for age-sex differences in survival status eliminates most of the age-related increase in expenditures, especially the very high expenditures in the group aged 85-and-over. It also eliminates the excess of male over female expenditures at given ages. The only reason why older men use more medical care than older women at any given age is because a higher proportion of the men are in their last year of life. I do not claim that there is *no* effect of aging on health care utilization apart from the proximity to death, but much of the apparent effect is attributable to the relationship between age and mortality. This observation would be of little consequence if mortality rates were constant over time, but they are not. Between 1965 and 1978 the age-adjusted death rate of persons aged 65 and older fell from 65 per 1,000 to 53 per 1,000. If age-specific death rates continue to fall at this rate, 75-year-olds in 1987 will face the same probability of death as 71-year-olds faced in 1965.

How much health care will 75-year-olds utilize in 1987? The answer will depend on many factors, including changes in medical technology, the strengthening or weakening of family support systems, and revisions in Medicare reimbursement policies.

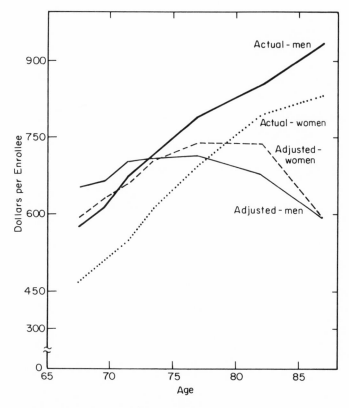

Figure 16.1 Medicare reimbursement per enrollee by age and sex, actual and adjusted for survival status, 1976.

But to the extent that fewer 75-year-olds will be in the last or next to last year of life, a simple extrapolation from past utilization of 75-year-olds is inappropriate.

Kenneth G. Manton (1982, p. 205) reaches a similar conclusion from a model that emphasizes the distinction between the hypothetical age trajectory of mortality risk for individuals and the age trajectory for a cohort. He writes: "As mortality rates decline at a given age, there would be some compensating decline in the rate of utilization of certain health services (e.g., nursing home care) before that age. In fact, such models might be used as the basis for improving projections of health service utilization by providing estimates of the likely change in health-service-utilization rates associated with a given mortality reduction."

The relationships between utilization, age, and survival status will depend on the *reasons* for the lower death rate. If mortality falls because people are living healthier lives or because of more effective preventive measures, the conventional extrapolations will overestimate health care utilization, as demonstrated earlier. On the other hand, if the lower death rates are a result of ever more complex technological interventions, the rising cost of such interventions will tend to offset the fact that fewer persons are in the last year of life.

Labor Force Participation

Between 1950 and 1980 the labor force participation rate of men aged 65 and over fell from 46 percent to 19 percent. Participation rates of men aged 55 to 64 have also dropped sharply in recent years, from 83 percent in 1965 to 72 percent in 1980. What accounts for these striking declines? Many explanations have been offered, including poor health, mandatory retirement rules, age discrimination, rising wages, and improved Social Security benefits.

Health

When older men are surveyed about their labor force status, those not participating frequently cite ill health as the reason. These replies have been viewed with some skepticism, because ill health may be offered as a socially acceptable reason for not working when the true explanation lies elsewhere. A longitudinal analysis of retirement patterns, however, revealed that poor health is a good predictor of which men currently at work will not be working four years later (Fuchs, 1982b). This relationship does *not*, however, explain why participation by older men is so much lower now than it was 30 years ago. As noted, the health of the elderly has probably improved, and the occupational structure has shifted away from blue-collar jobs requiring heavy physical exertion. Thus, at any given age probably fewer men are compelled to leave the labor force for health reasons now than in earlier decades. Therefore, we must look to other factors.

Mandatory Retirement and Age Discrimination

According to some popular discussions, men stop working because of mandatory retirement or because they are victims of age discrimination. In my judgment neither of these explanations has been a significant factor in the long-term downward trend in labor force participation. First, about half of all currently retired men were never subject to mandatory retirement rules (Schulz, 1976). Furthermore, many workers retire before the mandatory age, many retire willingly at the mandatory age, and some are not working for other reasons such as ill health.

Mandatory retirement rules are usually part of a total labor contract, either explicit or implicit, that provides workers with stable or even rising wages until retirement, even though their productivity may decline during their last years of employment. If older workers are being paid more than they are currently worth, when they lose their jobs through mandatory retirement they obviously have difficulty obtaining a new job at their old wage rate.

The gap that develops between the wages of some older workers and their productivity is one reason why we hear complaints about "age discrimination." It is obvious that many employers prefer younger to older workers, but this is not discrimination in an economic sense if age affects productivity or labor costs. For instance, the older worker may expect a higher wage even though his productivity does not justify the wage differential. Even if there is no wage-productivity gap, the fringe benefits of older workers are often relatively high, especially for health insurance, life insurance, and pension benefits. As the share of fringe benefits in the total compensation package increases, it becomes increasingly uneconomic for firms to hire older workers. If there appears to be more age discrimination now than there was 30 years ago, it is probably because of the changes in wages and fringe benefits that make it less attractive to hire older workers.

Decline of Self-employment

One factor that probably does contribute to the downward trend in participation by older men is the declining importance of self-employment. Self-employed men are more likely to continue working at older ages than are wage-and-salary workers, holding constant education, age, health, wages, and other relevant variables (Fuchs, 1982b). Wage-and-salary workers typically face more rigidity in hours and wages, while the self-employed find it easier to reduce their hours of work without changing their occupation or job. The proportion of workers who are self-employed has declined drastically throughout the twentieth century because of the shift of employment from agriculture to industry and service. Even within each sector, self-employment has declined in relative importance as small farms and small businesses find it increasingly difficult to compete with larger enterprises.

Real Wages

Some economists argue that the growth of real wages in the economy as a whole is a major reason for the decline in labor force participation of older men, although this conclusion does not flow directly from economic theory. An *increase* in participation would be equally consistent with theory because the higher the wage, the higher the price of not working. But higher wages also mean higher income, and the income effect increases the demand for leisure. It is difficult to predict whether the price or income effect will dominate.

For women of prime working age, higher real wages have resulted in more labor force participation, not less. In the case of older men, however, it appears that the income effect is larger than the price effect. This would explain why the labor force participation of older men has declined in the United States as real income has risen. One problem with this explanation is that participation rates of older men in Europe are as low as in the United States, even though real income is not as high. To be sure, European countries typically have generous public pension plans that facilitate retirement. But why do they have such plans? The increasing number of elderly may be the answer, partly because of the political power that numerical strength confers and partly because younger workers want the older ones to leave the labor market.

Number of Elderly

The growth in the proportion of elderly probably contributes to their low participation rate in the labor force. When there are relatively few older people, the population has a pyramid-like age structure similar to the hierarchical structure of most organizations; the relatively few older workers can more easily progress up the organizational ladder. Currently in the United States and in most European countries the age distribution is more rectangular in shape, but organizations still have a pyramid-like hierarchy with fewer and fewer openings the higher up one goes. Thus, if most older workers stayed in the labor force, they would find it impossible to move up within their organizations.

Social Security

Probably one of the most important reasons for the rapid decline in the labor force participation of older men is the unusual growth of Social Security benefits. Between 1970 and 1980, average retirement benefits (adjusted for inflation) increased by more than 3 percent per annum, while hourly earnings did not even keep pace with inflation. There is no doubt that public policy has made it increasingly attractive for older people to stop work—by increasing retirement benefits relative to wages, by offering an early retirement option at 62, and by withholding benefits from eligible retirees at the rate of 50 cents per dollar of earnings on earnings above a prescribed rate. The trend toward earlier retirement, combined with greater life expectancy, will place a tremendous burden on those workers who remain in the labor force. To reverse this trend, however, major changes would probably be required in the structure of jobs and labor markets, as well as changes in the structure of Social Security retirement benefits.

Income

From a purely financial perspective, today's older Americans are much better off than their predecessors: they have more income and more wealth (adjusted for inflation) than any previous generation of elderly. Their real income has risen not only in absolute terms but also relative to the income of the working population, primarily because of the rapid growth of Social Security retirement benefits. It is true that household income, when the householder is age 65 or over, is only half of that in the age range 45 to 64, but this figure must be adjusted for household size. In 1980 the households of the elderly had on average only 1.74 persons, compared with 2.83 persons when the householder is 45 to 64. Taxes also make a big difference. The taxes of elderly persons (federal and state individual income taxes, property taxes on owner-occupied housing, and payroll taxes) are estimated to be only 13 percent of their income, while the members of the 45–64 age group pay taxes equal to about 25 percent of income (U.S. Bureau of the Census, 1983). Thus, the *after-tax* income *per household member* of the elderly is almost equal to that of the 45–64 age group.

Not only does the average older person receive an after-tax income comparable to the one he or she received at younger ages, but income is more *equally* distributed after age 65 than before that age. Consider the following analysis of incomes based on the Retirement History Survey, a longitudinal study of approximately 11,000 individuals (Hurd and Shoven, 1985). In 1968, when the respondents were 58 to 63 years of age and most were still in the labor force, the wealthiest 10 percent of the sample had a mean income of $65,363 (all figures in 1982 dollars), while the poorest 10 percent received only $1,838. By 1978, however, at ages 68 to 73, with most of the sample in retirement, the mean income of the wealthiest 10 percent had fallen to $52,117 while the poorest 10 percent showed a *rise* in income to $4,070. The principal reason for the narrowing of inequality after age 65 is that Social Security benefits become more important and labor income less important, and the former is distributed much more equally than the latter.

The improvement in the income position of the poor elderly has been particularly striking. As recently as 1970 one out of four persons aged 65 and over was below the poverty level, while the proportion among persons under 65 was about one in eight. In 1982 the proportion was the same for both age groups—about one in seven.

To be sure, money income is only one measure of economic well-being, but consideration of other factors tends to strengthen the impression that the elderly are, on average, about as well-off as other age groups. For instance, persons over age 65 are more likely to own a house free and clear of any mortgage. In addition, the elderly receive a disproportionate share of noncash transfers such as subsidized housing, transportation, and medical care. Because they are typically not in the labor force, they have more time for home production activities such as gardening, repair, and maintenance; they experience fewer work-related expenses, such as commuting and meals away from home; and they have the opportunity to move to a less costly area of the country.

One disadvantage faced by the elderly is the small size of the typical household. In 1980, 44 percent of their households had only one person, and 46 percent had only two. Small households are usually not as efficient as larger ones in the use of space, equipment, food, heat, and light. The difficulties and disadvantages of doubling up with another older person in order to gain the economies of a larger household are, however, apparently considerable. Fewer than 2 percent of elderly households include members who are unrelated, despite efforts by social agencies to encourage shared housing.

Although most of the elderly receive an after-tax income that compares favorably with what they earned while at work, there is a dramatic change in the *source* of income after age 65. From ages 25 to 54, earnings account for more than 90 percent of the total, and between 55 and 64 they still account for 78 percent of income. For people over 65, however, earnings provide only 20 percent. Social Security retirement benefits are the most important other source, with capital income such as interest and dividends next in importance, followed by government employee pensions, private pensions, and public assistance.

Does the source of income matter? I think it does. Social Security retirement benefits and other annuity-like income do not flow from *assets* that the older person can pass on to children or consume at a pace that he or she determines. In an earlier era the elderly had less total income relative to younger people than they do today, but more of it came from farms or small businesses or bits of real estate that they owned. Ownership usually contributes to a sense of power and control and can affect intrafamily relationships. A recent analysis of frequency of visits by children to their elderly parents found that the number of visits was positively related to the parents' bequeathable wealth (such as stocks, bonds, bank accounts, real estate), but not to nonbequeathable wealth (for example, Social Security, private pensions) (Bernheim, Shleifer, and Summers, 1983). If seniors today are "doing better and feeling worse," it may be in part because of this loss of control over their economic assets.

Living and Dying

A wide variety of demographic, social, and economic forces have resulted in major changes in how the elderly live and die. For instance, the male-female differential in death rates and the tendency of older widowed and divorced men to choose younger wives when they remarry create a large surplus of unmarried women above the age of 65. This surplus has grown in recent decades because female life expectancy has grown much more rapidly than male. In 1980 there were almost four unmarried women aged 65 and over for every unmarried man of that age, a steep increase from a ratio of less than two to one in 1940. The greatest change occurred among the widowed. In 1940 there were approximately two elderly widows for every widower, but by 1980 there were more than five. The huge rise in the number of elderly widows has been accompanied by a dramatic change in their living arrangements. In 1950 one in four was living alone; the other three were living with children, other relatives, or friends. By 1980 two out of three widows aged 65 and over were living alone, and only one in three was sharing living quarters with someone else. Most elderly men, however, are married. Even at ages 75 and above, two out of three men are living with their wives, while only one woman in five has a husband.

There has been a great deal of hand-wringing about the decline of three-generation households, but historians have hastened to point out that in Western Europe and the United States the three-generation household has always been the exception, not the rule. We can accept their conclusion that most households did not contain an aged mother or father, but it does not follow that only a small fraction of aged men and women lived with their children. When mortality is high and the population is growing rapidly, it is possible for *most of the elderly* to live with their children even though only a *minority of children* have elderly parents living with them. For example, if each woman has two daughters, and if half of the women survive into old age, only one daughter in four would have her mother living with her, even if every one of the survivors were living with a daughter. As an indication of how longer life expectancy and falling birth rates have raised the mother-to-daughter ratio, the number of women aged 65 and over relative to those aged 35 to 44 doubled between 1950 and 1980.

In addition to these demographic changes, rising real income contributes to the decrease in the number of mothers who double up with their children (Michael, Fuchs, and Scott, 1980).

Americans of all ages have always put a high value on autonomy; therefore, the rising income of recent decades and the particularly rapid rise in the income of the elderly have made it possible for an ever-higher percentage of them to maintain their own households, health permitting.

Health is also an important factor in living arrangements. In earlier times, poor health was often the reason why older men and women moved in with their children. At present, poor health often results in a move to a nursing home. The number of elderly in nursing homes increased at an astonishing 7 percent per annum between 1963 and 1977, to a total of more than 1.1 million. On any given day 5 percent of all elderly live in nursing homes, and between 20 and 25 percent will do so at some point in their lives. Of those who do enter, only one in four returns to a private or semiprivate residence; one-half are transferred to another health facility (usually a short-term general hospital), possibly to die or to return to the nursing home.

Why have nursing homes become so important? Rising income, the increased propensity to live alone, higher mother-to-daughter ratios, and higher labor force participation rates by young and middle-aged women are all part of the answer. There are many more elderly people who need care and attention, and relatively fewer children who are providing it within the home. Public policy also influences the decision because nursing home care is frequently paid for by the government (57 percent of the total in 1981), while the cost of home care is borne mostly by the family through out-of-pocket expenditures and the foregone earnings of the caregiver.

Economic and social factors also affect the location and manner of death. According to a report from the National Center for Health Statistics (1982b), 62 percent of deaths of persons aged 65 and over occur in a hospital or medical center, often at great cost. In some cases the patient is hospitalized because there is a reasonable chance to postpone the death through the kinds of medical intervention that are only possible within a hospital setting. In other cases, however, the patient is taken to the hospital to die because public and private insurance pays more fully than if the dying person is cared for at home. And in still other cases, there is no one close enough, either geographically or emotionally, to offer any alternative to hospitalization.

The cost of caring for very ill patients can vary enormously, depending on the patient and the physician (see Chapter 7). In some cases the intensive application of modern technology can prolong life for one or two months, or perhaps even more. This type of decision has traditionally been left to the patient and his or her physician, but exploding costs may lead to a reexamination of that position. At a minimum, there will be a search for less costly alternatives, and a closer examination of the factors that influence such decisions.

A Final Note

The data presented in this chapter and the accompanying discussion are meant to be suggestive, not definitive. Large gaps in our understanding of the aging process and of the determinants of labor force participation, health care utilization, and other key variables make it difficult to draw firm conclusions. It may be useful, however, to state explicitly some of the major themes that are implicit in the preceding pages. Most important is the need to recognize that the "Medicare problem" reflects the intersection of two larger sets of issues. First, there is a range of questions concerning the elderly in general: questions of retirement benefits, age of eligibility, wages and hours of work, and the like. Second, there are questions concerning the financing, organization, and delivery of health care for persons of all ages. Any Medicare "solution" that fails to consider these larger issues will probably turn out to be counterproductive.

Also implicit in this chapter is the need to recognize that resources devoted to the elderly are resources that could be used to help children, teenagers, minorities, and other groups with special claims to public attention. To say this is not to deny that there are many elderly who are poor, sick, lonely, or otherwise disadvantaged. But the growing political power of the elderly suggests the possibility of disproportionate attention to this group at a time when many small children are neglected or abused, when the schools are at a low ebb, and when teenage suicide is at epidemic proportions. Twenty years ago the plight of the elderly was palpable. Today the most pressing social needs may lie elsewhere. The "good society" needs to balance its efforts, to make hard choices among many worthwhile objectives.

These considerations, and the data presented in this chapter, lead me to hazard three inferences that have direct relevance for policy. First, we need to revise periodically our definition of *who is old*. One way to do this is to focus on changes in life expectancy at older ages. For instance, in 1935 when the age of eligibility for Social Security retirement benefits was set at 65, life expectancy at that age was 12.5 years. In 1984 the average 72-year-old has that same life expectancy. From this point of view it is not unreasonable to say that if age 65 marked the entry into old age in 1935, in 1984 old age begins at 72.

Second, we need to develop *more flexible labor market arrangements* to facilitate the continued labor force participation of older men and women. Unless this happens, the ratio of workers to retirees will become so small as to pose a grave threat to our economy and our society. Simply passing laws against mandatory retirement and age discrimination will not solve the problem; we need to develop more flexibility in hours of work, in wages (to accommodate possible age-related declines in productivity), and in amount of responsibility (to speed the movement of younger men and women into positions of leadership within organizations).

Finally—and this may prove to be the most difficult task of all—we need to reach a social consensus concerning what is *appropriate care for the dying*. At present the United States spends about 1 percent of the gross national product on health care for elderly persons who are in their last year of life. This is much more than the nation spends on institutional care for the mentally ill and the mentally retarded of all ages, more than private and public expenditures for basic and applied research in all fields, and more than the total expenditures of all the private colleges and universities in the country. On the other hand, it is less than is spent on alcohol, and not much more than is spent on tobacco.

How much *should* be spent on care for the 1.3 million elderly persons who die each year? For most goods and services, our society answers this question by saying "Let the market decide." According to economic theory, the free choice of kowledgeable buyers paying with their own money for services rendered by competitive suppliers should result in a socially efficient allocation of resources. It will not necessarily be a "fair" allocation, but this problem is supposed to be addressed through redistribution of income, not direct subsidization of particular services.

This free-market approach is not likely to work well for the seriously ill. Patients and their families are often under great emotional stress, and they typically have little previous experience with the complex technical choices that must be made. The hospitals and physicians who serve them often have considerable monopoly power. Furthermore, even in the absence of public subsidies, private insurance would push utilization beyond the point where benefits are equal to cost. The problem of distributive justice is not amenable to solution through conventional income-redistribution methods because the amount society would want to give to an individual would depend on how much care they needed. Some economists would prefer an indemnification plan that provides old people with additional income when they become sick and lets them decide how much to spend for medical care. This plan may be a delight to some theorists, but it would be a nightmare for most patients and physicians.

It is possible to nibble at the edges of the problem by providing more information to patients, by fostering more competition among providers, by financing alternative modes of care for the dying, and by increasing deductibles and coinsurance. The fundamental problem, however, will remain. One of the biggest challenges facing policymakers for the rest of this century will be how to strike an appropriate balance between care for the dying and health services for the rest of the population.

In order to formulate good public policy for the elderly, what is needed is a balanced appraisal, one that neither ignores nor exaggerates their circumstances. The British poet Alfred Lord Tennyson strikes the right note when he has the aged Ulysses say, "Though much is taken, much abides."

17 | Paying the Piper, Calling the Tune

The financing of health care in the United States has undergone three revolutions since the end of World War II. First, there was the extraordinarily rapid diffusion of private health insurance between 1945 and 1960. In only 15 years the number of persons with hospital insurance jumped from 32 million to 122 million, and the number with insurance for physicians' services soared from fewer than 5 million to more than 83 million. Second, there was the 1965 legislation that created Medicare and Medicaid. This stroke of the pen provided substantial health insurance coverage to many additional millions of Americans among the elderly and the poor.

The third major change began in the 1970s, when a few states started experimenting with regulation of hospital reimbursement. This movement accelerated in the early 1980s as both the private and public sectors embraced large-scale, radical alterations in the reimbursement of hospitals and physicians. Medicare's prospective payment system based on diagnosis-related groups (DRGs), the state of California's hospital-specific contracts for Medi-Cal patients, deductibles and coinsurance, health maintenance organizations (HMOs), and preferred-provider organizations (PPOs) are well-known symbols of a new era in health care financing.

This third transformation is more difficult to define than the previous two, and it is far from completed. It may, however, prove to be the most revolutionary of the three. Certainly from the point of view of health care providers, the new methods of reimbursement have implications far greater than those stemming from the spread of private insurance or the introduction of Medicare and Medicaid. Although the latter two movements increased demand for medical care, regularized payment and made it more secure, and increased equality of access, neither movement threatened the traditional system of organization and delivery of care. Private insurance companies were extremely reluctant to challenge the behavior of physicians or hospitals, and the Medicare and Medicaid legislation stated specifically that there was to be no interference with traditional practice.

The current revolution in reimbursement starts from a different premise. The third parties (government and business) who have been paying the piper have decided to call the tune. Far from promising *not* to change the system, they frequently have change as a major objective. My primary purpose in this chapter is to consider the economic and ethical implications of these changes—their possible effects on patients as well as providers, and on medical education and research as well as patient care. I will also discuss implications for efficiency in the allocation of resources, for equity in their distribution, and for other ethical problems.

Background and Characteristics of Recent Changes

Health policy traditionally encompasses three major areas: *access* to care, the *health* of the population, and the *cost* of care. In the 1950s and 1960s the first two concerns were dominant. Numerous health policy initiatives, ranging from expansion of medical education and research to the introduction of Medicare and Medicaid, were undertaken with the goals of eliminating barriers to access and improving the health of the population. Costs were secondary, and frequently were not considered at all.

Considerable progress was achieved. Disparities in access to care across income groups and between whites and nonwhites were sharply reduced. Delays in admission to hospitals were virtually eliminated; indeed, most hospitals now report excess capacity. As surpluses of medical and surgical specialists in the larger cities developed, more physicians began to move to smaller cities and towns. Many of these changes are directly attributable to specific health policy initiatives.

There have also been extraordinary improvements in the health of the population during the last 20 years, including a 60 percent reduction in infant mortality (to 10 deaths per 1,000 live births) and very large declines in age-adjusted death rates from influenza and pneumonia, heart disease, and stroke. It is more difficult to tie these advances in health to specific policies or programs, but it is likely that the numerous public policy initiatives played some positive role.

As these gains were unfolding in the 1970s, the nation became increasingly aware of the high and rapidly rising cost of medical care. The health sector, which in 1950 had used only 4.4 percent of the nation's output, had grown to 6.1 percent by 1965, to 9.4 percent by 1980, and to 10.8 percent by 1983. The cost problem became critical in the late 1970s and early 1980s: the economy as a whole was growing very slowly, while expenditures on health kept increasing at an extremely rapid pace. Figure 17.1 shows that the annual rates of change in gross national product (GNP) and expenditures on health tend to follow the

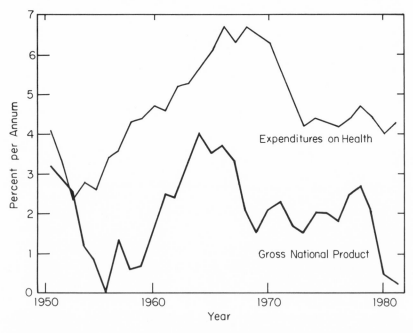

Figure 17.1 Changes in expenditures on health and GNP, adjusted for inflation and population growth, 1951–1981 (five-year moving average).

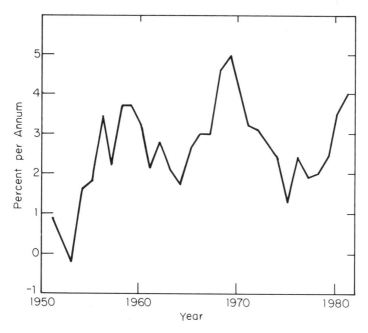

Figure 17.2 Difference between changes in expenditures on health and GNP, 1951–1981 (five-year moving average).

same pattern. (Both have been adjusted for inflation and population growth and smoothed with a five-year moving average.) In the late 1970s and early 1980s, however, the rate of growth of the GNP fell to less than 1 percent per annum, while real expenditures on health per capita continued to increase at more than 4 percent. The health care system is like an 80,000-ton ocean liner going full speed ahead—it cannot be turned around on a dime. But sooner or later health spending must reflect the country's underlying economic capacity.

The problem can be seen even more clearly in Figure 17.2, which shows the *difference* between changes in health spending and changes in the GNP. This gap is a measure of the rate at which labor and capital flow to the health sector away from the rest of the economy. When this gap reached 4 percent per annum in the late 1970s and early 1980s, the health sector's share of the GNP grew from 9 percent to 10 percent in less than three years. If the overall economy resumes and maintains a more rapid rate of growth, as it did in 1983 and 1984, the gap should decrease.

There is a second problem with respect to cost, however: the size of the gap in the long run. Over the past 30 years the gap has averaged 2.7 percent per annum. If a gap of this magnitude were to continue for another 30 years, health spending would grow to more than 20 percent of the GNP. It seems highly likely that the other sectors of the economy will make strenuous efforts to prevent that from happening.

Resistance to the expansion of the health sector tends to increase as long as its rate of growth exceeds that of the economy as a whole, because the larger the health sector gets, the more it will take away from the other sectors. When the health sector was only 5 percent of the GNP, the large gap in growth rates increased its share to 10 percent, thus taking away 5 percentage points from the rest of the economy. Now that the health sector's share is 10 percent of the GNP, the same gap over the same number of years would raise that share to almost 20 percent, thus taking away 10 percentage points from the rest of the economy. The larger any sector is relative to the total economy, the more difficult it is for it to grow faster than the whole. Even a 2 percent gap for 30 years would put health at 17 percent of the GNP. A smaller gap means a slower rate of growth for the health sector, unless the GNP grows very rapidly.

These macroeconomic considerations have had special force within the federal government and have contributed to a sense of panic, as Table 17.1 illustrates. On the fifth line of the table one can see the familiar increase in health spending as a percentage of GNP. One can also note the federal government's increased share of health spending (line 6) and, perhaps most important of all, the rise in federal health spending as a share of total federal spending (line 7). The federal government faces a tremendous deficit, now and for several years ahead; it must therefore either hold down spending or raise taxes appreciably. One step has been a strenuous effort to curb federal spending on health.

The private sector also feels the squeeze, as may be seen in Table 17.2, which highlights the growth of private health insurance premiums. Increases in these premiums in the short run are paid mostly by business corporations as employee benefits. In that sense, they come out of profits in the short run. In 1950 health insurance premiums were less than 6 percent of profits, but by 1980 they were 40 percent. In the long run,

Table 17.1 Federal and national health expenditures, total federal outlays, and gross national product (in billions of 1983 dollars)

	3-year averages centered on selected years						
	1950	1955	1960	1965	1970	1975	1980
(1) Federal expenditures on health	6	7	9	16	42	63	87
(2) National expenditures on health	52	63	84	119	176	228	302
(3) Total federal outlays	170	248	295	359	463	547	695
(4) Gross national product	1,175	1,404	1,589	2,015	2,369	2,686	3,224
(2) as percentage of (4)	4.4	4.5	5.3	5.9	7.4	8.5	9.4
(1) as percentage of (2)	12.5	11.2	11.2	13.4	24.2	27.6	28.7
(1) as percentage of (3)	3.8	2.9	3.2	4.4	9.2	11.5	12.5

Sources: Council of Economic Advisers, *Economic Report of the President* (Washington, D.C.: Government Printing Office, 1984), tables B-1 and B-73; Robert M. Gibson, Daniel R. Waldo, and Katharine R. Levit, "National Health Expenditures, 1982," *Health Care Financing Review* 5 (Fall), 1983, table 1.

Table 17.2 Health insurance premiums, corporate profits, and disposable personal income (in billions of 1983 dollars)

	3-year averages centered on selected years						
	1950	1955	1960	1965	1970	1975	1980
(1) Health insurance premiums	8	15	23	35	47	65	91
(2) Corporate profits before taxes	134	147	152	226	188	196	227
(3) Disposable personal income	833	975	1,105	1,382	1,639	1,879	2,226
(1) as percentage of (2)	5.9	10.3	15.4	15.4	25.1	32.9	40.0
(1) as percentage of (3)	0.9	1.6	2.1	2.5	2.9	3.4	4.1

Sources: Council of Economic Advisers, *Economic Report of the President* (Washington, D.C.: Government Printing Office, 1984), tables B-23 and B-82; Health Insurance Association of America, *Source Book of Health Insurance Data* (Washington, D.C.: HIAA, 1982–1983), table 3.1.

these payments come out of the real compensation of employees (in the form of lower wages or higher prices). It is also relevant, therefore, to note how rapidly these premiums have risen as a share of disposable personal income. In short, there is widespread concern about health spending because it looms so large in both public and private budgets.

To be sure, an increase in a sector's share of the GNP need not automatically be cause for alarm. There is nothing sacred about 5 percent of GNP, or 10 percent. Why not 20 percent? In a dynamic market economy, some sectors will grow and some will shrink as a result of changes in demand and supply. Thus if the health sector grows, so what? In general, economic theory supports this view, but there is something special about health spending—namely, the importance of third-party payers. Both theory and empirical research suggest that private and public insurance programs bias the system toward overutilization.

When consumers pay for goods and services directly, they tend to balance the costs of what they buy against the benefits they expect to receive. When insurance is present, however, the patient will want, and the responsive physician will choose, an amount of care such that the cost to society of the additional care exceeds its benefit to the patient. Deductibles and coinsurance can alleviate this problem a little, but most Americans want to be insured against large health care expenditures. Thus a fundamental problem of health care policy is how to provide insurance without pushing utilization far beyond the point where the additional benefit is equal to the additional cost.

Another reason for the recent changes in reimbursement—though probably a less important one from a long-range perspective—is that the country is currently pausing in, or even retreating from, its thrust toward more equal access to care. Some, but not all, of the cutbacks in funding and changes in methods of reimbursement can be interpreted as a weakening of the commitment to provide high-quality care to the poor. This aspect will be discussed further in later sections.

Since 1980 significant changes in health care financing have occurred in almost every sector of the economy. The federal government has radically altered hospital reimbursement for Medicare patients; several state governments regulate hospital rates for all types of patients; other states have installed special cost-containment programs for Medicaid patients; participation in HMOs has been growing at an unprecedentedly rapid rate; health care providers and health insurance companies are experimenting with a variety of new types of coverage that channel patients to preferred providers in exchange for discounts in fees and charges; and many conventional insurance policies are being changed to include larger deductibles and coinsurance.

With such diverse changes under way, it is not easy to summarize their characteristics. Indeed, apart from their desire to contain costs, there is probably no characteristic that is common to *all* new programs. There are, however, a few features that are sufficiently general to warrant brief discussion.

Lower costs for specific payers. Many previous policy proposals were aimed at containing costs for the health care system as a whole; examples are Alain Enthoven's Consumer Choice Health Plan and President Jimmy Carter's proposal to cap hospital expenditures. With the exception of the all-payer hospital regulations in a few states, however, this is not true of recent cost-containment initiatives. For example, Medicare's prospective payment system is designed to lower costs for Medicare. California's hospital-specific contracts for Medi-Cal (Medicaid) patients are designed to save the state money. The insurer-initiated PPOs and prudent buyer plans are explicitly intended to lower costs for the initiators of these plans.

There may be nothing wrong with this competitive, individualistic approach. Indeed, it may be the only way to obtain rapid change in a system that previously seemed rooted in "business as usual." Ever since Adam Smith, economists have been intrigued by the observation that an individual "by pursuing his own interest . . . frequently promotes that of the society more effectually than when he really intends to promote it" (Smith, 1776, p. 423). Economists have also discovered, however, that the individualistic approach does not always lead to socially optimal results. Later in the chapter I consider some possible adverse results of a free-market solution to problems of health insurance and health care.

Global payments. Payment for individual tests, visits, days in hospital, and the like are being replaced by global payments for an illness episode, a hospital admission, or a year of care, regardless of services used (capitation).

Prospective reimbursement. Reimbursement rates are set prospectively rather than retrospectively. This change is often described as "the end of cost-based reimbursement," but this is not entirely accurate. Costs of production will continue to play a major role in the determination of health care prices, as they do in virtually all markets, including the most competitive. What is disappearing is the willingness of payers to pay retrospectively based on cost; buyers are now negotiating prices for a particular package of services in advance.

Consumer choice. Consumers must make more choices and accept more financial responsibility for their choices. In the past, many employers offered a single health plan to their workers. Now it is not unusual for employees to be given a choice of conventional reimbursement insurance, a closed-panel prepaid group practice, a preferred-provider plan, and still other forms of payment and organization. Moreover, within the conventional reimbursement mode there are frequently choices to be made about the size of the deductible and the percentage of coinsurance. Those consumers who choose a preferred-provider plan frequently have the option of obtaining care outside the plan if they are willing to pay a larger coinsurance percentage.

Implications of Changes in Reimbursement

Just as it is difficult to generalize about the characteristics of recent changes in reimbursement, it is difficult to generalize about their probable effects. Each innovation in organization and finance has its own special impetus and its own special economic and ethical implications. Furthermore, most of the changes are very recent; not enough time has elapsed to collect and analyze reliable measures of their impact. This section, therefore, is primarily speculative: I infer from economic theory the likely effects of changing from retrospective to prospective payment and from reimbursement for individual services to global reimbursement. I also consider the implications that increased competition in insurance and medical care markets and greater use of deductibles and coinsurance may have for efficiency and equity. Inferences from theory are supplemented by the results of demonstrations and experiments in health care reform.

Economic Implications

The primary purpose of recent changes in organization and financing is to slow the rate of increase in health care spending. It seems likely that they will have this effect, at least in the short run. This slowdown will come about primarily because the incentives and constraints facing key decision makers—physicians, hospital administrators, insurance buyers, and patients—will be different from those facing them in the past.

The most important impact on physicians will probably come from the shift to global forms of reimbursement. As long as physicians are reimbursed for each service individually, there is less incentive for them to question the incremental benefit of each visit, test, x-ray, and so on. Global reimbursement for an episode of illness or for a year of care, regardless of services provided (as in capitation payment), will encourage physicians to consider the incremental benefit of what they do. Furthermore, as physicians begin to assume some financial responsibility for the hospitalization, prescriptions, and other dimensions of care that they order, they will begin to question the value of that care.

The best example of this phenomenon is the lower hospital utilization in prepaid group practice plans (see Luft, 1981). In the past, skeptics argued that lower hospital utilization in Kaiser Permanente, the Group Health Cooperative of Puget Sound, and other prepaid group practices was the result of patients' self-selection; they claimed that patients who needed or wanted less hospitalization sought out the prepaid plans. However, a prospective, controlled experiment that assigned patients at random to a prepaid plan or conventional insurance demonstrated the same difference in hospital utilization (Manning et al., 1984).

Although there is no completely satisfactory model of a nonprofit hospital or of the behavior of hospital administrators, there are a few generalizations that command wide agreement. The primary job of a hospital administrator is to keep other people happy—or, if not happy, at least not *too* unhappy. The "other people" are the physicians, the patients, the employees of the hospital, and the trustees; each of these constituencies has different and sometimes conflicting goals. The physician wants the hospital to have the most modern technical facilities, a large, high-quality staff of nurses, technicians, and other personnel, and enough excess capacity to reduce the possibility of delays in admission and in services for patients once admitted. Patients typically want high-quality care and amenities; price is rarely a concern, because hospital insurance is widespread and usually comprehensive. The nurses, technicians, and other employees want good wages and working conditions, and the opportunity to provide high-quality care. Trustees typically want to be associated with a hospital that delivers excellent care and that enjoys a good reputation in the community (the latter may entail providing care for persons who cannot pay for it). All groups want the hospital to remain solvent, but in the past that was usually taken for granted.

Under the traditional system of retrospective reimbursement based on incurred costs, most of the pressures on the administrator were in the direction of improving quality regardless of cost. A reimbursement system like Medicare's prospective payment system dramatically changes the situation: there is a real possibility that the hospital will not have enough revenue to cover its costs. The need to stay solvent was always an implicit pressure on the administrator, but now it has become explicit. Physicians are beginning to realize that the cost of new equipment and additional personnel will not necessarily be matched by increased revenue; if the hospital is forced out of business, it will not be there to receive their patients. Employees are beginning to realize that higher wages and more fringe benefits cannot automatically be covered by higher charges. Faced with the prospect of deficits and even bankruptcy, trustees are changing the questions they ask and the pressures they put on the administrator. (Nothing can match red ink for attracting the attention of trustees.)

Increased competition in the health insurance market will also tend to restrain the growth of expenditures for health care. Both public and private insurers are abandoning their laissez-faire attitude toward physicians and hospitals: they are bargaining about price, and they are insisting on controls over utilization. Individual insurance companies now have little choice in the matter—if they do not move to restrain costs, they will lose business to those companies that do.

Patients who continue to have "wall-to-wall" coverage under conventional insurance will continue to want "everything possible." An increasing proportion of patients, however, will be paying for some of their care directly, through deductibles and coinsurance. The basic law of demand says that an increase in the price of a commodity results in a decrease in the demand for it. The Rand health insurance experiment demonstrated conclusively that medical care is not an exception (see Newhouse et al., 1981): families with complete insurance coverage (no deductibles or coinsurance) used substantially more physicians' services and had more hospital admissions than did families who had to pay for a portion of the bill at the time of utilization.

The growing use of deductibles and coinsurance in private insurance and government programs is likely to decrease the demand for medical care. How this will affect the quantity and price of care will depend on the sensitivity of supply to price change. In the short run, when supply is likely to be quite inelastic, the decrease in demand will result in a small decrease in quantity and heavy downward pressure on price. In the long run, when supply is more elastic, the primary effect of a decrease in demand will be on quantity, with a smaller effect on price. All of the above assumes no shifting of demand. If suppliers, faced with decreasing demand, can partially offset the decrease by recommending more care, the declines in quantity and price will be smaller. Global reimbursement and direct controls on utilization, however, will tend to restrain the ability of suppliers to shift demand.

Differential impacts.   While the general effect of changes in reimbursement is to restrain the growth of expenditures, the impact will vary for hospitals, physicians, and nurses. Most of the belt-tightening is likely to be felt by hospitals, for several reasons. First, it is tempting to try to control hospital costs because they are such a large part of the total (over 40 percent) and have been rising especially rapidly. Second, it is easier to control payments to a few thousand hospitals than to hundreds of thousands of physicians. Third, most of the demand for hospital services is generated by physicians' decisions. As physicians begin to realize that money spent for hospital care is money that could be spent for *their* services, they are likely to recommend less hospital care. At first, it will be possible to do this without seriously jeopardizing patients' health as has been demonstrated with shorter lengths of stay and ambulatory surgery. Hospitals are likely to try to adapt to cost controls and the decreased demand for inpatient care by diversifying into other activities, including "captive" physicians' groups, home health care services, and community-based health promotion activities.

Although physicians collectively have the opportunity to protect their incomes by directing most of the restraint on spending toward hospitals, equipment manufacturers, and drug companies, they too will have to adapt in ways that many will find unpleasant. In particular, they will probably have to give up some of their independence and autonomy. They will increasingly feel the need to join group practices or other such practice organizations in order to be able to bargain with insurance companies and other purchasers of care. They will also need professional managers to help them function in a more competitive environment. In the process, some of their power and decision-making authority will be lost.

Changes in methods of hospital reimbursement are also likely to affect the goals of nurses. For instance, in the past many hospital nurses were working toward a goal of separate billing for their professional services, believing that this approach would increase their prestige and status as well as their pay. Given the trend toward global reimbursement, however, whether on a capitation or an admission basis, there is no scope for separate billing by nurses. Indeed, separate billing by physicians may well be on its way out. Another goal of hospital nurses was to transfer to other personnel responsibilities that were considered peripheral to nursing or below their level of skill. With lessened demand for hospital care, however, nurses will become more concerned about protecting their jobs. In the future, more nurses are likely to argue that it is better to have most patient services provided by the same person—the professional nurse.

Long-term effects.   Although many of the changes in behavior and ways of thinking induced by the changes in incentives may be short-term or one-time, some effects will emerge only over a longer period of time and are likely to be cumulative. For instance, even though physicians will have an immediate incentive to consider the incremental benefit of services in relation to their incremental cost, they may not know what the incremental value is. In the long run there is likely to be more research on this problem, both informally within health care institutions and more formally at medical schools and research organizations. Similarly, the education and training of physicians are likely to change, in order to make them better able to evaluate and assimilate this type of research. To cite another example: in the short run, hospital administrators may want to take account of marginal costs in their decision making, but the relevant information may not be available. In the long run, these data will be developed and used.

Another likely long-term consequence is a shift in the character of innovative activity. Innovations in medical care, as in other fields, typically take one of two forms. One is "product" innovation, which consists of introducing new services that improve the quality of care (for example, organ transplants and neonatal intensive care); these innovations usually increase the cost of care as well. The other kind is "process" innovation (for example, automated testing), which enables health professionals to continue doing what they have been doing but at lower cost. There have always been both kinds of innovation in medical care, but the cost-based reimbursement of the past tended to encourage product innovation. With prospective, closed-end reimbursement, the emphasis is likely to shift to process innovations that lower cost.

Distributional effects. One likely effect of Medicare's prospective payment system is redistribution of resources among institutions and among regions of the country. The implications of this redistribution for efficiency and equity vary, depending on the reasons for the original disparity in costs. Suppose that hospital A treats patients in a particular diagnosis-related group (DRG) at an average cost of $5,000 per admission, while hospital B has an average cost of $3,000 for patients in the same DRG. Under the old system each hospital would be paid its cost; under the new system each will get $4,000, thus redistributing resources from A to B. The desirability of this redistribution depends entirely on the *reason* for the difference in cost.

One possibility is that B is simply more efficient than A—that is, the patient mix is identical, input prices are identical, and patient outcomes are identical, but B does a better job of producing care. In this case it is both efficient and equitable to redistribute resources—to reward the efficient and punish the inefficient.

A second possibility is that there is no difference in patient mix, output, or efficiency, but hospital A pays higher prices for its inputs. It may be, for example, that a strong union in A has negotiated higher wages or the administrators in A are paid higher salaries. In that case there are no great gains in efficiency from redistributing resources, since there are no differences in efficiency. The redistribution does seem to be equitable, however, unless the wage differential simply offsets a difference in the cost of living.

A third possibility is that the difference in costs are due to differences in output. Although the patient mix is the same, hospital A uses more inputs to produce higher-quality care, more amenities, and the like. In this case the redistribution may be judged equitable, because there is nothing in the Medicare legislation to suggest that patients in hospital A ought to get a higher standard of care than patients in hospital B. The implications for efficiency are not as obvious, but the system is probably moving toward greater efficiency since the value of the marginal output of the additional resources is probably greater in B than in A.

Still another possibility is that the difference in cost is the result of differences in patient mix within the DRG. To the extent that this is the reason for the cost differential, there may be no gains in efficiency or equity from redistributing resources; there may even be losses. Teaching hospitals, for instance, claim that differences in patient mix contribute to their higher costs. Some studies suggest that education and research also contribute to higher costs in academic-center hospitals (Ament, Kobrinski, and Wood, 1981; Sloan, Feldman, and Steinwald, 1983).

Education and research. One special area of concern is the future of support for medical education and research. In the past, some of the funding for these efforts probably came from reimbursement for patient care. The new methods of reimbursement are designed, in part, to do away with this type of cross-subsidization. The buyers of care are saying: We want to pay for only the care we use; if we want to support education or research, we will do that separately. This argument has considerable appeal: buyers like to know what they are paying for and do not like to be forced to buy package deals.

It is also desirable to distinguish between the funding of medical education (undergraduate and postgraduate) and the funding of research. In too many discussions these activities are treated as if they were inseparable. This may well be true with respect to production, but it certainly need not be true of the funding. Indeed, economic theory suggests that they should be treated differently. Medical research often has large positive externalities; that is, it confers benefits on society as a whole that are far greater than the return to those carrying on the research. Because of these externalities, the private market will do less research than is socially optimal. The case for government subsidy, therefore, is very strong. With respect to medical education, however, the case for government subsidy is much weaker. Most of the benefits of this education are realized by those who receive the training; there is no obvious case for subsidization to achieve a socially optimal amount. As a matter of equity, society may want to help poor students obtain access to medical education, but this can be accomplished through sharply focused loans and scholarships.

Specialization: Hospitals. The new systems of reimbursement are likely to lead hospitals to specialize in the diagnosis and treatment of particular health problems. Such specialization would raise the quality of care and increase efficiency, but it would pose a problem for academic medical centers with traditional teaching programs. It would be more difficult to provide a complete educational experience for medical students in a specialized hospital; some changes in educational programs would be necessary.

Specialization may also bring one type of payment system into conflict with another. For instance, the Medicare system, which is based on diagnosis-related groups, clearly favors the growth of specialization, whereas preferred-provider organizations would tend to lose bargaining power as a result of hospital specialization. Suppose the XYZ Corporation enters into a preferred-provider arrangement with a local hospital whereby the corporation will send all its employees to that hospital in exchange for a price discount and utilization controls. If the hospital becomes specialized in certain types of care, those employees who need other types of care will not be well served by the PPO. The XYZ Corporation could presumably adapt by making arrangements with all the local hospitals, but that would dull the PPO's cutting edge.

Although many patients might benefit from the higher quality and lower costs resulting from hospital specialization, there would be disadvantages to patients as well. A major disadvantage is being hospitalized in an unfamiliar institution or in one that is inconveniently located. In a system of specialized hospitals, patients would have to weigh these disadvantages against the advantages of receiving more specialized care.

Specialization: Physicians. Although hospitals are likely to become more specialized, the proportion of physicians who are specialists or subspecialists is likely to fall. Surgery is a good example. Under the traditional fee-for-service system, with surgeons practicing alone or in small groups, the typical community has a large number of surgeons relative to the demand for operations. The average surgeon has a light work load but high enough fees per procedure to yield a good income. The new reimbursement systems, however, will shift medical practice toward large groups or other large-scale, organized systems of care. The Mayo Clinic and Kaiser Permanente, for example, hire only as many surgeons as are needed at a full work load. Their surgeons earn a good income, but their implicit fee per procedure is much lower than it would be in traditional practice. The light work load/high fee pattern will cease to be economically viable for most surgeons, and young physicians will be less likely to enter surgery.

Surgeons are not the only ones who will be affected. Much the same story could be told about many internal medicine subspecialties, and much the same pattern of change will emerge. This decrease in the number of specialists who have light work loads in their specialty could simultaneously lower costs and raise the quality of care.

Ethical Implications

The financing and delivery of health care have always posed ethical problems for health professionals and for society as a whole. Some existing problems will be exacerbated by the changes in reimbursement that are now under way, and some new problems are likely to arise. Problems will be encountered at every level: the individual physician, groups of physicians and hospitals, and the community and nation.

Physician-patient relations. The pressure to make physicians more conscious of costs, to make them practice more "cost-effective" medicine, will force them to make decisions that are contrary to the immediate interests of individual patients, even though the decisions may be optimal for society as a whole. The outlines of the conflict can be seen in Figure 17.3, which shows

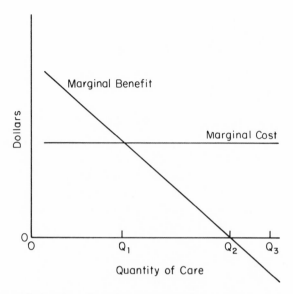

Figure 17.3 Choosing the "appropriate" amount of care.

the marginal (additional) benefits and marginal costs associated with varying amounts of care. The vertical axis is scaled in dollars; the horizontal axis may be thought of as measuring additional tests, prescriptions, days in the hospital, physician visits, and the like for any given medical condition. The downward slope of the marginal benefit curve indicates the assumption that the *additional* benefit of care gets smaller as the quantity of care increases. Beyond some point (where the curve crosses the horizontal axis), additional care does the patient more harm than good. The marginal cost curve is horizontal, representing the simplifying assumption that each additional unit of care increases total cost by about the same amount as the preceding unit. To be sure, for any given patient there will always be great uncertainty about the benefit of any particular intervention, and there may be uncertainty about marginal costs as well; these curves should be regarded as average or expected or best-guess results.

Given the situation portrayed in Figure 17.3, what is the optimal amount of care? From a social point of view, the optimum is clearly Q_1, where the marginal benefit is equal to the marginal cost (under the assumption that the marginal cost reflects the value of the resources in some alternative use). If more care than Q_1 is provided, the additional cost is greater than the additional benefit. If less than Q_1 is provided, the benefit of additional care is greater than its cost.

From the patient's point of view, Q_1 is best if the patient is not insured (that is, if the patient must pay the full marginal cost), but Q_2 is best if the patient is fully insured. Any pressure on the physician to move from Q_2 to Q_1 creates a dilemma: the physician must choose between what is good for society as a whole (and what competitive pressures may require for the survival of his or her group or hospital) and what is best for the individual patient. For instance, the physician may believe that an extra day in the hospital would slightly reduce the probability of a complication, but that the value of this reduction is far less than the cost of the extra day. Under the old system of reimbursement, the physician had little incentive to discharge the patient a day earlier; the cost of the extra day was widely diffused among all health insurance buyers or all taxpayers. If, however, the hospital is receiving global reimbursement for each admission, or if it is on a prospective global budget, or if the physician belongs to an HMO with capitation reimbursement or to a PPO with utilization controls, there will be considerable pressure on the physician to avoid that extra day of hospitalization.

Assuming the physician chooses Q_1, what does he or she tell the patient: that Q_1 is "best," or that Q_2 is better but Q_1 is recommended because it is more cost-effective? Most patients follow their physician's suggestions with regard to tests, hospitalizations, and the like because they assume that the physician has a professional commitment to putting their interests first. Confidence in the integrity and intentions of the physician frequently makes a positive contribution to patients' health. If insured patients begin to believe that their physician is recommending Q_1 rather than Q_2, they may become less honest in describing their symptoms and conditions, and this loss of candor will make the physician's task more difficult.

Under the old system there was frequently an economic incentive for the physician to recommend Q_3, especially for services that produced income for the physician. According to some observers, widespread insurance coverage led some (many?) physicians to recommend Q_3, which is clearly not in the best interests of either the patient (even if fully insured) or society. These observers see the current cost-containment effort as pushing physicians back from Q_3 to Q_2. If this is the case, there is no conflict for the ethical physician.

Relations among physicians and hospitals. Compared to relations among competitors in most other industries, relations among physicians and among hospitals in the same community have been marked by an unusual degree of cooperation and openness. Although they were ostensibly competing with one another, physicians have freely exchanged information, helped one another, and covered for one another; hospitals, especially the nonprofit community hospitals, have behaved in much the same way. Indeed, one of the complaints of outside observers was that physicians and hospitals did not compete enough. Whatever rivalry existed was largely expressed in efforts to raise the quality of care, leaving the community to pick up the tab.

One of the objectives of the new reimbursement methods is to increase competition among physicians and among hospitals—to transform health care into a competitive industry. There are unquestionably advantages to competition, but what will happen to the free exchange of information, the cooperation, and the mutual assistance that characterized health care in the past? Will physicians in one group be reluctant to share information with physicians in a competing group? How will physicians reconcile profession-wide obligations with obligations to their group and hospital? Will hospitals be willing to make data freely available if by doing so they may give other hospitals a competitive advantage? The virtues of competitive markets are considerable, but it is questionable whether the transformation of the health care industry into an approximation of the used car industry represents social progress. Even if more competition is, on balance, good for society, the health professionals caught in the competitive maelstrom are likely to feel great conflict about what constitutes appropriate behavior.

Collective responsibility for health care. The citizens of most countries feel a responsibility for meeting the medical-care needs of their fellow citizens. In developed countries this is typically done through some form of national health insurance. Altruism is only one motive, to be sure. National health insurance may be desired to eliminate "free riders" (but this concept itself presupposes an unwillingness to let sick people go without care), or to gain more control over physicians and hospitals, or to pursue other goals.

The United States has never had national health insurance, for several reasons. We are more heterogeneous than most other nations; we are less sanguine about the beneficence of government; and we have a more comprehensive network of private institutions to pay for health care for those in need. Community-rated insurance premiums, for instance, keep insurance affordable for those who use a great deal of care. The heavy users are, in effect, cross-subsidized by those who use less care. Non-profit hospitals also have typically been an instrument of cross-subsidization: they charge less than full cost to some patients (sometimes charging or collecting nothing at all), while making up the difference through charges to other patients. The pattern of coverage that emerged in the United States in the late 1960s and 1970s was patchy in many respects, but it came closer to providing universal coverage for a single standard of care than anything experienced previously in this country.

The new methods of reimbursement are designed to change this pattern. Competitive purchase of health insurance on a selective basis will erode community rating, as groups with low utilization demand and obtain lower premiums. Cross-subsidization by hospitals will be eliminated as competitive buyers refuse to pay more than their true costs.

The normative inferences to be drawn from these changes vary with circumstances and values. For instance, many people believe that if cigarette smokers use more medical care than nonsmokers, it is appropriate that they pay a higher premium for health insurance. But what if old people use more care than the young, women more than men, blacks more than whites, or persons with congenital abnormalities more than those without such limitations? Legislation that prohibits insurance companies from explicitly considering specific characteristics in setting individual premiums does not have much effect. Most insurance is bought by groups and is usually experience-rated or self-insured. The current trend is for each group to try to get the lowest possible premium for itself, regardless of what happens to the rest of the community.

The ethical dilemma is clear. On the one hand, it is socially desirable to reward healthful behavior and efficiency and to punish excessive use of care. On the other hand, the fragmentation of the insurance market raises the possibility of very high premiums for some groups. Society could deal with this problem by explicitly subsidizing those groups with high utilization; however, this may be more difficult to accomplish (for political and administrative reasons) than the previous method of implicit subsidies through community-wide or nationwide premiums.

What Is To Be Done?

Politicians, academicians, health professionals, and policy experts have been offering "solutions" to the problems of health care for decades. Competition, regulation, more government subsidy, less government subsidy, increasing the supply of hospitals and physicians, decreasing the supply—most of these strategies have been adopted at one time or another, but none has been or is likely to be *the* solution. Why not? Are they flawed in theory? In execution? Not necessarily. The time has come to acknowledge candidly that some problems defy solution, that the most one can hope for is alleviation and amelioration.

Health policy, like so many other major areas of public concern, requires trade-offs between such highly valued goals as efficiency and justice, freedom and security. Even the best solution must fall short in one direction or another, and the more effective the solution is for one goal, the greater the shortfall is likely to be for another. This is the principal reason why there is so much controversy over policy: people differ in the values they place on the various goals. Some are prepared to see society give up a good deal of efficiency to get more justice or more security, while others feel that freedom is paramount.

The financing of health care is a classic example of an insoluble dilemma, the need to choose between the Scylla of financial risk and the Charybdis of excessive utilization. Most people do not want to run the risk of having to pay very large bills for medical care. They seek health insurance, but once they have the insurance they consume more medical care than they would have without it—and more than is socially optimal. The cost of this additional care makes health insurance more expensive than it would otherwise be. All of this is true regardless of whether insurance is obtained privately or provided collectively through government.

A theoretical solution is for individuals, while well, to make an arrangement with the insurance company or the providers of care, or both, that only the socially optimal amount of care will be provided during illness, *even though the insurance nominally covers all necessary care.* Prepaid group practices (such as Kaiser Permanente) and the British National Health Service can be regarded as being organized on that principle. It works, and sometimes it works very well, but it requires either a little deception or a great deal of restraint. It is rational for a person who is well to want to be part of such a system, but once that person is sick it is equally rational to want all the care that might provide some benefit. The challenge to the system is to keep the patient from getting that additional care.

It may not have been too difficult to meet that challenge in the past, because much of the additional care delivered in other systems was of questionable value. But as competitive pressures drive all systems toward more stringent evaluation of the cost-effectiveness of care, it will become more difficult to convince patients that they are getting the best possible care. Low-yield medicine is not no-yield medicine.

A partial solution lies in changing our perceptions of what constitutes appropriate care. Once the leading medical centers change their approach and the leading medical schools change what they teach their students, most physicians will adapt to prevailing practice, just as they have in the past. Patients will then adapt to their physicians' recommendations.

As discussed earlier, competition among physicians and hospitals may inhibit the flow of socially useful information. A partial solution to this problem can be found in the approach of other industries. The public utility companies, for instance, sponsor and generously fund the Electric Power Research Institute to conduct long-term economic, social, and technical research that benefits the individual companies and society as a whole. Several highly competitive electronics companies have created a consortium to carry on research on a scale greater than would be possible for any of them individually. The key to such industry undertakings is widespread agreement that all companies will contribute funds, data, personnel, and so on. Such agreement is necessary to keep each company from thinking that cooperation on its part will put it at a competitive disadvantage.

The problem of ensuring medical care for all, regardless of income or other circumstances, is primarily a matter of *will* rather than method of reimbursement. When government agencies change their method of paying for care for the elderly or the poor or any other group and at the same time reduce the amount they are prepared to pay, there is a high probability that there will be some reduction in the quantity or quality of care received. It is not the change in reimbursement method per se that is responsible for reducing care; the change is simply the means whereby a weakening of commitment to the poor is given expression. If society wants to provide care for the poor, virtually any system of reimbursement can be used.

The situation is actually more complicated than this. Much of the pressure for change in reimbursement is motivated not by a desire to see the poor get less care, but by a desire to make the system more cost-effective. In that case, there is an urgent need to find ways to halt and reverse the erosion of support for the least fortunate in our society. It seems highly unlikely that this can be accomplished without substantial intervention of government through taxes and subsidies. Such intervention need not involve a takeover of medicine by government or an abandonment of the movement toward more cost-effective medicine. If it is not done in a timely fashion, however, a back-lash may develop.

Every revolution carries within it the seeds of its own destruction through excessive preoccupation with one goal. The present revolution in health care financing is no exception. The problems it addresses are palpable: overutilization of medical serv-ices, inadequate evaluation of new technologies, inefficient and inequitable cross-subsidization, excess supplies of specialists and hospital beds. But the problems it may create are also significant: inadequate insurance coverage for millions, erosion of profes-sional ethics as an instrument of control, loss of trust between physicians and patients, a decrease in activities with large positive externalities. The challenge is to capture and preserve the ben-efits of the revolution while minimizing its costs. Now that society has decided it can call the tune, it must think carefully about what tune it wants the piper to play.

NOTES
REFERENCES
ACKNOWLEDGMENTS
SOURCES
INDEX

Notes

1. Health Care and the United States Economic System

1. Health might be measured by life expectancy, absence of disabilities, speed of recovery after surgery, and so forth. Health care inputs might refer to the size of a health care program, or the total amount of care given to a particular patient or a particular aspect of care, such as number of tests or number of days in the hospital.

2. This assumes that some input—for example, the state of technology—is fixed at any given point in time.

3. This point is well recognized in the theoretical literature on socialist planning (see Lange, 1956) and in the attempts of the Soviet government and other Eastern European governments to make greater use of the market mechanism.

4. The flow of resources (and the reciprocal flow of goods and services) in the United States is currently at a rate of approximately one trillion dollars per annum. About 7 percent of these resources flow to "firms" producing health care. Fifteen years ago only about 4.5 percent of such smaller resource flow went in that direction. The resource flow, measured in dollars, depends on the quantities of various resources and their prices. Over long periods of time, prices of equivalent resources usually change at about the same rate in all sectors of the economy. Thus the increased share in dollar terms reflects a substantial increase in the share of real resources as well. This large shift of resources over a relatively short period of time is the most important element in the present "health care crisis."

5. The fact that these services proliferate contrary to what economies of scale would indicate is the result of other problems, such as the absence of appropriate incentives and constraints for physicians and hospital administrators.

6. For a pioneering article, see Stigler, 1961.

7. The firm or household will presumably equate *its* marginal cost and *its* marginal benefit. The social optimum requires taking into account the costs or benefits imposed on others.

8. When medical care keeps an employed head of family alive and well, a type of external benefit is created because society does not have to provide for his or her dependents. Much medical care, however, goes to the young or the elderly or to keeping people alive but not well enough to work, so it is doubtful if on balance a positive externality exists in this sense.

9. What would constitute a "fair" distribution of income has never been satisfactorily answered by economists or anyone else. One feature of the market system that makes it attractive to some is that a household's share of goods and services will be roughly proportional to its contribution to total output as evaluated by all households collectively.

10. Note the analogy with the individual household's decision regarding vaccination.

11. However, where medical care for the poor is tied to using them for teaching and research purposes, significant externalities are probably present.

12. But there would be no a priori case for favoring health over other commodities. The choice should depend on relative costs and benefits.

4. Determinants of Expenditures for Physicians' Services

1. For comparisons of our formulations and conclusions with those of other investigators, see Andersen and Benham, 1970; Benham, Maurizi, and Reder, 1968; Fein, 1967; M. Feldstein, 1970; P. Feldstein, 1964; Klarman et al., 1970; Rimlinger and Steele, 1965; Sloan, 1970.

2. This would be the case if all physicians had solo practices.

3. Differences in actual medical practice across states are undoubtedly larger than differences in the frontier of medical knowledge. Our interpretation of the technological factor in demand, however, is predicated on the assumption that the demand for physicians' services increases with an expansion in the range of services physicians are *technically* able to offer. Variations in actual medical practice across states are viewed primarily as the consequence of variations in demand rather than as their cause.

4. The range of variation in per capita disposable income was substantially less in that year for the 33 states in our sample, having a high value of $3,185 in Connecticut and a low of $1,586 in Mississippi. The coefficients of variation for per capita physician expenditures and per capita income were 24.0 percent and 16.0 percent, respectively. State data for 1965 and 1967 show about the same degree of variation as in 1966.

5. Endogenous variables are determined within the system ("jointly determined"), while exogenous variables are determined outside the system ("predetermined").

6. Some of the excluded exogenous variables were significant in equations in which they appeared (for example, race as a determinant of health status), but because the endogenous variable health was found to be insignificant in the demand equation, both health and race factored out of the system.

7. A hat over a variable indicates that its predicted value is used in estimating the equation. An asterisk indicates that the variable is phrased in per capita terms.

8. It would, of course, be possible to combine the two dimensions of supply into one overall supply equation, but to do so would be to discard much valuable information regarding the behavior of physicians.

9. Physician behavior might conceivably be affected if the source of payment were governmental, because of the consequent red tape and the physician's personal political philosophy. However, only private insurance is considered in this analysis; data on governmental expenditures for physicians' services are unavailable on a state basis.

10. Our measure of physician output weights hospital inpatient visits higher than outpatient visits because of differences in their relative prices.

11. All series refer to 1966 unless otherwise indicated.

12. These correlations are weighted by 1966 state population. The unweighted correlations are 0.760 and 0.824, respectively.

13. Simple regressions across states of the annual change in total expenditures EXP_{t+1}/EXP_t on the annual change in physicians filing returns IRS_{t+1}/IRS_t show the independent variable to be highly significant and the explanatory power of the equation fairly high. IRS_{t+1}/IRS_t, however, bears almost no relation to the percentage change in private practitioners MD_{t+1}/MD_t, as recorded by the AMA, even though the correlation between IRS and MD for any given year is on the order of 0.99.

Dependent variable	Independent variable	Coefficient (standard error)	R^2
$\dfrac{EXP_{67}}{EXP_{66}}$	$\dfrac{IRS_{67}}{IRS_{66}}$	0.50 (0.13)	0.40
$\dfrac{EXP_{66}}{EXP_{65}}$	$\dfrac{IRS_{66}}{IRS_{65}}$	0.66 (0.10)	0.63
$\dfrac{IRS_{67}}{IRS_{66}}$	$\dfrac{MD_{67}}{MD_{66}}$	1.82 (1.99)	0.03
$\dfrac{IRS_{66}}{IRS_{65}}$	$\dfrac{MD_{66}}{MD_{65}}$	1.09 (2.69)	0.01

14. The AMA figures refer to private practice physicians only.

15. Office of Research and Statistics, Social Security Administration, U.S. Department of Health, Education, and Welfare, "Current Medicare Survey Report," *Health Insurance Statistics*, CMS-12, January 27, 1970.

16. Both figures are derived from survey data published in *Medical Economics*.

17. The one exception is *MED SCLS*, which is phrased as a linear variable because it sometimes takes on the value zero.

18. Plots of the residuals from unweighted regressions demonstrate an inverse relationship between population and the size of the unexplained residual.

19. t-statistics are ordinarily obtained by dividing each coefficient by its standard error, but this procedure is not valid when the predicted values of endogenous variables appear on the right-hand side of an equation. In such cases the following adjustment is necessary: (1) Recompute the residuals for each observation by applying the estimated second-stage regression coefficients

to the *actual* values of the included endogenous variables. (2) Obtain the ratio of the sum of squared residuals from the recomputed equation to the sum of squared residuals from the estimated regression. (3) Multiply each of the original *t*-statistics for a particular regression equation by this factor (which may be equal to, greater than, or less than 1.0) in order to arrive at a set of adjusted *t*-statistics applicable to the second-stage regression. We are grateful to Christopher Sims for bringing this to our attention.

20. Andersen and Benham, in their calculations for physician use, employ an estimate of "permanent income" as the independent variable rather than measured income, but this does not imply incomparability with our results since the transitory component of income is largely eliminated by using grouped data.

21. Other demand elasticities reported in the literature are 0.62 and 0.21, respectively, in Feldstein (1964) and Fein (1967). The elasticity implicit in Fein's book was computed by Herbert Klarman (1969).

22. Morris Silver (1972) postulates a *positive* relationship between earnings and *expenditures* for physicians' services, and his results bear this out. But such a finding can be readily explained by the close association between earnings and price. It does not necessarily contradict our view that high earnings have a negative impact on the quantity component of expenditures.

23. Visit-relatives for women 65 to 75 and 75 and over rise rapidly, as predicted, over low income classes, but then fall even more steeply, for some unknown reason, over high income classes.

24. This is not to say that all, or even most, physicians' services are technically essential for health. To *believe* in their efficacy is sufficient to make the average individual treat them as a necessity in his budget.

25. Feldstein's study pertained to physician visits by families in 1953.

26. The same argument can be made with regard to "negative inputs" in the production of health, including consumption items such as tobacco, alcohol, narcotics, and (occasionally) motor vehicles.

27. Paul Feldstein (1964) uses an insurance variable (the ratio of benefits to expenditures) in his demand analysis. Contrary to his expectations, the elasticity is negative, though insignificant. Regrettably, no discussion of this finding appears in the text.

28. Because the total number of practicing physicians in the country (MD_t) is constant in cross section, an analysis such as this can only throw light on the reasons for geographic variation in this total. Given the presence of substantial barriers to entry into medicine, it is wholly unwarranted to conclude that the same behavioral patterns observed for physicians in cross section will also apply over time in the determination of MD_t. In all probability, a proportional change in INC^* across all states would have no effect on MD_t or on the particular state levels of MD^*_{it}. It follows that only variations in *relative* income are potentially influential in determining the geographic distribution of a given number of physicians. The relative attractiveness of a state is best represented by $INC^*_i/\overline{INC}^*$, where the denominator represents mean per capita income for the sample. Replacing our INC^* variables with this relative income measure would have no effect on the estimated elasticities because the corresponding values of both variables are proportional in any one year. But it

is best kept in mind that the *INC** variable of Table 4.3B should only be interpreted in a relative sense.

29. Because of some collinearity between these variables and *UNION**, the significance level of each of the three is diminished in D.6, and the coefficients are somewhat lower as well.

30. It may be argued that insurance purchases are sensitive both to their price and to anticipated expenditures levels, and that *AP* therefore serves in a dual capacity in the *BEN** regression. If this is correct, the *AP* coefficient we observe should be on the order of -0.6 ($+1.0$ for the expenditures theory and -1.6 for the price theory). This possibility is tested and rejected in D.5, for the *PRM/BEN* and *AP* coefficients are essentially unchanged from their values in D.3, while Q^* is now negative.

31. In a reduced form, individual regression equations are solved so that Q^* and *AP* can be expressed wholly in terms of the exogenous variables.

32. Two-stage regressions with health as the dependent variable are not feasible within the context of the present model, because the exogenous determinants of health do not appear in the model. Their exclusion was based on the insignificance of health itself in the demand equation. To reintroduce health would necessitate bringing back into the model several exogenous variables that bear no demonstrable relationship to the market for physicians' services, and, as explained earlier, this in turn would impart a bias to all of the first-stage predicted endogenous variables.

33. Our analysis implicitly assumes causality to run only from education to health, but this is not necessarily the case. See Michael Grossman (1975).

5. The Utilization of Surgical Operations

1. For each hospitalization, only first operations were included; the number of second and third operations was small. Deliveries, abortions, and all other obstetrical surgical procedures were excluded from our analysis because they are primarily a function of conception rates.

2. The results reported in the text are based on regressions with observations weighted by $(1/N_c)^{-1/2}$, where N_c is the number of persons observed in cell c. Alternative estimates of the parameters of the model were obtained by weighting instead by $[\hat{R}_c(1000 - \hat{R}_c)/N_c]^{-1/2}$, where $\hat{R}_c$ is the surgical rate adjusted for age and sex from a prior regression weighted by $(1/N_c)^{-1/2}$. Numerical estimates of coefficients were very close (within $2/1000$), and statistical significance tests were qualitatively identical.

3. Cells with none of the 11 procedures were necessarily deleted from the analysis. These cells accounted for 2.7 percent of individuals in 1970 and 2.4 percent in 1963.

6. The Supply of Surgeons and the Demand for Operations

1. For a fuller discussion of physician-maximizing behavior, see Evans (1974), Sloan and Feldman (1977), Reinhardt (1977), and Green (1978).

2. Let X_n = number of operations performed in nonmetropolitan areas; R_n = number of operations performed on residents of nonmetropolitan areas;

P_n = population of nonmetropolitan areas; and X_m, R_m, P_m = the same for metropolitan areas.

$$X = X_m/P_m \div X_n/P_n, \qquad R = R_m/P_m \div R_n/P_n, \qquad P = P_m/P_n,$$

given $X = 1.75$, $R = 1.10$, $P = 2.33$, and assuming that no metropolitan residents are operated on in nonmetropolitan areas. Solve for X_n/R_n:

$$R_m/R_n = RP,$$
$$X_m/X_n = XP,$$
$$(R_m + R_n)/R_n = 1 + RP,$$
$$(X_m + X_n)/X_n = 1 + XP,$$
$$X_n/R_n = (1 + RP)/(1 + XP) = (1 + 2.563)/(1 + 4.078) = 0.70.$$

3. The coefficient of rank correlation of surgical utilization (adjusted for demographic characteristics) between 1963 and 1970 across the divisions is only 0.42.

4. In-hospital procedures are typically monitored by hospital audit committees. Moreover, such procedures expose the patient to much greater risk.

5. The East North Central area is divided into an eastern section (Ohio and Michigan) and a western section (Indiana, Illinois, and Wisconsin). The South Atlantic area is divided into an upper section (Delaware, Maryland, District of Columbia, Virginia, and West Virginia) and a lower section (North Carolina, South Carolina, Georgia, and Florida).

6. Nevada was excluded because its huge gambling-based receipts did not seem relevant.

7. The number shown for the Middle Atlantic division is larger than the division's population.

8. All regressions use population weights.

9. Equality of slope coefficients between 1963 and 1970 was tested for both S^* and Q^* regressions, and the null hypothesis was not rejected in any equation.

10. The 11 selected operations are appendectomy, cataract removal, cholecystectomy, dilation and curettage (excluding abortions), hemorrhoidectomy, hernia repair, hysterectomy, lumbar laminectomy for disk, prostatectomy, tonsillectomy, and varicose-vein stripping.

11. The coefficients of rank correlation across the nine divisions are: IOV and FOV, 0.77; IOV and FHV, 0.67; FOV and FHV, 0.90.

12. $r = 0.78$ for undeflated price, and 0.71 when the surgical price index is deflated by the Williamson-BLS index.

13. This explanation was suggested by Sherwin Rosen.

9. Some Economic Aspects of Mortality in Developed Countries

1. For a concise discussion of some of the difficulties encountered in analyzing mortality differentials, see Benjamin (1965).

2. See McKeown (1967). For a contrary, but not particularly convincing, argument see Stolnitz (1955, 1956).

3. Let A = age-specific death rate from causes A
        B = age-specific death rate from causes B
       M = $A + B$ = age-specific death rate from all causes
       a = elasticity of A with respect to income per capita
       b = $(a + k)$ = elasticity of B with respect to income per capita
      m = elasticity of M with respect to income per capita
      α = A/M = share of causes A in total death rate
      Y = income per capita
subscript 0 = initial period
       g = $Y \div Y_0$

(9.1) $$m = \alpha a + (1 - \alpha)b.$$

(9.2) $$m(Y) = \frac{\alpha_0 a Y_o^b Y^a + (1 - \alpha_0)b Y_o^a Y^b}{\alpha_0 Y_o^b Y^a + (1 - \alpha_0)Y_o^a Y^b}.$$

This can be rewritten:

(9.3) $$m(g) = \frac{\alpha_0 a + (1 - \alpha_0)(a + k)g^k}{\alpha_0 + (1 - \alpha_0)g^k}.$$

As income per capita grows, the B cause gets more weight if $k > 0$ and less if $k < 0$. Either way, the entire term becomes less negative or more positive.

If we let $c = A_1 \div A_0$ and $d = B_1 \div B_0$ where A_1 and B_1 are the death rates in period 1, holding income constant but taking account of the shifts, we can rewrite Eq. (9.3) to take account of the shifts as follows:

(9.4) $$m(g, t = 1) = \frac{c\alpha_0 a + d(1 - \alpha_0)(a + k)g^k}{c\alpha_0 + d(1 - \alpha_0)g^k}.$$

4. There are probably many errors in the reports of occupation on death certificates.

5. This conclusion applies, of course, only over the observed range of variation. If inputs of care were reduced significantly below the lowest levels now observed, the marginal contribution might be much larger.

6. The influence of genetic factors on longevity is not considered here.

7. For some of the hazards of speculating about marital-status differentials, see Sheps (1961).

11. Time Preference and Health

1. For an excellent summary of present knowledge in this field, as well as many useful bibliographies, see *Healthy People: The Surgeon General's Report on Health Promotion and Disease Prevention, Background Papers*, U.S. Department of Health, Education, and Welfare (PHS) no. 79-55071A (Washington, D.C.: Government Printing Office, 1979).

2. There are, to be sure, many other possible explanations for this correlation. For instance, persons with better health endowments may be more efficient in schooling activities, or their expected rate of return to schooling

may be higher because of their greater life expectancy. Conversely, the rate of return to investment in health may be greater for those who have had more schooling.

3. "When habits are once formed, they regulate the tenor of the future life, and make slaves of their former masters." John Rae, *The Sociological Theory of Capital*, ed. C. W. Mixtor (1834; reprint ed., New York: Macmillan, 1905) as quoted in Maital and Maital (1978).

4. William Hazlitt wrote in *The Round Table* (1817), "Persons without education . . . see their objects always near, and never in the horizon." And Robert Penn Warren wrote in the poem "Brother to Dragons," "Without the fact of the past, we cannot dream the future."

5. I am grateful to Alan Garber and Richard Zeckhauser for helpful comments on this point.

6. Temporal orientation refers to the point in time around which a person's thoughts center and to the volume of those thoughts.

7. The questionnaire was administered by psychologists at Perceptronics in Eugene, Oregon.

8. Stephen Cole also made many contributions to the design of the questionnaire.

9. A digit-raising technique was used to ensure inclusion of unlisted numbers.

10. See the appendix at the end of the chapter for a list of time-preference questions.

11. I am grateful to Amos Tversky for advice on this point.

12. Approximately one-quarter of the respondents classified as consistent chose "now" for all six questions, and another one-quarter always chose to wait. Their replies, while not inconsistent, are not as informative about consistency as the replies of those respondents who chose "now" for some questions and "wait" for others.

13. Given six questions, every possible set of replies can be made consistent with a maximum of three reversals.

14. This hypothesis was suggested by Phillip Farrell.

15. Ceteris paribus, individuals with low rates of time discount might accumulate more savings, might choose occupations with larger on-the-job investment opportunities, and so forth.

16. For example, a respondent who answered "now" to the first four questions in Table 11.1 and "wait" to the next two was assigned a rate of 35.35 percent.

17. A different set of values, based on a regression with a different sample, yielded almost identical results to those reported here.

18. Grossman's regression (for middle-aged males), comparable to regression (2) in the top part of Table 11.9, had a coefficient of .035 for schooling and −.017 for age.

19. No hospitalization in past year, no prescription drugs in past week, no medical condition requiring regular visits to physician, and fewer than three visits to physician in past six months. To be sure, medical care utilization may reflect factors such as income and insurance coverage as well as health status.

20. The weak effect of schooling is attributable to the "symptoms" and "utilization" measures of health status. When these measures are used as

dummy dependent variables in regressions equivalent to (3) in Table 11.9, schooling is negatively (albeit not significantly) related to good health.

12. Schooling and Health: The Cigarette Connection

1. For example, see Auster et al. (1969), Grossman (1972b), Newhouse and Friedlander (1980), and Taubman and Rosen (1982).

2. Spells of nonsmoking by ever regular smokers were ignored, since their duration and timing were not recorded in the survey. For our purposes the error thus introduced in determination of smoking status at age 17 or 24 is negligible.

3. Approximately 17 percent of the white survey respondents did not give father's schooling; the median years of completed father's schooling for their 10-year age cohort was assigned. Regressions were also tried excluding those missing father's years of completed schooling. The results were the same as the full sample with median values assigned to missing observations.

4. For example, Consumer's Union (1954), Lieb (1953), Miller and Monahan (1954), and Norr (1952).

5. In our subset of whites aged 24–75, the mean levels of expired air CO (ppm) and blood thiocyanate (micromoles/liter) for self-reported smokers and nonsmokers varied by years of schooling as follows (standard errors of the means in parentheses):

Amount of schooling	Smokers		Nonsmokers	
	Men	Women	Men	Women
		CO		
12 years	28.7	25.6	6.26	4.08
	(1.95)	(1.86)	(0.62)	(0.12)
16+ years	26.0	17.9	4.79	3.80
	(2.24)	(2.02)	(0.24)	(0.12)
		Thiocyanate		
12 years	154.1	166.3	65.6	48.9
	(6.26)	(5.68)	(4.04)	(1.57)
16+ years	155.1	135.2	62.3	49.3
	(8.83)	(11.32)	(2.57)	(1.73)

6. To estimate the maximum survivorship bias, use our cohort of 17-year-olds in 1921–1941 (born 1904–1924). Assume that all were born in 1915 and experienced the age-specific death rates of successive decennial cross sections (for example, the number surviving to 1920 estimated from death rates for 0- to 5-year-olds observed in 1920, and so forth). Further assume that at every age after 25, persons smoking by age 25 experience an age-specific mortality rate twice that of those who were not smoking by age 25 (this surely overstates differential mortality because of later starting and stopping behavior). Finally, assume that the ratio of survival rates of smokers and nonsmokers in this cohort to the year 1979 (defined as the variable C) is independent of years of schooling. Using U.S. Life Tables for decennial years and apportioning deaths between initial smokers and nonsmokers according to the observed

proportions of smokers at age 24 in this cohort and the 2 to 1 mortality rate assumption, C is calculated at 0.81 for white men and 0.87 for white women. Let T_a be the true proportion of smokers at age a and O_a be the observed proportion from a survey of cohort survivors. Then, $T_a = O_a/(C + O_a - CO_a)$. Using the predicted probabilities of smoking at ages 17 and 24 for specific sex/cohort/schooling cells that we obtain from estimating our regression model (see Table 12.2) as the "observed" proportions, the "true" proportions, adjusted for effects of differential survivorship, can be calculated from the formula just given. For men, T_{17} ranges from 14% to 16% higher than O_{17} for years of schooling from 12 to 18; T_{24} ranges from 6% to 9% higher than O_{24}. For women, T_{17} is 11% higher than O_{17} for all schooling categories; T_{24} varies from 8% to 9% higher than O_{24}. These are the maximum effects of survivorship bias, which diminishes rapidly for the younger cohorts. The bias in the coefficient of schooling can be approximated by considering the change in slope (between "observed" and "true" proportions) of a straight line drawn between the smoking probabilities for the 12th and 18th graders. For men, the true slope is 10% higher than the observed slope at age 17, and 6% lower at age 24. For women, the true slope is 13% higher than the observed slope at age 17, and 4% higher at age 24. Differences of this size are practically and statistically insignificant, considering the very small schooling coefficients estimated for this cohort.

7. Estimation was done by the method of maximum likelihood using the iterative procedure *LOGIST* of the Statistical Analysis System, version 79.5, on an IBM 370/3081 processor.

8. To specify an exact test for the significance of the differences in the schooling coefficients between the two ages, one would need a model that accounted for the paired nature of the observations and the correlations of the error terms from the two age regressions. A conservative test of the hypothesis of no difference is possible by simply pooling the observations at ages 17 and 24 and then reestimating the regressions by cohort and sex with interaction terms for the age of the observation. The standard error of the interaction (difference) coefficient for schooling will be biased downward. A difference that is not significant in this test will thus not be significant with correctly estimated unbiased standard errors. In this simple test, the significance level (two-tailed) for a difference in the schooling coefficient by age is greater than 0.2 for all sex/cohort regressions.

The finding of no change in the schooling coefficients between the two ages in the logistic model means that realizing additional years of schooling results in no change in the relative odds of smoking as a function of eventual schooling. This is not the same as asserting that realizing additional schooling will give no change in the relative proportions of smokers as a function of eventual schooling. But the logistic model is clearly the more appropriate one. To illustrate, use as an example two groups of men from our 1953-1963 cohort: those who eventually complete 18 years of schooling, and those who eventually complete only 12 years of schooling. Using the predicted probabilities of smoking from Table 12.2 (which correspond closely to the observed proportions of smokers), we see that the relative odds of smoking for the eventual 18th graders versus the eventual 12th graders at age 17 are:

$$(0.08/0.92)/(0.62/0.38) = 0.053$$

The relative odds of smoking for the two groups at age 24, after they have differentiated on the schooling dimension, equals 0.051. These relative odds at the two ages are nearly identical. However, the relative proportions of smokers for eventual 18th graders versus eventual 12th graders rises from 0.129 to 0.25 between the ages of 17 and 24. These relative proportions are clearly different. But how could one expect them to be the same? The proportion of smokers at those two ages is affected by other factors besides eventual schooling (not the least of which is simply the passage from adolescence to adulthood, with greater income and freedom). Thus, it is not surprising to see a 260% increase in the proportion smoking for the group of eventual 18th graders between ages 17 and 24 (of whom only 8% were smoking at 17), but such a percentage increase between ages 17 and 24 in the proportion smoking would have been mathematically impossible for the group of eventual 12th graders, of whom 62% were already smoking at age 17.

9. This chapter does not explicitly address the possibility that differences in quality of schooling prior to the 12th grade could be the cause of the observed differences in smoking behavior at age 17. Differences in quality, however, are similar to additional years of schooling because both reflect differences in the quantity of education inputs into the individual. We find no causal relationship between education inputs after the 12th grade (in the form of additional years of schooling) and smoking. To assert a strong causal role for education inputs up to the 12th grade (in the form of "quality" differences) would then require that causality diminish with increasing schooling and finally cease by the 12th grade. It seems implausible to us to suppose that schooling can increase knowledge, change preference, increase ability for self-control, or otherwise exert strong influence over smoking behavior until the 12th grade and not thereafter.

13. From Bismarck to Woodcock

1. For a discussion of why the United States is the last to adopt national health insurance, see the section "Why Is the United States Last?" near the end of this chapter.

2. I am grateful to Sherman Maisel for suggestions concerning this section.

3. I am grateful to Seth Kreimer for suggestions concerning this section.

4. Maurice LeClair (1975, p. 16) writes that the experience in Saskatchewan clearly indicated economies of scale in the administration of a virtually universal plan. See also further comments on this point by LeClair (1975, p. 24).

14. Economics, Health, and Postindustrial Society

1. The change in quantity is equal to the product of the change in price and the elasticity of demand, where the changes between period 1 and period

2 are measured as percentages according to the following formula:
$(2 - 1) \div (2 + 1) \div 2$.

16. Though Much Is Taken

1. Let X = expenditures per person
   N = number of persons
   P = predicted expenditures per person
   X' = expenditures adjusted for age-sex differences in survival status
   g = age-sex group g
   t = all age-sex groups
   s = survival status s
   u = all survival statuses

$$X'_{ug} = \frac{X_{ug}}{P_{ug}} X_{ut}, \quad \text{where} \quad P_{ug} = \frac{\sum_{s} X_{st} N_{sg}}{\sum_{s} N_{sg}}.$$

References

Abel-Smith, Brian. 1964. Major patterns of financing and organization of medical care in countries other than the United States. *Bulletin of the New York Academy of Medicine* 40 (2nd ser.).

Acton, Lord. 1907. History of freedom in Christianity. In *History of freedom and other essays,* ed. J. N. Figgis and R. V. Laurence. (Reprinted: 1971, Arno Publishers, New York.)

Aday, L. A., and R. Andersen. 1975. *Access to medical care.* Ann Arbor, Mich.: Health Administration Press.

Adelman, Irma. 1963. An econometric analysis of population growth. *American Economic Review* 53 (June):314–339.

Altman, Stuart H. 1970. The structure of nursing education and its impact on supply. In *Empirical studies in health economics,* ed. Herbert E. Klarman. Baltimore: Johns Hopkins Press.

Ament, Richard P., Edward J. Kobrinski, and Walter R. Wood. 1981. Case mix complexity differences between teaching and nonteaching hospitals. *Journal of Medical Education* 56 (November):894–903.

American Board of Medical Specialists. 1970–71. *Directory of medical specialties,* vol. 14.

American College of Surgeons and the American Surgical Association. 1971. The study on surgical services for the United States. *Bulletin of the American College of Surgeons* 56 (March):14–21.

Andersen, Ronald, and Lee Benham. 1970. Factors affecting the relationship between family income and medical care consumption. In *Empirical studies in health economics,* ed. Herbert Klarman. Baltimore: Johns Hopkins Press.

Antonovsky, A. 1967. Social class, life expectation and overall mortality. *Milbank Memorial Fund Quarterly* 45 (April) 31–37.

Antonovsky, A., and J. Bernstein. 1977. Social class and infant mortality. *Social Science Medicine* 11:453–470.

Arrow, Kenneth J. 1969. The organization of economic activity: Issues pertinent to the choice of market vs. non-market allocations. In *The analysis and evaluation of public expenditures: The P.P.B. system,* Subcommittee on

Economy in Government of the Joint Economic Committee, 91st Congress of the United States, First Session, vol. 1, pp. 47–66.

────── 1973. Government decision making and the preciousness of life. In *Ethics of health care,* ed. Laurence R. Tancredi. Washington, D.C.: Institute of Medicine.

Auster, Richard, Irving Leveson, and Deborah Sarachek. 1969. The production of health: An exploratory study. *Journal of Human Resources* 4 (Fall):412–436.

Barnes, Allan C. 1970. The missing evidence. *Perspectives in Biology and Medicine* 14 (Autumn):53–62.

Becker, E. R., and B. Steinwald. 1981. Determinants of hospital casemix complexity. *Health Services Research* 16:439–458.

Becker, Gary S. 1964. *Human capital.* New York: National Bureau of Economic Research and Columbia University Press.

────── 1965. A theory of the allocation of time. *Economic Journal* 75 (September):493–517.

Becker, Gary S., and Robert T. Michael. 1973. On the new theory of consumer behavior. *Swedish Journal of Economics* 75:378–396.

Becker, Gary S., and Nigel Tomes. 1976. Child endowments, and the quantity and quality of children. *Journal of Political Economy* 84 (August):S143–S162.

Bell, D. 1973. *The coming of post-industrial society.* New York: Basic Books.

Benham, Lee. 1971. The effect of advertising on prices. Graduate School of Business, University of Chicago (mimeo).

Benham, Lee, and Alexandra Benham. 1975a. The impact of incremental medical services on health status, 1963–1970. In *Equity in health services: Empirical analyses in social policy,* ed. R. Andersen, J. Kravits, and O. W. Anderson. Cambridge, Mass.: Ballinger.

────── 1975b. Utilization of physician services across income groups, 1963–1970. In *Equity in health services: Empirical analyses in social policy,* ed. R. Andersen, J. Kravits, and O. W. Anderson. Cambridge, Mass.: Ballinger.

Benham, Lee, A. Maurizi, and M. W. Reder. 1968. Migration, location, and remuneration of medical personnel: Physicians and dentists. *Review of Economics and Statistics* 50 (August):332–347.

Benjamin, B. 1965. *Social and economic factors affecting mortality.* Paris: Mouton.

Berlin, Isaiah. 1970. *Four essays on liberty.* New York: Oxford University Press.

Bernheim, B. D., A. Shleifer, and L. H. Summers. 1983. The manipulative bequest motive (mimeo).

Bombardier, Claire, Victor R. Fuchs, Lee A. Lillard, and Kenneth E. Warner. 1977. Socioeconomic factors affecting the utilization of surgical operations. *New England Journal of Medicine* 297 (29 September):699–705. [Chapter 5 of this volume.]

Borland, Barry L., and Joseph P. Rudolph. 1975. Relative effects of low socioeconomic status, parental smoking and poor scholastic performance on smoking among high school students. *Social Science and Medicine* 9:27–30.

Breslow, Lester, and Anne R. Somers. 1977. The lifetime health-monitoring program. *New England Journal of Medicine* 296 (17 March):601–608.

Breton, Albert. 1974. *The economic theory of representative government.* London: Macmillan.

Brooks, C. H. 1975. The changing relationship between socioeconomic status and infant mortality: An analysis of state characteristics. *Journal of Health and Social Behavior* 16:291–303.

Bunker, John P. 1970. Surgical manpower: A comparison of operations and surgeons in the United States and in England and Wales. *New England Journal of Medicine* 282 (15 January):135–144.

Bunker, John P., Benjamin A. Barnes, and Frederick Mosteller. 1977. *Costs, risks, and benefits of surgery*. New York: Oxford University Press.

Bureau of Medical Care Insurance, The Council Committee on Economics. 1965. *1965 relative value scale*. Medical Society, State of New York.

Buxbaum, R. C., and T. Colton. 1966. Relationship of motor vehicle inspection to accident mortality. *Journal of the American Medical Association* 197 (4 July):31–36.

Calabresi, G. C., and P. Bobbitt. 1978. *Tragic choices*. New York: W. W. Norton.

Carnegie Commission on Higher Education. 1970. *Higher education and the nation's health*. New York: McGraw-Hill.

Clark, Colin. 1960. *The conditions of economic progress*. London: Macmillan.

Committee on Fees of the Commission on Medical Services. 1960. *1960 relative value studies*, 3rd ed. San Francisco: California Medical Association.

Committee on Relative Value Studies. 1969. *1969 California relative value*, 4th ed. San Francisco: California Medical Association.

Consumer's Union. 1954. Cigarette smoking and lung cancer. *Consumer Reports* 19 (February):54–92.

Cyert, Richard M., and James G. March. 1964. The behavioral theory of the firm: A behavioral science-economics amalgam. In *New perspectives in organization research*, ed. W. W. Cooper. New York: John Wiley and Sons.

Davis, C., and M. Feshbach. 1978. Life expectancy in the Soviet Union. *Wall Street Journal*, 20 June.

Davis, Karen, and Roger Reynolds. 1976. The impact of Medicare and Medicaid on access to medical care. In *The role of health insurance in the health services sector*, ed. Richard N. Rosett. New York: National Bureau of Economic Research and Neale Watson Academic Publications.

Dorfman, R. (ed.). 1965. *Measuring benefits of government investments*. Washington, D.C.: The Brookings Institution.

Dubos, R. 1959. *The mirage of health*. New York: Harper.

Eisner, V., M. W. Pratt, A. Hexter, M. J. Chabot, and N. Sayal. 1978. Improvement in infant and perinatal mortality in the United States, 1965–1973. I. Priorities for intervention. *American Journal of Public Health* 68 (April):359–364.

Evans, Robert G. 1974. Supplier-induced demand: Some empirical evidence and implications. In *The economics of health and medical care*, ed. Mark Perlman. London: Macmillan.

Farquhar, John W., Nathan Maccoby, P. D. Wood, J. K. Alexander, H. Breitrose, B. W. Brown, Jr., W. L. Haskell, A. L. McAlister, A. J. Meyer, J. D. Nash, and M. P. Stern. 1977. Community education for cardiovascular health. *Lancet* 1 (4 June):1192–1195.

Farrell, Phillip, and Victor R. Fuchs. 1982. Schooling and health: The cigarette connection. *Journal of Health Economics* 1 (December):217–230. [Chapter 12 of this volume.]

Fein, Rashi. 1967. *The doctor shortage: An economic diagnosis.* Washington, D.C.: The Brookings Institution.

Feldstein, Martin S. 1970. The rising price of physicians' services. *Review of Economics and Statistics* 52 (May):121–133.

———— 1971. Hospital cost inflation: A study of nonprofit price dynamics. *American Economic Review* 61:853–872.

———— 1973. The welfare loss of excess health insurance. *Journal of Political Economy* 81, no. 2, part 1 (March/April):251–280.

Feldstein, Paul J. 1964. The demand for medical care. In *Commission on the cost of medical care: General report,* vol. 1. Chicago: American Medical Association.

Ferguson, C., L. Maw, and R. Wallace. 1976. Effects of Medicare on hospital use: A disease-specific study. *Medical Care* 14:574–589.

Field, Mark G. 1967. *Soviet socialized medicine.* New York: Free Press.

Ford, G. R. 1971. Innovations in care: Treatment of hernia and varicose veins. In *Portfolio for health,* ed. G. McLachlan. London: Oxford University Press, for Nuffield Provincial Hospitals Trust.

Friedman, Gary D., Diana B. Petitti, Richard D. Bawol, and A. B. Siegelaub. 1981. Mortality in cigarette smokers and quitters. *New England Journal of Medicine* 304 (4 June):1407–1410.

Friedman, Milton. 1975. Leonard Woodcock's free lunch. *Newsweek* (21 April), p. 84.

Fries, James F. 1980. Aging, natural death, and the compression of morbidity. *New England Journal of Medicine* 303 (17 July):130–135.

Fuchs, Victor R. 1965. Some economic aspects of mortality in the United States (mimeo).

———— 1967. The basic forces influencing costs of medical care. Address given at the National Conference on Medical Care Costs, Washington, D.C., 27 June. In *Essays in the Economics of Health and Medical Care,* ed. Victor R. Fuchs. New York: National Bureau of Economic Research and Columbia University Press.

———— 1968a. *The service economy.* New York: National Bureau of Economic Research and Columbia University Press.

———— 1968b. The growing demand for medical care. *New England Journal of Medicine* 279 (25 July):190–195.

———— 1969a. *Production and productivity in the service industries* (ed.). NBER Conference on Research in Income and Wealth, vol. 34. New York: National Bureau of Economic Research and Columbia University Press.

———— 1969b. Improving the delivery of health services. *Journal of Bone and Joint Surgery* 51-A (March):407–412.

———— 1972a. *Essays in the economics of health and medical care* (ed.). New York: National Bureau of Economic Research and Columbia University Press.

———— 1972b. Health care and the United States economic system: An essay in abnormal physiology. *Milbank Memorial Fund Quarterly* 50, no. 2, part 1 (April):211–237. [Chapter 1 of this volume.]

———— 1974a. *Who shall live? Health, economics, and social choice.* New York: Basic Books.

———— 1974b. Some economic aspects of mortality in developed countries. In *The economics of health and medical care*, ed. Mark Perlman. London: Macmillan. [Chapter 9 of this volume.]

———— 1976. From Bismarck to Woodcock: The "irrational" pursuit of national health insurance. *Journal of Law and Economics* 19 (August):347–359. [Chapter 13 of this volume.]

———— 1978a. The service industries and U.S. economic growth since World War II. In *Economic growth or stagnation?*, ed. Jules Backman. Indianapolis: Bobbs-Merrill.

———— 1978b. The supply of surgeons and the demand for operations. *Journal of Human Resources* 13 (suppl.):35–56. [Chapter 6 of this volume.]

———— 1979. Economics, health, and post-industrial society. *Milbank Memorial Fund Quarterly/Health and Society* 57 (Spring):153–182. [Chapter 14 of this volume.]

———— 1981a. The coming challenge to American physicians. *New England Journal of Medicine* 304 (11 June):1487–1490.

———— 1981b. Low-level radiation and infant mortality. *Health Physics* 40 (June):847–854. [Chapter 10 of this volume.]

———— 1982a. Time preference and health: An exploratory study. In *Economic aspects of health*, ed. Victor R. Fuchs. Chicago: University of Chicago Press. [Chapter 11 of this volume.]

———— 1982b. Self-employment and labor force participation of older males. *Journal of Human Resources* 17 (Summer):339–357.

———— 1982c. The battle for control of health care. *Health Affairs* 1 (Summer):5–13. [Chapter 15 of this volume.]

———— 1983. Setting priorities in health education and promotion. *Health Affairs* 2 (Winter):56–69. [Chapter 2 of this volume.]

———— 1984. "Though much is taken": Reflections on aging, health, and medical care. *Milbank Memorial Fund Quarterly/Health and Society* 62 (Spring):143–166. [Chapter 16 of this volume.]

———— 1986. Paying the piper, calling the tune: Implications of changes in reimbursement. *Frontiers of Health Services Management* 2 (February). [Chapter 17 of this volume.]

Fuchs, Victor R., and Marcia J. Kramer. 1972. *Determinants of expenditures for physicians' services in the United States, 1948–1968*. Washington, D.C.: DHEW publication no. (HSM) 730–3013 (December). [Chapter 4 of this volume.]

Fuchs, Victor R., and Irving Leveson. 1967. Motor accident mortality and compulsory inspection of vehicles. *Journal of the American Medical Association* 201 (28 August):657–661. [Chapter 8 of this volume.]

Galbraith, J. K. 1958. *The affluent society*. Boston: Houghton Mifflin.

Garber, Alan M., Victor R. Fuchs, and James F. Silverman. 1984. Case mix, costs, and outcomes: Differences between faculty and community services in a university hospital. *New England Journal of Medicine* 310 (10 May):1231–1237. [Chapter 7 of this volume.]

Garrison, Louis P. 1981. Studies in the economics of surgery. Ph.D. dissertation, Stanford University.

Ginzberg, Eli. 1966. Physician shortage reconsidered. *New England Journal of Medicine* 275 (14 July):85–87.

—— 1969. *Men, money, and medicine.* New York: Columbia University Press.

Godber, Sir George. 1981. Disease prevention and health promotion. In *Getting better: A report on health care from the Salzburg Seminar,* ed. Herbert P. Gleason. Cambridge, Mass.: Oelgeschlager, Gunn, and Hain.

Gordon, H. S. 1971. Social institutions, change and progress. The E. S. Woodward Lectures in Economics. Vancouver, Canada: University of British Columbia.

Grahn, D., and J. Kratchman. 1963. Variation in neonatal death rate and birth weight in the United States and possible relations to environmental radiation, geology and altitude. *American Journal of Human Genetics* 15:329–352.

Green, Jerry. 1978. Physician-induced demand for medical care. *Journal of Human Resources* 13 (suppl.):21–34.

Gronau, Reuben. 1973. The intrafamily allocation of time: The value of the housewives' time. *American Economic Review* 63:634–651.

Grossman, Michael. 1972a. *The demand for health: A theoretical and empirical investigation.* New York: National Bureau of Economic Research and Columbia University Press.

—— 1972b. On the concept of health capital and the demand for health. *Journal of Political Economy* 80 (March/April):223–255.

—— 1975. The correlation between health and schooling. In *Household production and consumption,* ed. Nestor E. Terleckyj. NBER Studies in Income and Wealth, no. 40. New York: National Bureau of Economic Research and Columbia University Press.

Harris, Jeffrey E. 1979. Cigarette smoking in the United States, 1950–1978. In *Smoking and health: Report of the Surgeon General.* USDHEW, Public Health Service. DHEW publication no. (PHS) 79-50066. Washington, D.C.: Government Printing Office.

—— 1980. Patterns of cigarette smoking. In *The health consequences of smoking for women: Report of the Surgeon General.* U.S. Department of Health and Human Services. Washington, D.C.: Government Printing Office.

—— 1981. On the mortality risk of cigarette smoking. Presented at the International Workshop on the Analysis of Actual versus Perceived Risks, Washington, D. C., June 1–3.

Hirschfield, Daniel S. 1970. *The lost reform: The campaign for compulsory health insurance in the United States.* Cambridge, Mass.: Harvard University Press.

Holen, Arlene S. 1965. Effects of professional licensing arrangements on interstate labor mobility and resource allocation. *Journal of Political Economy* 73 (October):492–498.

Hornbrook, M. C. 1982. Hospital case mix: Its definition, measurement and use. II. Review of alternative measures. *Medical Care Review* 39:73–123.

Hospital Physician. 1970. Where four specialties are concentrated. *Hospital Physician* 6 (January):75–79.

Hughes, Edward F. X., Victor R. Fuchs, John E. Jacoby, and Eugene M. Lewit. 1972. Surgical work loads in a community practice. *Surgery* 71 (March):315–327. [Chapter 3 of this volume.]

Hurd, Michael, and John Shoven. 1985. The economic status of the elderly: 1969–79. In *Horizontal equity, uncertainty, and measures of well-being,* ed. M. David and T. Smeeding. Chicago: University of Chicago Press.

Iglehart, John K. 1982. The new era of prospective payment for hospitals. *New England Journal of Medicine* 307 (11 November):1288–1292.

——— 1983. Medicare begins prospective payment of hospitals. *New England Journal of Medicine* 308 (9 June):1428–1432.

Jewkes, John, and Sylvia Jewkes. 1963. *Value for money in medicine.* Oxford: Blackwell.

Journal of the American Medical Association. 1970. The need for more physicians (editorial). *J.A.M.A.* 213 (10 August):1027–1028.

Kahnemann, Daniel, and Amos Tversky. 1979. Prospect theory: An analysis of decision under risk. *Econometrica* 47 (March):263–291.

Kessel, Reuben A. 1958. Price discrimination in medicine. *Journal of Law and Economics* 1 (October):20–53.

Klarman, Herbert E. 1965. *The economics of health.* New York: Columbia University Press.

——— 1969. Economic aspects of projecting requirements for health manpower. *Journal for Human Resources* 4 (Summer):360–376.

Klarman, Herbert E., Dorothy P. Rice, Barbara S. Cooper, and Louis H. Stettler III. 1970. Sources of increase in expenditures for selected health services, 1929–69. U.S. Department of Health, Education, and Welfare, Social Security Administration, Office of Research and Statistics. Staff paper no. 4 (April).

Lalonde, M. 1974. *A new perspective on the health of Canadians.* Ottawa: Government of Canada.

Lange, Oscar. 19!6. On the economic theory of socialism. In *On the economic theory of socialism,* ed. B. E. Lippincott. Minneapolis: University of Minnesota Press.

Lave, Charles A. 1978. The costs of going 55. *Newsweek* (23 October).

Lave, J. R., and L. B. Lave. 1971. The extent of role differentiation among hospitals. *Health Services Research* 6:15–38.

Lave, J. R., L. B. Lave, and S. Leinhardt. 1975. Medical manpower models: Need, demand and supply. *Inquiry* 12 (June):97–125.

LeClair, Maurice. 1975. The Canadian health care system. In *National health insurance: Can we learn from Canada?,* ed. Spyros Andreopoulos. New York: John Wiley.

LeRiche, H., and W. B. Stiver. 1959. The work of specialists and general practitioners in Ontario. *Canadian Medical Association Journal* 81:37.

Lieb, C. W. 1953. Can the poisons in cigarettes be avoided? *Reader's Digest* 63 (December):45–47.

Linder, Staffan B. 1970. *The harried leisure class,* trans. Staffan B. Linder and Keith Bradfield. New York: Columbia University Press.

Lindop, P. J., and J. Rotblat. 1969. Strontium-90 and infant mortality. *Nature* 224:1257–1260.

Lindsay, Cotton M. 1969. Medical care and the economics of sharing. *Economica* 36 (November):351–362.

Lippmann, Walter. 1955. *Essays in the public philosophy.* Boston: Little, Brown.

Lohrenz, F. N., and R. Payne. 1968. The physician-assistant—surgical. *Group Practice* 17 (April):13–16.

Longmire, W. P. 1965. Problems in the training of surgeons and in the practice of surgery. *American Journal of Surgery* 110 (July):16–20.

Lubitz, J., and R. Prihoda. 1982. Use and costs of Medicare services in the last years of life. Baltimore: Office of Research and Office of Statistics and Data Management, Health Care Finance Adminstration (mimeo).

Luft, Harold S. 1981. Health maintenance organizations: Dimensions of performance. New York: Wiley and Sons.

Maccoby, Nathan, and Douglas S. Solomon. 1981. Health disease prevention: Multi-community studies. In *Public communication campaigns,* ed. R. E. Rice and W. J. Paisley. Beverly Hills, Calif.: Sage Publications.

Macrae, N. 1976. *America's third century.* New York: Harcourt Brace Jovanovich.

Maital, Shlomo, Sharona Maital. 1978. Time preference, delay of gratification, and the intergenerational transmission of economic inequality: A behavioral theory of income distribution. In *Essays in labor market analysis,* ed. Orley Ashenfelter and Wallace Oates. New York: John Wiley.

Maloney, J. V., Jr. 1970. A report on the role of economic motivation in the performance of medical school faculty. *Surgery* 68 (July):1–19.

manning, Willard G., Arleen Leibowitz, George Goldberg, William Rogers, and Joseph P. Newhouse. 1984. A controlled trial of the effect of a prepaid group practice on use of services. *New England Journal of Medicine* 310 (7 June):1501–1507.

Manton, K. G. 1982. Changing concepts of morbidity and mortality in the elderly population. *Milbank Memorial Fund Quarterly/Health and Society* 60 (Spring):183–244.

Martz, E. W., and R. Ptakowski. 1978. Educational costs to hospitalized patients. *Journal of Medical Education* 53:383–386.

Masson, P. G., T. C. Moody, and J. D. Stubbs. 1971. Planning and control for community hospitals: A case study of the Cambridge Hospital. Cambridge, Mass.: Sloan School of Management, Massachusetts Instutute of Technology.

McAlister, Alfred L. 1979. Tobacco, alcohol, and drug abuse: Onset and prevention. In *Healthy people,* Surgeon General's report on health promotion and disease prevention, background papers. Washington, D.C.: Government Printing Office.

McDermott, Walsh. 1969. Demography, culture, and economics and the evolutionary stages of medicine. In *Human ecology and public health,* 4th ed., ed. Edwin D. Kilbourne and Wilson G. Smillie. London: Collier-Macmillan.

McKeown, Thomas, and R. G. Record. 1967. Reasons for the decline of mortality in England and Wales during the nineteenth century. *Population Studies* 16 (November):94–122.

Medical Society of New York. 1968–69. *Medical directory of New York State,* 52.

Metcalf, Charles E. 1974. Predicting the effects of permanent programs from a limited duration experiment. *Journal of Human Resources* 9 (Fall):530–555.

Michael, Robert T., Victor R. Fuchs, and Sharon R. Scott. 1980. Changes in the propensity to live alone: 1950–1976. *Demography* 17 (February):39–56.

Miller, L. M., and J. Monahan. 1954. The facts behind the cigarette controversy. *Reader's Digest* 65 (July):1–6.

Mills, W. A. 1969. Preface to E. Tompkins and M. L. Brown. Evaluation of possible causal relationship between fallout deposition of Strontium-90 and infant and fetal mortality trends. USDHEW, Public Health Service, DBE 69-2, October.

Multiple Risk Factor Intervention Trial Research Group. 1982. Multiple risk factor intervention trial. *Journal of the American Medical Association* 248 (24 September):1465–1477.

National Center for Health Statistics. 1965. Reporting of hospitalization in the Health Interview Survey (PHS publication no. 1000, series 2, no. 6). Washington, D.C.: Government Printing Office.

———— 1981. *Vital and health statistics*, series 11, no. 221, Hypertension in adults 25–74 years of age, United States, 1971–1975. Washington, D.C.: Government Printing Office.

———— 1982a. *Advancedata*, no. 84, Blood pressure levels and hypertension in persons ages 65–74 years: United States, 1976–80. Hyattsville, Md.: Public Health Service.

———— 1982b. *Monthly Vital Statistics Report* 31 (6):supplement. Advance report of final mortality statistics, 1979. Hyattsville, Md.: Public Health Service.

National Safety Council. 1961. *Accident facts*. Chicago: National Safety Council.

Nelson, Richard R. 1972. Issues and suggestions for the study of industrial organizations in a regime of rapid technical change. In *Policy issues and research opportunities in industrial organization,* ed. Victor R. Fuchs. New York: National Bureau of Economic Research and Columbia University Press.

Newhouse, Joseph P., and L. J. Friedlander. 1980. The relationship between medical resources and measures of health: Some additional evidence. *Journal of Human Resources* 15 (Spring):200–218.

Newhouse, Joseph P., Willard G. Manning, Carl N. Morris, Larry L. Orr, Naihua Duan, Emmett B. Keeler, Arleen Leibowitz, Kent H. Marquis, M. Susan Marquis, Charles E. Phelps, and Robert H. Brook. 1981. Some interim results from a controlled trial of cost sharing in health insurance. *New England Journal of Medicine* 305 (17 December):1501–1507.

Newhouse, Joseph P., Charles E. Phelps, and W. B. Schwartz. 1974. Policy options and the impact of national health insurance. *New England Journal of Medicine* 290 (13 June):1345–1359.

Norr, R. 1952. Cancer by the carton. *Reader's Digest* 61 (December):7–8.

Okun, Arthur M. 1975. *Equality and efficiency: The big tradeoff*. Washington, D.C.: The Brookings Institution.

Owens, A. 1970. General surgeons: Too many in the wrong places. *Medical Economics* 47:128.

Paradise, Jack L., Charles D. Bluestone, Ruth Z. Bachman, Georgann Karantonis, Ida H. Smith, Carol A. Saez, D. Kathleen Colborn, Beverly S. Bernard, Floyd H. Taylor, Robert H. Schwarzbach, Herman Felder, Sylvan E. Stool, Andrea M. Fitz, and Kenneth D. Rogers. 1978. Limitation of sore-throat history as an indication for tonsillectomy. *New England Journal of Medicine* 298 (23 February):409–413.

Pauly, Mark V. 1971. *Medical care at public expense: A study in applied welfare economics*. New York: Praeger.

———— 1980. *Doctors and their workshops*. Chicago: University of Chicago Press.

Pauly, Mark V., and M. Redisch. 1969. The not-for-profit hospital as a physicians' cooperative. Northwestern University (mimeo).

Phillips, R. 1968. Analysis of a rural surgical practice. *American Journal of Surgery* 115 (June):795–798.

Preston, Samuel H. 1980. Causes and consequences of mortality declines in less developed countries during the twentieth century. In *Population and economic change in developing countries,* ed. Richard Easterlin. Chicago: University of Chicago Press.

Rafferty, J. 1975. Enfranchisement and rationing: Effects of Medicare on discretionary hospital use. *Health Services Research* 10 (Spring):51–62.

Reed, Louis S., and Willine Carr. 1970. *The benefit structure of private insurance.* U.S. Department of Health, Education, and Welfare, Social Security Administration, Office of Research and Statistics. Research report no. 32.

Reinhardt, Uwe. 1977. Parkinson's law and the demand for physicians' services. Princeton University (mimeo).

Relman, Arnold S. 1980. The new medical–industrial complex. *New England Journal of Medicine* 303 (23 October):963–970.

Rice, Dorothy P. 1966. *Estimating the cost of illness.* Health Economics Series no. 6. Washington, D.C.: U.S. Public Health Service.

Riley, G. J., C. R. Wille, and R. J. Haggerty. 1969. A study of family medicine in upstate New York. *Journal of the American Medical Association* 208 (23 June):2307–2314.

Rimlinger, G. V., and H. B. Steele. 1965. Income opportunities and physician location trends in the United States. *Western Economic Journal* (Spring):182–194.

Roe, Benson B. 1981. The UCR boondoggle: A death knell for private practice? *New England Journal of Medicine* 305 (2 July):41–45.

Roemer, M. I., and D. M. Duboise. 1969. Medical costs in relation to the organization of ambulatory care. *New England Journal of Medicine* 280 (1 May):988–993.

Roemer, M. I., and W. Shonick. 1973. HMO performance: The recent evidence. *Milbank Memorial Fund Quarterly* 51 (Summer):271–317.

Sagan, L. A. 1969. A reply to Sternglass. *New Scientist* 44:14.

Samuelson, Paul. 1970. *Economics.* New York: McGraw-Hill.

Schneider, E. L., and J. A. Brody. 1983. Aging, natural death, and the compression of morbidity: Another view. *New England Journal of Medicine* 309 (6 October):854–855.

Schulz, J. H. 1976. *The economics of aging.* Belmont, Calif.: Wadsworth.

Schumpeter, J. S. 1942. *Capitalism, socialism and democracy.* New York: Harper and Brothers.

Schwartzman, David. 1969. The growth of sales per man-hour in retail trade, 1929–1963. In *Production and productivity in the service industries,* ed. Victor R. Fuchs. New York: National Bureau of Economic Research and Columbia University Press.

Scitovsky, Anne A., Lee Benham, and Nelda McCall. 1979. Use of physician services under two prepaid plans. *Medical Care* 17 (May):441–460.

Shapiro, S., E. R. Schlesinger, and R. E. L. Nesbitt. 1968. *Infant, perinatal, childhood mortality in the United States.* Cambridge, Mass.: Harvard University Press.

Shefrin, H. M., and Richard Thaler. 1977. An economic theory of self-control. Working Paper 208. Cambridge, Mass.: National Bureau of Economic Research.

Sheps, Mindel C. 1961. Marriage and mortality. *American Journal of Public Health* 51 (April):547–555.

Silver, Morris. 1972. An economic analysis of variations in medical expenses and work loss rates. In *Essays in the economics of health and medical care,* ed. Victor R. Fuchs. New York: National Bureau of Economic Research and Columbia University Press.

Simborg, D. W. 1981. DRG creep: A new hospital-acquired disease. *New England Journal of Medicine* 304 (25 June):1602–1604.

Simon, Herbert A. 1962. New developments in the theory of the firm. *American Economic Review* 52 (May):1–15.

Sloan, Frank A. 1970. Economic models of physician supply. Ph.D. dissertation, Harvard University.

Sloan, Frank A., and Roger Feldman. 1977. Monopolistic elements in the market for physicians' services. Paper presented at Conference on Competition in the Health Care Sector, Federal Trade Commission, Washington, D.C., June 1–2.

Sloan, Frank A., Roger D. Feldman, and A. Bruce Steinwald. 1983. Effects of teaching on hospital costs. *Journal of Health Economics* 2 (March): 1–28.

Smith, Adam. 1776. *An inquiry into the national cause of the wealth of nations.* 1937 edition: Edwin Cannan, New York, Modern Library.

SOSSUS. 1976. *Surgery in the United States: A summary report of the study on surgical services for the United States,* I. Sponsored jointly by the American College of Surgeons and the American Surgical Association.

Sternglass, E. J. 1969a. Infant mortality and nuclear tests. *Bulletin for Atomic Scientists* 25:18–20.

——— 1969b. Evidence for low-level radiation effects on the human embryo and fetus. *Proceedings of the Hanford Symposium on the Radiation Biology of the Fetal and Juvenile Mammal,* May 5–8.

Stigler, George J. 1958a. The goals of economic policy. *Journal of Business* 31 (July):169–176.

——— 1958b. The economies of scale. *Journal of Law and Economics* 1 (October):54–71.

——— 1958c. *Medical care at public expense: A study in applied welfare economics.* New York: Praeger.

——— 1961. The economics of information. *Journal of Political Economy* 69 (June):213–225.

——— 1975. *The citizen and the state: Essays on regulation.* Chicago: University of Chicago Press.

Stolnitz, G. J. 1955, 1956. A century of international mortality trends. *Population Studies* 9 (July):24–55, 10 (July):17–42.

Strickler, J. H. 1968. How many surgeons are needed? *Minnesota Medicine* 51:331.

Taubman, Paul, and Sherwin Rosen. 1982. Healthiness, education and marital status. In *Economic aspects of health,* ed. Victor R. Fuchs. Chicago: University of Chicago Press.

Tawney, R. H. 1926. *Religion and the rise of capitalism.* New York: Harcourt Brace.

Taylor, H. C. 1965. Objectives and principles in the training of the obstetrician–gynecologist. *American Journal of Surgery* 110 (July):35–42.

Thaler, Richard. 1979. Individual intertemporal choice: A preliminary investigation. Research memorandum (mimeo).

Thaler, Richard, and Sherwin Rosen. 1975. The value of saving a life: Evidence from the labor market. In *Household production and consumption,* ed. Nestor E. Terleckyj. New York: National Bureau of Economic Research and Columbia University Press.

Thaler, Richard A., and H. M. Shefrin. 1981. An economic theory of self control. *Journal of Political Economy* 89 (April):392–406.

Thomas, Ewart A. C., and Wanda E. Ward. 1979. Time orientation, optimism, and quasi-economic behavior. Stanford University (mimeo).

Thompson, J. D., R. B. Fetter, and M. D. Mross. 1975. Case mix and resource use. *Inquiry* 12:300–312.

Thompson, J. D., R. B. Fetter, and Y. Shin. 1978. One strategy for controlling costs in university teaching hospitals. *Journal of Medical Education* 53:167–175.

Thurow, Lester C. 1974. Cash versus in-kind transfer. *American Economic Review* 64, part 2. Papers and Proceedings (May):190–195.

Tompkins, E., and M. L. Brown. 1969. Evaluation of possible causal relationship between fallout deposition of Strontium-90 and infant and fetal mortality trends. USDHEW, Public Health Service, DBE 69-2, October.

Townsend, Peter. 1974. Inequality and the health service. *Lancet* 1 (15 June):1179–1190.

U.S. Bureau of the Census. 1966. *Statistical abstract of the United States: 1966.* Washington, D.C.: Government Printing Office, p. 574, table 825.

———— 1982. *Statistical abstract of the United States, 1982–83.* Washington, D.C.: Government Printing Office.

———— 1983. *Current Population Reports.* Series P-23, no. 126, Estimating after-tax money income distributions using data from the March Current Population Survey, table 1, p. 12. Washington, D.C.: Government Printing Office.

U.S. Department of Health, Education, and Welfare. 1964. *Smoking and health: Report of the Advisory Committee to the Surgeon General,* Public Health Service publication no. 1103. Washington, D.C.: Government Printing Office.

———— 1976. Adult use of tobacco—1975. USDHEW National Clearinghouse for Smoking and Health. Washington, D.C.: Government Printing Office.

———— 1979. *Healthy people: The Surgeon General's report on health promotion and disease prevention, background papers.* Public Health Service, no. 79-55071A. Washington, D.C.: Government Printing Office.

U.S. Department of Health and Human Services. 1980. *Promoting health/Preventing disease.* Washington, D.C.: Government Printing Office.

Usher, Dan. 1971. An imputation to the measure of economic growth for changes in life expectancy. In *The measurement of economic and social performance,* ed. Milton Moss. New York: National Bureau of Economic Research and Columbia University Press.

Viscusi, W. Kip. 1978. Labor market valuations of life and limb: Empirical evidence and policy implications. *Public Policy* (Summer):359–386.

Vogt, T. M., S. Selvin, G. Widdowson, and S. B. Hulley. 1977. Expired air carbon monoxide and serum thiocyanate as objective measures of cigarette exposure. *American Journal of Public Health* 67:545–549.

Warner, Kenneth E. 1977a. Treatment decision making in catastrophic illness. *Medical Care* 15 (January):19–33.

———— 1977b. The effects of the anti-smoking campaign on cigarette consumption. *American Journal of Public Health* 67 (July):645–650.

Watkins, Richard N., Edward F. X. Hughes, and Eugene M. Lewit. 1976. Time utilization of a population of general surgeons in a prepaid group practice. *Medical Care* 14 (October):824–838.

Watts, C. A., and T. D. Klastorin. 1980. The impact of case mix on hospital cost: A comparative analysis. *Inquiry* 17:357–367.

Wechsler, Henry, Sol Levine, Roberta K. Idelson, Mary Rohman, and James O. Taylor. 1983. The physician's role in health promotion: A survey of primary-care practitioners. *New England Journal of Medicine* 308 (13 January):97–100.

Weisbrod, Burton A. 1971. Costs and benefits of medical research: A case study of poliomyelitis. *Journal of Political Economy* 79 (May-June):527–544.

West, Richard W. 1978. The rate of time preference of families in the Seattle and Denver income maintenance experiment. Research Memorandum 51. Menlo Park, Calif.: SRI International.

Williamson, Jeffrey G. 1980. Unbalanced growth, inequality, and regional development: Some lessons from U.S. history. In *Alternatives to confrontation*, ed. Victor L. Arnold. Lexington, Mass.: Lexington Books.

Williamson, Oliver E. 1970. *Corporate control and business behavior*. Englewood Cliffs, N.J.: Prentice-Hall.

Wolfe, S., R. F. Badgley, and R. V. Kasius. 1968. The work of a group of doctors in Saskatchewan. *Milbank Memorial Fund Quarterly*, part 1, 46 (January):103–129.

Yett, Donald E. 1970. The chronic shortage of nurses: A public policy dilemma. In *Empirical studies in health economics*, ed. Herbert E. Klarman, Baltimore: Johns Hopkins Press.

Acknowledgments

This book resulted from a suggestion of Michael Aronson of Harvard University Press, and I am grateful to him for valuable advice at all stages of its development. Also at the Press, Mary Ellen Geer edited the manuscript with great care and understanding, and Maria Ascher made helpful comments on the introduction.

The National Bureau of Economic Research has provided a splendid environment for my research in health economics. I have benefited from fruitful interaction with numerous colleagues, including several collaborators who are specifically identified at relevant points in this book. For the past twelve years Claire Gilchrist has done an outstanding job as administrator/secretary of the health project. I would like to express special thanks to her for preparing this manuscript for publication and for many useful suggestions along the way. I also want to thank my research assistant, Leslie Perreault, for her perceptive comments and conscientious checking of references, figures, and tables.

During the nearly two decades of my work in health economics, I have received funds from several organizations, including the Commonwealth Fund, the National Center for Health Services Research, the Carnegie Corporation, and the Henry J. Kaiser Family Foundation. I again express my thanks to them for their support. I particularly want to acknowledge the backing of the trustees and officers of The Robert Wood Johnson Foundation. Their flexible funding over more than a decade has played a key role in enabling me to study and write about the health economy.

Sources

Chapter 1 Reprinted from "Health Care and the United States Economic System: An Essay in Abnormal Physiology," *Milbank Memorial Fund Quarterly*, 50 (April 1972):211–237.

Chapter 2 Reprinted from "Setting Priorities in Health Education and Promotion," *Health Affairs*, 2 (Winter 1983):56–69.

Chapter 3 Reprinted from Edward F. X. Hughes, Victor R. Fuchs, John E. Jacoby, and Eugene M. Lewit, "Surgical Work Loads in a Community Practice," *Surgery*, 71 (March 1972):315–327, by permission of the C. V. Mosby Company.

Chapter 4 Reprinted from Victor R. Fuchs and Marcia J. Kramer, "Determinants of Expenditures for Physicians' Services in the United States 1948–1968," DHEW Publication no. (HSM)73-3013, Department of Health, Education, and Welfare Health Services and Mental Health Administration, National Center for Health Services, December 1972.

Chapter 5 Reprinted from Claire Bombardier, Victor R. Fuchs, Lee A. Lillard, and Kenneth E. Warner, "Socioeconomic Factors Affecting the Utilization of Surgical Operations," *New England Journal of Medicine*, 297 (29 September 1977):699–705.

Chapter 6 Reprinted from "The Supply of Surgeons and the Demand for Operations," *Journal of Human Resources*, 13 (1978 suppl.):35–56.

Chapter 7 Reprinted from Alan M. Garber, Victor R. Fuchs, and James F. Silverman, "Case Mix, Costs, and Outcomes," *New England Journal of Medicine*, 310 (10 May 1984):1231–1237.

Chapter 8 Reprinted from Victor R. Fuchs and Irving Leveson, "Motor Accident Mortality and Compulsory Inspection of Vehicles," *Journal of the American Medical Association*, 201 (28 August 1967):657–661. Copyright 1967, American Medical Association.

Chapter 9 Reprinted from "Some Economic Aspects of Mortality in Developed Countries," in *The Economics of Health and Medical Care*, ed. Mark Perlman

(London: Macmillan, 1974). Proceedings of a conference held by the International Economic Association, Tokyo, April 1973.

Chapter 10 Reprinted from "Low-Level Radiation and Infant Mortality," *Health Physics,* 40 (June 1981):847–854, by permission of the Health Physics Society.

Chapter 11 Reprinted from "Time Preference and Health: An Exploratory Study," in *Economic Aspects of Health,* ed. Victor R. Fuchs (Chicago: University of Chicago Press, 1982), pp. 93–120. Copyright 1982 by the University of Chicago.

Chapter 12 Reprinted from Phillip Farrell and Victor R. Fuchs, "Schooling and Health: The Cigarette Connection," *Journal of Health Economics,* 1 (December 1982):217–230, by permission of North-Holland Publishing Company, Amsterdam.

Chapter 13 Reprinted from "From Bismarck to Woodcock: The 'Irrational' Pursuit of National Health Insurance," *Journal of Law and Economics,* 19 (August 1976):347–359. Copyright 1976 by the University of Chicago.

Chapter 14 Reprinted from "Economics, Health, and Post-Industrial Society," *Milbank Memorial Fund Quarterly/Health and Society,* 57 (Spring 1979):153–182. The E. S. Woodward Lectures in Economics, delivered at The University of British Columbia, Vancouver, Canada, November 1–2, 1978.

Chapter 15 Reprinted from "The Battle for Control of Health Care," *Health Affairs,* 1 (Summer 1982):5–13.

Chapter 16 Reprinted from " 'Though Much Is Taken': Reflections on Aging, Health, and Medical Care," *Milbank Memorial Fund Quarterly/Health and Society,* 62 (Spring 1984):143–166.

Chapter 17 Reprinted from "Paying the Piper, Calling the Tune: Implications of Changes in Reimbursement," *Frontiers of Health Services Management,* 2 (February 1986). Copyright 1986 by the Regents of The University of Michigan. Funding from the W. K. Kellogg Foundation is gratefully acknowledged.

Index

Abel-Smith, Brian, 257, 270
Abortions: and infant-mortality decrease, 192, 213; and government intervention, 287–288
Academic medical centers: vs. community centers, 305–306, 308–309; and reimbursement revolution, 347, 348
Accidents, as cause of youthful death, 5, 194
Accidents from motor vehicles, cost of, 178–179. *See also* Motor accident/inspection study
Accreditation, and surgical work load, 57–58, 63
Acton, Lord, 298
Aday, L. A., 108
Adelman, Irma, 182
Adverse seletion, 26, 290, 311
Age: and health problems, 4–5; and surgical utilization, 118, 121, 122, 124; and hospital admission, 152, 153; and time preference, 225. *See also* Elderly
Age discrimination, 321–322
Altman, Stuart H., 22
Ament, Richard P., 148, 347
Anderson, Ronald, 87, 108, 360n.1, 362n.20
Antonovsky, A., 209, 243
Arrow, Kenneth, 19–20, 265
Auster, Richard, 106, 107, 124, 182, 189, 215, 367n.1

Barnes, Allan C., 68
Barnes, Benjamin A., 147
Becker, E. R., 149, 159
Becker, Gary S., 12, 27–28, 216, 264
Behavior, personal. *See* Life-style; Personal behavior; Way of life
Bell, D., 273
Benham, Alexandra, 108
Benham, Lee, 22, 72, 87, 99, 108, 360n.1, 362n.20
Benjamin, B., 364n.1
Berlin, Isaiah, 36
Bernheim, B. D., 326
Bernstein, J., 209
Bevan, Aneurin, 257
Beveridge, William, 257
Birth control, and infant mortality decrease, 192, 213
Birth order, and infant mortality, 192
Bismarck, Otto von, 257, 262, 263, 269, 271
Blacks, and death rate/infant mortality, 104–105, 107. *See also* Race
Bobbitt, Phillip, 287
Border-crossing, by surgical patients, 130
Borland, Barry L., 254
Breslow, Lester, 39, 40
Breton, Albert, 265
Britain (England), and Leftist critique, 296

Radioactive fallout, and infant mortality, 200–213
Rae, John, 366n.3
Rafferty, J., 109
Rand health insurance experiment, 344
Rand study on medical care and health, 274–275
Rate of return. See Discounted future earnings approach; Time preference
Real wages, growth of, 323
Reder, M.W., 72, 99, 360n.1
Redisch, M., 18
Redistribution: through in-kind vs. cash transfers, 24–25, 265; as market corrective, 25, 330–331; as government aim, 290, 298; in institutional reimbursement, 346–347. See also Egalitarianism; Equal access to health care
Reed, Louis S., 95
Reimbursement: prospective, 5, 148, 164–165, 341, 343; fee-for-service, 41–42, 349; by Medicare, 318, 320; global, 340, 342, 344, 345; consumer choice in, 341; retrospective, 343. See also Expenditures for health care; Health care financing
Reimbursement revolution, 5–6, 332–333, 339–341; background, 333–339; economic implications, 341–349; ethical implications, 349–354; and financing trade-offs, 354–355; and care for the poor, 355–356; challenges to, 356
Reinhardt, Uwe, 363n.1
Religion: decline in, 1, 268–269, 291, 298; and health insurance need, 268–269; and growth of health care, 284–286; government as substitute for, 290; government impact on, 299
Research. See Medical research; Technological change
Resource allocation: and scarcity, 12; and equality at the margin,

13, 16, 30; in market system, 16–17; and technological change, 30; and health education, 33; and technological innovation, 283–284; decentralization in, 293, 295; and elderly, 329; and care for dying, 330–331
Retirement History Survey, 325
Retrospective reimbursement, 343
Reverse causality (operations leading to lower income), 112, 124
Reynolds, Roger, 108
Rice, Dorothy, 178
Right (political), on government role, 292–295, 299
Riley, G.J., 50, 64
Rimlinger, G.V., 360n.1
Risk. See Uncertainty
Roe, Benson, 307
Roemer, M.I., 49, 108
Rosen, Sherwin, 38, 364n.13, 367n.1
Rotblat, J., 200
Rudolph, Joseph P., 254

Sagan, L.A., 200
Samuelson, Paul, 12
Sarachek, Deborah, 106, 107, 124, 182, 189, 215
Schneider, E.L., 315
Schooling. See Educational level
Schulz, J.H., 322
Schumpeter, Joseph, 293
Schwartzman, David, 71
Science, advances in, 5. See also Medical science; Technological change
Scitovsky, Anne A., 42
Scott, Sharon R., 327
Seat belt usage, 231, 234
Seattle-Denver income maintenance experiment, 219
Self-employment, decline of, 322–323
Sex differentials: in mortality, 193–194, 195; in smoking-schooling relation, 250, 251, 252; in elderly health expenditures, 318, 319,